MCAT®

Psychology and Sociology Review

4th Edition

The Staff of The Princeton Review

Penguin
Random
House

The Princeton Review
110 E. 42nd Street
New York, NY 10017

ISBN: 978-0-593-51622-5
ISSN: 2332-8495

MCAT is a registered trademark of the Association of American Medical Colleges.

The Princeton Review is not affiliated with Princeton University.

Editor: Patricia Murphy
Production Artist: Jennifer Chapman
Production Editor: Sarah Litt and Liz Dacey

Manufactured in China.

10 9 8 7 6 5 4 3 2 1

4th Edition

The Princeton Review Publishing Team

Rob Franek, Editor-in-Chief

David Soto, Senior Director, Data Operations

Stephen Koch, Senior Manager, Data Operations

Deborah Weber, Director of Production

Jason Ullmeyer, Production Design Manager

Jennifer Chapman, Senior Production Artist

Selena Coppock, Director of Editorial

Aaron Riccio, Senior Editor

Meave Shelton, Senior Editor

Chris Chimera, Editor

Orion McBean, Editor

Patricia Murphy, Editor

Laura Rose, Editor

Alexa Schmitt Bugler, Editorial Assistant

Random House Publishing Team

Tom Russell, VP, Publisher

Alison Stoltzfus, Senior Director, Publishing

Brett Wright, Senior Editor

Emily Hoffman, Assistant Managing Editor

Ellen Reed, Production Manager

Suzanne Lee, Designer

Eugenia Lo, Publishing Assistant

For customer service, please contact
editorialsupport@review.com,
and be sure to include:

- full title of the book

- ISBN

- page number

CONTRIBUTORS

Nadia L. Johnson, M.A., M.S.
Senior Author
Rizwan Ahmad, M.A.
Senior Author
Tomislav Kurtović, M.A.
Senior Author

TPR MCAT Psychology and Sociology Team:
Matthew Dempsey, Ph.D., Lead Developer and Senior Editor
Christine Lindwall, M.A., J.D.

Edited for Production by:
Judene Wright, M.S., M.A.Ed.
National Content Director, MCAT Program, The Princeton Review

The TPR MCAT Psychology and Sociology Team and Judene would like to thank the following people for their contributions to this book :

Erika C. Castro, B.A., Maria S. Chushak, M.S., Guenevieve O. del Mundo, B.A., B.S., C.C.S., Jon Fowler, M.A., Michelle E. Fox, B.S., Kevin Keogh, Anthony Krupp, Ph.D., Christine Lindwall, M.A., J.D., Ali Landreau, B.A., Toni Lupro, Mike Matera, Jennifer A. McDevitt, Paola A. Munoz , M.A., B.A., Jonathan Nasrallah, Bikem Ayse Polat, Shalom Shapiro, Andrew D. Snyder, M.S., M.A., Gordy Steil, M.A., M.F.T., David Stoll, Chelsea K. Wise, M.S., Alexandra Vinson, Betsy Walli, M.S., Ph.D.

JOURNAL ARTICLE PERMISSIONS

PERIODIC TABLE OF THE ELEMENTS

1																	18
1 **H** 1.0	**2**												**13**	**14**	**15**	**16**	**17**	**2** **He** 4.0
3 **Li** 6.9	**4** **Be** 9.0												**5** **B** 10.8	**6** **C** 12.0	**7** **N** 14.0	**8** **O** 16.0	**9** **F** 19.0	**10** **Ne** 20.2
11 **Na** 23.0	**12** **Mg** 24.3	**3**	**4**	**5**	**6**	**7**	**8**	**9**	**10**	**11**	**12**	**13** **Al** 27.0	**14** **Si** 28.1	**15** **P** 31.0	**16** **S** 32.1	**17** **Cl** 35.5	**18** **Ar** 39.9
19 **K** 39.1	**20** **Ca** 40.1	**21** **Sc** 45.0	**22** **Ti** 47.9	**23** **V** 50.9	**24** **Cr** 52.0	**25** **Mn** 54.9	**26** **Fe** 55.8	**27** **Co** 58.9	**28** **Ni** 58.7	**29** **Cu** 63.5	**30** **Zn** 65.4	**31** **Ga** 69.7	**32** **Ge** 72.6	**33** **As** 74.9	**34** **Se** 79.0	**35** **Br** 79.9	**36** **Kr** 83.8
37 **Rb** 85.5	**38** **Sr** 87.6	**39** **Y** 88.9	**40** **Zr** 91.2	**41** **Nb** 92.9	**42** **Mo** 95.9	**43** **Tc** (98)	**44** **Ru** 101.1	**45** **Rh** 102.9	**46** **Pd** 106.4	**47** **Ag** 107.9	**48** **Cd** 112.4	**49** **In** 114.8	**50** **Sn** 118.7	**51** **Sb** 121.8	**52** **Te** 127.6	**53** **I** 126.9	**54** **Xe** 131.3
55 **Cs** 132.9	**56** **Ba** 137.3	**57** *****La** 138.9	**72** **Hf** 178.5	**73** **Ta** 180.9	**74** **W** 183.9	**75** **Re** 186.2	**76** **Os** 190.2	**77** **Ir** 192.2	**78** **Pt** 195.1	**79** **Au** 197.0	**80** **Hg** 200.6	**81** **Tl** 204.4	**82** **Pb** 207.2	**83** **Bi** 209.0	**84** **Po** (209)	**85** **At** (210)	**86** **Rn** (222)
87 **Fr** (223)	**88** **Ra** (226)	**89** **†Ac** (227)	**104** **Rf** (267)	**105** **Db** (268)	**106** **Sg** (271)	**107** **Bh** (270)	**108** **Hs** (269)	**109** **Mt** (278)	**110** **Ds** (281)	**111** **Rg** (282)	**112** **Cn** (285)	**113** **Nh** (286)	**114** **Fl** (289)	**115** **Mc** (289)	**116** **Lv** (293)	**117** **Ts** (294)	**118** **Og** (294)

*Lanthanoids	**58** **Ce** 140.1	**59** **Pr** 140.9	**60** **Nd** 144.2	**61** **Pm** (145)	**62** **Sm** 150.4	**63** **Eu** 152.0	**64** **Gd** 157.3	**65** **Tb** 158.9	**66** **Dy** 162.5	**67** **Ho** 164.9	**68** **Er** 167.3	**69** **Tm** 168.9	**70** **Yb** 173.0	**71** **Lu** 175.0
†Actinoids	**90** **Th** 232.0	**91** **Pa** (231)	**92** **U** 238.0	**93** **Np** (237)	**94** **Pu** (244)	**95** **Am** (243)	**96** **Cm** (247)	**97** **Bk** (247)	**98** **Cf** (251)	**99** **Es** (252)	**100** **Fm** (257)	**101** **Md** (258)	**102** **No** (259)	**103** **Lr** (266)

CONTENTS

CONTENTS

Get More (Free) Content

at **PrincetonReview.com/prep**

As easy as **1•2•3**

1 Go to PrincetonReview.com/prep or scan the **QR code** and enter the following ISBN for your book:
9780593516225

2 Answer a few simple questions to set up an exclusive Princeton Review account. *(If you already have one, you can just log in.)*

3 Enjoy access to your **FREE** content!

Once you've registered, you can...

- Take **3** full-length practice MCAT exams

- Find useful information about taking the MCAT and applying to medical school

- Check to see if there have been any corrections or updates to this edition

- Get our take on any recent or pending updates to the MCAT

Need to report a potential **content** issue?

Contact **EditorialSupport@review.com** and include:

- full title of the book
- ISBN
- page number

Need to report a **technical** issue?

Contact **TPRStudentTech@review.com** and provide:

- your full name
- email address used to register the book
- full book title and ISBN
- Operating system (Mac/PC) and browser (Firefox, Safari, etc.)

Chapter 1
MCAT Basics

SO YOU WANT TO BE A DOCTOR.

So...you want to be a doctor. If you're like most premeds, you've wanted to be a doctor since you were pretty young. When people asked you what you wanted to be when you grew up, you always answered "a doctor." You had toy medical kits, you bandaged up your dog or cat, and you played "hospital." You probably read your parents' home medical guides for fun.

When you got to high school you took the honors and AP classes. You studied hard, got straight As (or at least really good grades!), and participated in extracurricular activities so you could get into a good college. And you succeeded!

At college you knew exactly what to do. You took your classes seriously, studied hard, and got a great GPA. You talked to your professors and hung out at office hours to get good letters of recommendation. You were a member of the premed society on campus, volunteered at hospitals, and shadowed doctors. All that's left to do now is get a good MCAT score.

Just the MCAT.

Just the most confidence-shattering, most demoralizing, longest and most brutal entrance exam for any graduate program. At about 7.5 hours (including breaks), the MCAT tops the list...even the closest runners-up, the LSAT and GMAT, are only about 4 hours long. The MCAT tests significant science content knowledge along with the ability to think quickly, reason logically, and read comprehensively, all under the pressure of a timed exam.

The path to a good MCAT score is not as easy to see as the path to a good GPA or the path to a good letter of recommendation. The MCAT is less about what you know, and more about how to apply what you know...and how to apply it quickly to new situations. Because the path might not be so clear, you might be worried. That's why you picked up this book.

We promise to demystify the MCAT for you, with clear descriptions of the different sections, how the test is scored, and what the test experience is like. We will help you understand general test-taking techniques as well as provide you with specific techniques for each section. We will review the science content you need to know as well as give you an overview of the Psychology/Sociology section of the MCAT. We'll show you the path to a good MCAT score and help you walk the path.

After all...you want to be a doctor. And we want you to succeed.

WHAT IS THE MCAT...REALLY?

Most test-takers approach the MCAT as though it were a typical college science test, one in which facts and knowledge simply need to be regurgitated in order to do well. They study for the MCAT the same way they did for their college tests, by memorizing facts and details, formulas and equations. And when they get to the MCAT, they are surprised...and disappointed.

It's a myth that the MCAT is purely a content-knowledge test. If medical school admission committees want to see what you know, all they have to do is look at your transcripts. What they really want to see, is how you *think*, especially how you think under pressure. That's what your MCAT score will tell them.

The MCAT is really a test of your ability to apply basic knowledge to different, possibly new, situations. It's a test of your ability to reason out and evaluate arguments. Do you still need to know your science content? Absolutely. But not at the level that most test-takers think they need to know it. Furthermore, your science knowledge won't help you on the Critical Analysis and Reasoning Skills (CARS) section. So how do you study for a test like this?

You study for the science sections by reviewing the basics and then applying them to MCAT practice questions. You study for the Psychology and Sociology section of the MCAT by reading this book, and by studying the people, and world, around you.

The book you are holding will review all the relevant MCAT Psychology and Sociology content you will need for the test, and a little bit more. Plus, it includes questions designed to make you think about the material in a deeper way, along with full explanations to clarify the logical thought process needed to get to the answer. It also comes with access to three full-length online practice exams to further hone your skills. For more information on accessing those online exams, please refer to the "Get More (Free) Content" spread on page viii.

MCAT NUTS AND BOLTS

Overview

The MCAT is a computer-based test (CBT) that is *not* adaptive. Adaptive tests base your next question on whether or not you've answered the current question correctly. The MCAT is *linear*, or *fixed-form*, meaning that the questions are in a predetermined order and do not change based on your answers. However, there are many versions of the test, so that on a given test day, different people will see different versions. The following table highlights the features of the MCAT exam.

Registration	Online via www.aamc.org. Begins as early as six months prior to test date; available up until week of test (subject to seat availability).
Testing Centers	Administered at small, secure, climate-controlled computer testing rooms.
Security	Photo ID with signature, electronic fingerprint, electronic signature verification, assigned seat.
Proctoring	None. Test administrator checks examinee in and assigns seat at computer. All testing instructions are given on the computer.
Frequency of Test	Many times per year distributed over January, April, May, June, July, August, and September.
Format	Exclusively computer-based. NOT an adaptive test.
Length of Test Day	7.5 hours
Breaks	Optional 10-minute breaks between sections, with a 30-minute break for lunch.
Section Names	1. Chemical and Physical Foundations of Biological Systems (Chem/Phys) 2. Critical Analysis and Reasoning Skills (CARS) 3. Biological and Biochemical Foundations of Living Systems (Bio/Biochem) 4. Psychological, Social, and Biological Foundations of Behavior (Psych/Soc)
Number of Questions and Timing	59 Chem/Phys questions, 95 minutes 53 CARS questions, 90 minutes 59 Bio/Biochem questions, 95 minutes 59 Psych/Soc questions, 95 minutes
Scoring	Test is scaled. Several forms per administration.
Allowed/ Not allowed	No timers/watches. Noise reduction headphones available. Noteboard booklet and wet-erase marker given at start of test and taken at end of test. Locker or secure area provided for personal items.
Results: Timing and Delivery	Approximately 30 days. Electronic scores only, available online through AAMC login. Examinees can print official score reports.
Maximum Number of Retakes	The MCAT can be taken a maximum of three times in one year, four times over two years, and seven times over the lifetime of the examinee. An examinee can be registered for only one date at a time.

Registration

Registration for the exam is completed online at www.aamc.org/students/applying/mcat/reserving. The AAMC opens registration for a given test date at least two months in advance of the date, often earlier. It's a good idea to register well in advance of your desired test date to make sure that you get a seat.

Sections

There are four sections on the MCAT, all of which consist of multiple-choice questions:

Section	Concepts Tested	Number of Questions and Timing
Chemical and Physical Foundations of Biological Systems (Chem/Phys)	Basic concepts in chemistry and physics, including biochemistry, scientific inquiry, reasoning, research and statistics skills.	59 questions in 95 minutes
Critical Analysis and Reasoning Skills (CARS)	Critical analysis of information drawn from a wide range of social science and humanities disciplines.	53 questions in 90 minutes
Biological and Biochemical Foundations of Living Systems (Bio/Biochem)	Basic concepts in biology and biochemistry, scientific inquiry, reasoning, research and statistics skills.	59 questions in 95 minutes
Psychological, Social, and Biological Foundations of Behavior (Psych/Soc)	Basic concepts in psychology, sociology, and biology, research methods and statistics.	59 questions in 95 minutes

Most questions on the MCAT (44 in the science sections, all 53 in the CARS section) are passage-based; the science sections have 10 passages each and the CARS section has 9. A passage consists of a few paragraphs of information on which several following questions are based. In the science sections, passages often include graphs, figures, and experiments to analyze. CARS passages come from literature in the social sciences, humanities, ethics, philosophy, cultural studies, and population health, and they do not test content knowledge in any way.

Some questions in the science sections are freestanding questions (FSQs). These questions are independent of any passage information and appear in four groups of about four to five questions interspersed throughout the passages. About 15 of the questions in the sciences sections are freestanding, and the remainder are passage-based.

Each section on the MCAT is separated by either a 10-minute break or a 30-minute lunch break:

Section	Time
Test Center Check-In	Variable, can take up to 40 minutes if center is busy.
Tutorial	10 minutes
Chemical and Physical Foundations of Biological Systems	95 minutes
Break (optional)	10 minutes
Critical Analysis and Reasoning Skills	90 minutes
Lunch Break (optional)	30 minutes
Biological and Biochemical Foundations of Living Systems	95 minutes
Break (optional)	10 minutes
Psychological, Social, and Biological Foundations of Behavior	95 minutes
Void Option	5 minutes
Survey (optional)	5 minutes

The survey includes questions about your satisfaction with the overall MCAT experience, including registration, check-in, etc., as well as questions about how you prepared for the test.

Scoring

The MCAT is a scaled exam, meaning that your raw score will be converted into a scaled score that takes into account the difficulty of the questions. There is no guessing penalty. All sections are scored from 118–132, with a total scaled score range of 472–528. Because different versions of the test have varying levels of difficulty, the scale will be different from one exam to the next. Thus, there is no "magic number" of questions to get right in order to get a particular score. Plus, some of the questions on the test are considered "experimental" and do not count toward your score; they are just there to be evaluated for possible future inclusion in a test.

At the end of the test (after you complete the Psychological, Social, and Biological Foundations of Behavior section), you will be asked to choose one of the following two options, "I wish to have my MCAT exam scored" or "I wish to VOID my MCAT exam." You have five minutes to make a decision, and if you do not select one of the options in that time, the test will automatically be scored. If you choose the VOID option, your test will not be scored (you will not now, or ever, get a numerical score for this test), medical schools will not know you took the test, and no refunds will be granted. You cannot "unvoid" your scores at a later time.

So, what's a good score? The AAMC is centering the scale at 500 (i.e., 500 will be the 50th percentile), and recommends that application committees consider applicants near the center of the range. To be on the safe side, aim for a total score of around 510. Remember that if your GPA is on the low side, you'll need higher MCAT scores to compensate, and if you have a strong GPA, you can get away with lower MCAT scores. But the reality is that your chances of acceptance depend on a lot more than just your MCAT scores. It's a combination of your GPA, MCAT scores, undergraduate coursework, letters of recommendation, experience related to the medical field (such as volunteer work or research), extracurricular activities, your personal statement, and so on. Medical schools are looking for a complete package, not just good scores and a good GPA.

GENERAL LAYOUT AND TEST-TAKING STRATEGIES

Layout of the Test

In each section of the test, the computer screen is divided vertically, with the passage on the left and the range of questions for that passage indicated above (e.g., "Passage 1 Questions 1–5"). The scroll bar for the passage text appears in the middle of the screen. Each question appears on the right, and you need to click "Next" to move to each subsequent question.

In the science sections, the freestanding questions are found in groups of 4–5, interspersed with the passages. The screen is still divided vertically; on the left is the statement "Questions [X–XX] do not refer to a passage and are independent of each other," and each question appears on the right as described above.

CBT Tools

There are a number of tools available on the test, including highlighting, strike-outs, the Flag for Review button, the Navigation and Review Screen buttons, the Periodic Table button, and of course, the noteboard booklet. All tools are available with both mouse control (buttons to click) or keyboard commands (Alt+ a letter). As everyone has different preferences, you should practice with both types of tools (mouse and keyboard) to see which is more comfortable for you personally. The following is a brief description of each tool.

1) **Highlighting:** This is done in the passage text (including table entries and some equations, but excluding figures and molecular structures), in the question stems, and in the answer choices (including Roman numerals). Select the words you wish to highlight (left-click and drag the cursor across the words), and in the upper left corner click the "Highlight" button to highlight the selected text yellow. Alternatively, press "Alt+H" to highlight the words. Highlighting can be removed by selecting the words again and in the upper left corner clicking the down arrow next to "Highlight." This will expand to show the "Remove Highlight" option; clicking this will remove the highlighting. Removing highlighting via the keyboard is cumbersome and is not recommended.

2) **Strike-outs:** This can be done on the answer choices, including Roman numeral statements, by selecting the text you want to strike out (left-click and drag the cursor across the text), then clicking the "Strikethrough" button in the upper left corner. Alternatively, press "Alt+S" to strikeout the words. The strike-out can be removed by repeating these actions. Figures or molecular structures cannot be struck out, however, the letter answer choice of those structures can.

3) **Flag for Review button:** This is available for each question and is found in the upper right corner. This allows you to flag the question as one you would like to review later if time permits. When clicked, the flag icon turns yellow. Click again to remove the flag. Alternatively, press "Alt+F."

4) **Navigation button:** This is found near the bottom of the screen and is only available on your first pass through the section. Clicking this button brings up a navigation table listing all questions and their statuses (unseen, incomplete, complete, flagged for review). You can also press "Alt+V" to bring up the screen. The questions can be sorted by their statuses, and clicking a question number takes you immediately to that question. Once you have reached the end of the section and viewed the Review screen (described below), the Navigation screen is no longer available.

5) **Review Screen button:** This button is found near the bottom of the screen after your first pass through the section and, when clicked, brings up a new screen showing all questions and their statuses (either incomplete, unseen, or flagged for review). Questions that are complete are assigned no additional status. You can then choose one of three options by clicking with the mouse or with keyboard shortcuts: Review All (Alt+A), Review Incomplete (Alt+I), or Review Flagged (Alt+R); alternatively, you can click a question number to go directly back to that question. You can also end the section from this screen.

6) **Periodic Table button:** Clicking this button will open the periodic table (or press "Alt+T"). Note that the periodic table is large, covering most of the screen. However, this window can be resized to see the questions and a portion of the periodic table at the same time. The table text will not decrease, but scroll bars will appear on the window so you can center the section of the table of interest in the window.

7) **Noteboard Booklet (Scratch Paper):** At the start of the test, you will be given a spiral-bound set of four laminated 8.5"×14" sheets of paper and a wet-erase black marker to use as scratch paper. You can request a clean noteboard booklet at any time during the test; your original booklet will be collected. The noteboard is only useful if it is kept organized; do not give in to the tendency to write on the first available open space! Good organization will be very helpful when/if you wish to review a question. Indicate the passage number, the range of questions for that passage, and a topic in a box near the top of your scratch work, and indicate the question you are working on in a circle to the left of the notes for that question. Draw a line under your scratch work when you change passages to keep the work separate. Do not erase or scribble over any previous work. If you do not think it is correct, draw one line through the work and start again. You may have already done some useful work without realizing it.

General Strategy for the Science Sections

Passages vs. FSQs in the Science Sections: What to Start With

Since the questions are displayed on separate screens, it is awkward and time consuming to click through all of the questions up front to find the FSQs. Therefore, go through the section on a first pass and decide whether to do the passage now or to save it for later, basing your decision on the passage text and the first question. Tackle the FSQs as you come upon them. More details are below.

Here is an outline of the procedure:

1) For each passage, write a heading on your noteboard with the passage number, the general topic, and its range of questions (e.g., "Passage 1, thermodynamics, Q 1–5" or "Passage 2, enzymes, Q 6–9"). The passage numbers do not currently appear in the Navigation or Review screens, thus having the question numbers on your noteboard will allow you to move through the section more efficiently.

2) Skim the text and rank the passage. If a passage is a "Now," complete it before moving on to the next passage (also see "Attacking the Questions" below). If it is a "Later" passage, first write "SKIPPED" in block letters under the passage heading on your noteboard and leave room for your work when you come back to complete that passage. (Note that the specific passages you skip will be unique to you; in the Bio/Biochem section, you might choose to do all Biology passages first, then come back for Biochemistry. Or in Chem/Phys you might choose to skip experiment-based or analytical passages. Know ahead of time what type of passages you are going to skip and follow your plan.)

3) Next, click on the "Navigation" button at the bottom to get to the Navigation screen. Click on the first question of the next passage; you'll be able to identify it because you know the range of questions from the passage you just skipped. This will take you to the next passage, where you will repeat steps 1–3.

4) Once you have completed your first pass through the section, go to the Review screen and click the first question for the first passage you skipped. Answer the questions, and continue going back to the Review screen and repeating this procedure for other passages you have skipped.

Attacking the Questions

As you work through the questions, if you encounter a particularly lengthy question, or a question that requires a lot of analysis, you may choose to skip it. This is a wise strategy because it ensures you will tackle all the easier questions first, the ones you are more likely to get right. If you choose to skip the question (or if you attempt it but get stuck), write down the question number on your noteboard, click the Flag for Review button and move on to the next question. At the end of the passage, click "Previous" to move back through the set of questions and complete any that you skipped over the first time through. Make sure that you have filled in an answer for every question.

General Strategy for the CARS Section

Ranking and Ordering the Passages: What to Start With

Ranking: Since the questions are displayed on separate screens, it is awkward and time consuming to click through all of the questions before ranking each passage as Now (an easier passage), Later (a harder passage), or Killer (a passage that you will randomly guess on). Therefore, rank the passage and decide whether or not to do it on the first pass through the section based on the passage text, skimming the first 2–3 sentences.

Ordering: Because of the additional clicking through screens (or, use of the Review screen) that is required to navigate through the section, the "Two-Pass" system (completing the "Now" passages as you find them) is likely to be your most efficient approach. However, if you find that you are continuously making a lot of bad ranking decisions, it is still valid to experiment with the "Three-Pass" approach (ranking all nine passages up front before attempting your first "Now" passage).

Here is an outline of the basic Ranking and Ordering procedure to follow.

1) For each passage, write a heading on your noteboard with the passage number and its range of questions (e.g., "Passage 1 Q 1–7"). The passage numbers do not currently appear in the Navigation or Review screens, thus having the question numbers on your noteboard will allow you to move through the section more efficiently.

2) Skim the first 2–3 sentences and rank the passage. If the passage is a "Now," complete it before moving on to the next. If it is a "Later" or "Killer," first write either "Later" or "Killer" and "SKIPPED" in block letters under the passage heading on your noteboard and leave room for your work if you decide to come back and complete that passage. Then click through each question, flagging each one for review and filling in random guesses, until you get to the next passage.

3) Once you have completed the "Now" passages, come back for your second pass and complete the "Later" passages, leaving your random guesses in place for any "Killer" passages that you choose not to complete. Go to the Review screen and use your noteboard notes on the question numbers. Click on the number of the first question for that passage to go back to that question, and proceed from there. Alternatively, if you have consistently flagged all the questions for passages you skipped in your first pass, you can use "Review Flagged" from the Review screen to find and complete your "Later" passages.

4) Regardless of how you choose to find your second pass passages, unflag each question after you complete it, so that you can continue to rely on the Review screen (and the "Review Flagged" function) to identify questions that you have not yet attempted.

Previewing the Questions

The formatting and functioning of the tools facilitates effective previewing. Having each question on a separate screen will encourage you to really focus on that question. Even more importantly, you can now highlight in the question stem and the answer choices.

Here is the basic procedure for previewing the questions:

1) Start with the first question, and if it has lead words referencing passage content, highlight them. You may also choose to jot them down on your noteboard. Once you reach and preview the last question for the set on that passage, THEN stay on that screen and work the passage (your highlighting appears and stays on every passage screen, and persists through the whole 90 minutes).

2) Once you have worked the passage and defined the Bottom Line—the main idea and tone of the entire passage—work **backward** from the last question to the first. If you skip over any questions as you go (see "Attacking the Questions" below), write down the question number on your noteboard. Then click **forward** through the set of questions, completing any that you skipped over the first time through. Once you reach and complete the last question for that passage, clicking "Next" will send you to the first question of the next passage. Working the questions from last to first the first time through the set will eliminate the need to click back through multiple screens to get to the first question immediately after previewing, and will also make it easier and more efficient to do the hardest questions last (see "Attacking the Questions" below).

3) Remember that previewing questions is a CARS-only technique. It is not efficient to preview questions in the science sections.

Attacking the Questions

The question types and the procedure for actually attacking each type is discussed in much greater detail in the *MCAT CARS Review*. However, it is still important **not** to attempt the hardest questions first (potentially getting stuck, wasting time, and discouraging yourself).

So, as you work the questions from last to first (see "Previewing the Questions" above), if you encounter a particularly difficult and/or lengthy question (or if you attempt a question but get stuck), write down the question number on your noteboard (you may also choose to Flag for Review) and move on backward to the next question. Then click **forward** through the set and complete any that you skipped over the first time through the set, unflagging any questions that you flagged that first time through and making sure that you have filled in an answer for every question.

Pacing Strategy for the MCAT

Since the MCAT is a timed test, you must keep an eye on the timer and adjust your pacing as necessary. It would be terrible to run out of time at the end only to discover that the last few questions could have been easily answered in just a few seconds each.

If you complete every question, in the science section you will have about one minute and thirty-five seconds (1:35) per question, and in the CARS section you will have about one minute and forty seconds (1:40) per question (not taking into account time spent reading the passage before answering the questions).

Section	# of Questions in passage	Approximate time (including reading the passage)
Chem/Phys, Bio/Biochem, and Psych/Soc	4	6.5 minutes
	5	8 minutes
	6	9.5 minutes
CARS	5	8.5 minutes
	6	10 minutes
	7	11.5 minutes

When starting a passage in the science sections, make note of how much time you will allot for it, and the starting time on the timer. Jot down on your noteboard what the timer should say at the end of the passage. Then just keep an eye on it as you work through the questions. If you are near the end of the time for that passage, guess on any remaining questions, make some notes on your noteboard, flag the questions for review, and move on. Come back to those questions later if you have time.

For the CARS section, keep in mind that many people will maximize their score by *not* trying to complete every question or every passage in the section. A good strategy for test-takers who cannot achieve a high level of accuracy on all nine passages is to randomly guess on at least one passage in the section, so that you can spend your time getting a high percentage of the other questions right. To complete all nine CARS passages, you have about ten minutes per passage. To complete eight of the nine, you have about 11 minutes per passage.

To help maximize your number of correct answer choices in any section, do the questions and passages within that section in the order *you* want to do them in. See "General Strategy" above.

Process of Elimination

Process of Elimination (POE) is probably the most useful technique you have to tackle MCAT questions. Since there is no guessing penalty, POE allows you to increase your probability of choosing the correct answer by eliminating those you are sure are wrong.

1) Strike out any choices that you are sure are incorrect or that do not address the issue raised in the question.
2) Jot down some notes to help clarify your thoughts if you return to the question.
3) Use the "Flag for Review" button to identify questions you may want to return to. (Note, however, that in the CARS section, you generally should not be returning to rethink questions once you have moved on to a new passage.)

4) Do not leave it blank! For the sciences, if you are not sure and you have already spent more than 60 seconds on that question, just pick one of the remaining choices. If you have time to review it at the end, you can always debate the remaining choices based on your previous notes. For CARS, if you have been through the choices two or three times, have re-read the question stem and gone back to the passage and you are still stuck, move on. Do the remaining questions for that passage, take one more look at the question you were stuck on, then pick an answer and move on for good.

5) Special Note: if three of the four answer choices have been eliminated, the remaining choice must be the correct answer. Don't waste time pondering *why* it is correct; just click it and move on. The MCAT doesn't care if you truly understand why it's the right answer, only that you have the right answer selected.

6) More subject-specific information on techniques is presented in the next chapter.

Guessing

Remember, there is NO guessing penalty on the MCAT. NEVER leave a question blank!

QUESTION TYPES

In the science sections of the MCAT, the questions fall into one of three main categories:

1) Memory questions: These questions can be answered directly from prior knowledge and represent about 25 percent of the total number of questions.

2) Explicit questions: These questions are those for which the answer is explicitly stated in the passage. To answer them correctly, for example, may just require finding a definition, or reading a graph, or making a simple connection. Explicit questions represent about 35 percent of the total number of questions.

3) Implicit questions: These questions require you to apply knowledge to a new situation; the answer is typically implied by the information in the passage. These questions often start "If.... Then...." (for example, "if we modify the experiment in the passage like this, then what result would we expect?"). Implicit style questions make up about 40 percent of the total number of questions.

In the CARS section, the questions fall into four main categories:

1) Specific questions: These either ask you for facts from the passage (Retrieval questions) or require you to deduce what is most likely to be true based on the passage (Inference questions).

2) General questions: These ask you to summarize themes (Main Idea and Primary Purpose questions) or evaluate an author's opinion (Tone/Attitude questions).

3) Reasoning questions: These ask you to describe the purpose of, or the support provided for, a statement made in the passage (Structure questions) or to judge how well the author supports his or her argument (Evaluate questions).

4) Application questions: These ask you to apply new information from either the question stem itself (New Information questions) or from the answer choices (Strengthen, Weaken, and Analogy questions) to the passage.

More detail on question types and strategies can be found in Chapter 2.

TESTING TIPS

Before Test Day

- Take a trip to the test center at least a day or two before your actual test date so that you can easily find the building and room on test day. This will also allow you to gauge traffic and see if you need money for parking or any other unexpected expenses. Knowing this type of information ahead of time will greatly reduce your stress on the day of your test.
- During the week before the test, adjust your sleeping schedule so that you are going to bed and getting up in the morning at the same times as on the day before and morning of the MCAT. Prioritize getting a reasonable amount of sleep during the last few nights before the test.
- Don't do any heavy studying the day before the test. This is not a test you can cram for! Your goal at this point is to rest and relax so that you can go into test day in a good physical and mental condition.
- Eat well. Try to avoid excessive caffeine and sugar. Ideally, in the weeks leading up to the actual test you should experiment a little bit with foods and practice tests to see which foods give you the most endurance. Aim for steady blood sugar levels during the test: sports drinks, peanut-butter crackers, trail mix, etc. make good snacks for your breaks and lunch.

General Test Day Info and Tips

- On the day of the test, arrive at the test center at least a half hour prior to the start time of your test.
- Examinees will be checked in to the center in the order in which they arrive.
- You will be assigned a locker or secure area in which to put your personal items. Textbooks and study notes are not allowed, so there is no need to bring them with you to the test center.
- Your ID will be checked, your palm vein will be scanned, and you will be asked to sign in.
- You will be given a noteboard booklet and a wet-erase pen, and the test center administrator will take you to the computer on which you will complete the test. You may not choose a computer; you must use the computer assigned to you.
- Nothing is allowed at the computer station except your photo ID, your locker key (if provided), and a factory sealed packet of ear plugs; not even your watch.
- If you choose to leave the testing room at the breaks, you will have your palm vein scanned again, and you will have to sign in and out.
- You are allowed to access the items in your locker, except for notes and cell phones. (Check your test center's policy on cell phones ahead of time; some centers do not even allow them to be kept in your locker.)
- Don't forget to bring the snack foods and lunch you experimented with in your practice tests.
- At the end of the test, the test administrator will collect your noteboard and pen.
- Definitely take the breaks! Get up and walk around. It's a good way to clear your head between sections and get the blood (and oxygen!) flowing to your brain.
- Ask for a clean noteboard at the breaks if you want a fresh one.

Chapter 2
Psychology and Sociology Strategy for the MCAT

2.1 SCIENCE SECTIONS OVERVIEW

There are three science sections on the MCAT:

- Chemical and Physical Foundations of Biological Systems
- Biological and Biochemical Foundations of Living Systems
- Psychological, Social, and Biological Foundations of Behavior

The Chemical and Physical Foundations of Biological Systems section (Chem/Phys) is the first section on the test. It includes questions from General Chemistry (about 30%), Physics (about 25%), Organic Chemistry (about 15%), Biochemistry (about 25%), and Biology (about 5%). Further, the questions often test chemical and physical concepts within a biological setting, for example, pressure and fluid flow in blood vessels. A solid grasp of math fundamentals is required (arithmetic, algebra, graphs, trigonometry, vectors, proportions, and logarithms), however, there are no calculus-based questions.

The Biological and Biochemical Foundations of Living Systems section (Bio/Biochem) is the third section on the test. Approximately 65% of the questions in this section come from biology, approximately 25% come from biochemistry, and approximately 10% come from Organic and General Chemistry. Math calculations are generally not required on this section of the test, however, a basic understanding of statistics as used in biological research is helpful.

The Psychological, Social, and Biological Foundations of Behavior section (Psych/Soc) is the fourth and final section on the test. About 65% of the questions will be drawn from Psychology (with about 5% of these having biological relevance), about 30% from Sociology, and about 5% from Biology. As with the Bio/Biochem section, calculations are generally not required, however, a basic understanding of statistics as used in research is helpful.

Most of the questions in the science sections (44 of the 59) are passage-based, and each section has ten passages. Passages consist of a few paragraphs of information and include equations, reactions, graphs, figures, tables, experiments, and data. Four to six questions will be associated with each passage.

The remaining 25% of the questions (15 of 59) in each science section are freestanding questions (FSQs). These questions appear in approximately four groups interspersed between the passages. Each group contains four to five questions.

95 minutes are allotted to each of the science sections. This breaks down to approximately one minute and 35 seconds per question.

2.2 SCIENCE PASSAGE TYPES

The passages in the science sections fall into one of three main categories: Information and/or Situation-Presentation, Experiment/Research Presentation, or Persuasive Reasoning.

Information and/or Situation Presentation

These passages either present straightforward scientific information or they describe a particular event or occurrence. Generally, questions associated with these passages test basic science facts or ask you to predict outcomes given new variables or new information. Here is an example of an Information/Situation Presentation passage:

Figure 1 shows a portion of the inner mechanism of a typical home smoke detector. It consists of a pair of capacitor plates which are charged by a 9-volt battery (not shown). The capacitor plates (electrodes) are connected to a sensor device, D; the resistor R denotes the internal resistance of the sensor. Normally, air acts as an insulator and no current would flow in the circuit shown. However, inside the smoke detector is a small sample of an artificially produced radioactive element, americium-241, which decays primarily by emitting alpha particles, with a half-life of approximately 430 years. The daughter nucleus of the decay has a half-life in excess of two million years and therefore poses virtually no biohazard.

Figure 1 Smoke detector mechanism

The decay products (alpha particles and gamma rays) from the ^{241}Am sample ionize air molecules between the plates and thus provide a conducting pathway which allows current to flow in the circuit shown in Figure 1. A steady-state current is quickly established and remains as long as the battery continues to maintain a 9-volt potential difference between its terminals.

However, if smoke particles enter the space between the capacitor plates and thereby interrupt the flow, the current is reduced, and the sensor responds to this change by triggering the alarm. (Furthermore, as the battery starts to "die out," the resulting drop in current is also detected to alert the homeowner to replace the battery.)

$$C = \varepsilon_0 \frac{A}{d}$$

Equation 1

Where ε_0 is the universal permittivity constant, equal to 8.85 $\times 10^{-32}$ $C^2/(N \cdot m^2)$. Since the area A of each capacitor plate in the smoke detector is 20 cm² and the plates are separated by a distance d of 5 mm, the capacitance is 3.5×10^{-12} F = 3.5 pF.

Experiment/Research Presentation

These passages present the details of experiments and research procedures. They often include data tables and graphs. Generally, questions associated with these passages ask you to interpret data, draw conclusions, and make inferences. Here is an example of an Experiment/Research Presentation passage:

The development of sexual characteristics depends upon various factors, the most important of which are hormonal control, environmental stimuli, and the genetic makeup of the individual. The hormones that contribute to the development include the steroid hormones estrogen, progesterone, and testosterone, as well as the pituitary hormones FSH (follicle-stimulating hormone) and LH (luteinizing hormone).

To study the mechanism by which estrogen exerts its effects, a researcher performed the following experiments using cell culture assays.

Experiment 1:

Human embryonic placental mesenchyme (HEPM) cells were grown for 48 hours in Dulbecco's Modified Eagle's Medium (DMEM), with media change every 12 hours. Upon confluent growth, cells were exposed to a 10 mg per mL solution of green fluorescent-labeled estrogen for 1 hour. Cells were rinsed with DMEM and observed under confocal fluorescent microscopy.

Experiment 2:

HEPM cells were grown to confluence as in Experiment 1. Cells were exposed to Pesticide A for 1 hour, followed by the 10 mg/mL solution of labeled estrogen, rinsed as in Experiment 1, and observed under confocal fluorescent microscopy.

Experiment 3:

Experiment 1 was repeated with Chinese Hamster Ovary (CHO) cells instead of HEPM cells.

Experiment 4:

CHO cells injected with cytoplasmic extracts of HEPM cells were grown to confluence, exposed to the 10 mg/mL solution of labeled estrogen for 1 hour, and observed under confocal fluorescent microscopy.

The results of these experiments are given in Table 1.

Table 1 Detection of Estrogen (+ indicates presence of Estrogen)

Experiment	Media	Cytoplasm	Nucleus
1	+	+	+
2	+	+	+
3	+	+	+
4	+	+	+

After observing the cells in each experiment, the researcher bathed the cells in a solution containing 10 mg per mL of a red fluorescent probe that binds specifically to the estrogen receptor only when its active site is occupied. After 1 hour, the cells were rinsed with DMEM and observed under confocal fluorescent microscopy. The results are presented in Table 2.

The researcher also repeated Experiment 2 using Pesticide B, an estrogen analog, instead of Pesticide A. Results from other researchers had shown that Pesticide B binds to the active site of the cytosolic estrogen receptor (with an affinity 10,000 times greater than that of estrogen) and causes increased transcription of mRNA.

Table 2 Observed Fluorescence and Estrogen Effects (G = green, R = red)

Experiment	Media	Cytoplasm	Nucleus	Estrogen effects observed?
1	G only	G and R	G and R	Yes
2	G only	G only	G only	No
3	G only	G only	G only	No
4	G only	G and R	G and R	Yes

Based on these results, the researcher determined that estrogen had no effect when not bound to a cytosolic, estrogen-specific receptor.

Persuasive Reasoning

These passages typically present a scientific phenomenon along with a hypothesis that explains the phenomenon, and may include counter-arguments as well. Questions associated with these passages ask you to evaluate the hypothesis or arguments. Persuasive Reasoning passages in the science sections of the MCAT tend to be less common than Information Presentation or Experiment-based passages. Here is an example of a Persuasive Reasoning passage:

Two theoretical chemists attempted to explain the observed trends of acidity by applying two interpretations of molecular orbital theory. Consider the pK_a values of some common acids listed along with the conjugate base:

acid	pK_a	conjugate base
H_2SO_4	< 0	HSO_4-
H_2CrO_4	5.0	$HCrO_4-$
H_2PO_4	2.1	H_2CrO_4-
HF	3.9	F–
HOCl	7.8	ClO–
HCN	9.5	CN–
HIO_3	1.2	IO_3-

Recall that acids with a $pK_a < 0$ are called strong acids, and those with a $pKa > 0$ are called weak acids. The arguments of the chemists are given below.

Chemist #1:

"The acidity of a compound is proportional to the polarization of the H—X bond, where X is some nonmetal element.

Complex acids, such as H_2SO_4, $HClO_4$, and HNO_3 are strong acids because the H—O bonding electrons are strongly drawn toward the oxygen. It is generally true that a covalent bond weakens as its polarization increases. Therefore, one can conclude that the strength of an acid is proportional to the number of electronegative atoms in that acid."

Chemist #2:

"The acidity of a compound is proportional to the number of stable resonance structures of that acid's conjugate base. H_2SO_4, $HClO_4$, and HNO_3 are all strong acids because their respective conjugate bases exhibit a high degree of resonance stabilization."

Mapping a Passage

"Mapping a passage" refers to the combination of on-screen highlighting and noteboard notes that you take while working through a passage. Typically, good things to highlight include the overall topic of a paragraph, familiar terms, unusual terms, italicized terms, numerical values, hypothesis, and experimental results. Noteboard notes can be used to summarize the paragraphs and to jot down important facts and connections that are made when reading the passage. More details on passage mapping will be presented in section 2.5.

2.3 SCIENCE QUESTION TYPES

Questions in the science sections are generally one of three main types: Memory, Explicit, or Implicit.

Memory Questions

These questions can be answered directly from prior knowledge, with no need to reference the passage or question text. Memory questions represent approximately 25 percent of the science questions on the MCAT. Usually, Memory questions are found as FSQs, but they can also be tucked into a passage. Here's an example of a Memory question:

> Which of the following acetylating conditions will convert diethylamine into an amide at the fastest rate?
>
> A) Acetic acid / HCl
> B) Acetic anhydride
> C) Acetyl chloride
> D) Ethyl acetate

Explicit Questions

Explicit questions can be answered primarily with information from the passage, along with prior knowledge. They may require data retrieval, graph analysis, or making a simple connection. Explicit questions make up approximately 35–40 percent of the science questions on the MCAT; here's an example (taken from the Information/Situation Presentation passage above):

> The sensor device *D* shown in Figure 1 performs its function by acting as:
>
> A) an ohmmeter.
> B) a voltmeter.
> C) a potentiometer.
> D) an ammeter.

Implicit Questions

These questions require you to take information from the passage, combine it with your prior knowledge, apply it to a new situation, and come to some logical conclusion. They typically require more complex connections than do Explicit questions, and may also require data retrieval, graph analysis, etc. Implicit questions usually require a solid understanding of the passage information. They make up approximately 35–40 percent of the science questions on the MCAT; here's an example (taken from the Experiment/ Research Presentation passage above):

If Experiment 2 were repeated, but this time exposing the cells first to Pesticide A and then to Pesticide B before exposing them to the green fluorescent-labeled estrogen and the red fluorescent probe, which of the following statements will most likely be true?

A) Pesticide A and Pesticide B bind to the same site on the estrogen receptor.
B) Estrogen effects would be observed.
C) Only green fluorescence would be observed.
D) Both green and red fluorescence would be observed.

2.4 PSYCHOLOGY AND SOCIOLOGY ON THE MCAT

This section will test your content knowledge of psychological, biological, and sociological factors that shape human thought, perception, behavior, attitude, and learning. Furthermore, you will be expected to have a basic understanding of mental illness, social structure, and global disparities in health, health care, and social class. The MCAT will test your knowledge and application of these subjects at approximately the level that you would be expected to understand them in an introductory psychology class (one semester), introductory sociology class (one semester), and an introductory biology class (two semesters, though you should be prepared for more advanced physiology concepts, like you would see on the MCAT Biological and Biochemical Foundations of Living Systems section). The application of this material is potentially vast; passages can discuss anything from the specifics about a psychological research study to the complexities of studying population dynamics to the nuances of an unusual neurological disease. Additionally, questions on the Psych/Soc section will require you to demonstrate your scientific inquiry, reasoning, and understanding of basic research and statistical methods as applied to concepts in the psychological, sociological, and biological sciences. Overall, this section is designed to test your knowledge and application of the behavioral, biological, and social determinants of health and wellness.

The science sections of the MCAT have 10 passages and 15 freestanding questions (FSQs). On the Psych/ Soc section, introductory biology will comprise approximately 5% of the questions, introductory sociology concepts will comprise roughly 30% of the questions, and introductory psychology concepts will comprise about 65% of the questions, with 5% having biological relevance.

2.5 TACKLING A PSYCH/SOC PASSAGE

In order to complete all of the passages and freestanding questions on the Psych/Soc section, it will be important to tackle this section strategically. An understanding about the types of passages you will encounter should help you accomplish this.

Experiment/Research Presentation

This type of passage on the Psych/Soc section will typically present some information about a relevant topic, and also present the details behind an experiment relating to that topic. Data will be presented in the tables, graphs, figures, and within the passage. These passages are challenging because they require an understanding of the reasoning and logic behind the experiment and research, the ability to analyze the results and form conclusions, and a basic understanding of statistics.

Information/Situation Presentation

This type of passage will generally present a basic concept with additional detail (that goes well beyond an introductory-level understanding) or a novel concept (like a rare neurological disease) that extrapolates information from more basic information. In order to tackle these passages, first, do not panic if you see information that you've never heard about! Rather, look for concepts that parallel what you *do* know about. For example, if you see a question about a rare neurological disorder, look for information that applies to your basic knowledge of the nervous system.

However, in order to answer passage questions and freestanding questions effectively and efficiently, you *will* need to know your basics. Don't waste time staring at a passage or question wondering, "Should I know this?" Instead, with a solid foundation in the basic core knowledge, you will be confident that you are *not* expected to know about this random, rare disease, and rather will find information in the passage and/or apply core concepts.

READING A PSYCH/SOC PASSAGE

Although tempting, try not to get too bogged down in reading all of the little details in a passage. While it is easy to get lost in the science or the glut of background information in a passage, it isn't necessary to read every nuance. Almost every psychology/sociology passage—including information/situation passages —will, in some way, describe research that was conducted. When skimming the passage, look for the key elements of any study: the methods, participants, hypotheses, and results. Your goal is to skim, and as quickly as possible get a gist for what the study was about and what the results suggested.

For Experiment/Research Presentation passages, you will need to read more closely and carefully. You will likely have questions concerning the experimental design and/or the data and results. Therefore, invest a little more time reading so you understand the experiment and the outcomes, but don't worry about completely absorbing the results until you see what types of questions are asked.

Information/Situation Presentation passages can be skimmed to get a general sense of where the information is located within the passage. The research that is described in these passages tends to be more of a general overview of findings and less detail about the methodology of the study is generally provided. Furthermore, these passages may contain a fair amount of detailed information that you may not need, so save your time—don't bother reading all of the details until you come to a question that asks about them; then go back and read more closely.

Advanced Reading Skills

To improve your ability to read and glean information from a passage, you need to practice. Be critical when you read the content; watch for vague areas or holes in the passage that aren't explained clearly. Remember that information about new topics will be woven throughout the passage; you may need to piece together information from several paragraphs and a figure to get the whole picture.

After you've read, highlighted, and mapped a passage (more on this in a bit), stop and ask yourself the following questions:

- What was this passage about? What was the conclusion or main point?
- Was there a paragraph that was mostly background?
- What question were the researchers trying to explore?
- Who were the participants?
- What groups did researchers divide the participants into, or what groups were present in the research that was described?
- What were the hypotheses?
- What were the results?
- Were there any unexpected results, or did they confirm the hypotheses?

This takes a while at first, but eventually becomes second nature and you will start doing it as you are reading the passage. With practice, you will begin to notice patterns in the way that passages are presented: they usually begin with background information (of varying complexity and utility), then frame a specific area of researchers that social scientists have been interested in. Once this frame is established, a research question is explored either through a study or information that has been gathered. Then, in some order, there are groups, hypotheses, results, and conclusions. This is more of a general guideline than a hard and fast rule, but identifying these patterns (and noticing exceptions and deviations when they arise) during abundant practice will greatly increase the efficiency and effectiveness with which you are able to skim the passage. If you have a study group you are working with, consider doing this as an exercise with your study partners. Take turns asking and answering the questions above. Having to explain something to someone else not only solidifies your own knowledge, but helps you see where you might be weak.

MAPPING A PSYCH/SOC PASSAGE

Mapping a Psych/Soc passage is a combination of highlighting and noteboard notes that can help you organize and understand the passage information.

Resist the temptation to highlight everything (everyone has done this: you're reading a psychology textbook with a highlighter, and then look back and realize that the whole page is yellow!). Restrict your highlighting to a few things:

2.5

- the main theme of a paragraph (does it describe background, methods, results, etc.?)
- an unusual or unfamiliar term that is defined specifically for that passage (e.g., something that is italicized)
- each of the important details of the study that we described earlier: methods, participants, groups, hypotheses, results, and conclusions

Your noteboard notes should be organized. Make sure the passage number, the range of questions for that passage, and a topic appear at the top of your notes. For each paragraph, note "P1," "P2," etc., on the noteboard, and jot down a few notes about that paragraph. Try to translate science-y jargon into your own words using everyday language (this is particularly useful for experiments). Also, make sure to jot down simple relationships (e.g., the relationship between two variables).

Pay attention to figures and tables to see what type of information they contain. Don't spend a lot of time analyzing at this point, but do jot down on your noteboard "Fig 1" and a brief summary of the data. Also, if you've discovered a list in the passage, note its topic and location down on your noteboard.

Let's take a look at how we might highlight and map a practice passage:

Psychotic disorders—most notably schizophrenia and bipolar disorder with psychotic features—affect approximately 2% of Americans. These disorders are extremely manageable with psychotropic medications—to relieve symptoms such as hallucinations and delusions—and behavioral therapy, such as social skills training and hygiene maintenance.

However, individuals with psychotic disorders have the lowest level of medication compliance, as compared to individuals with mood or anxiety disorders. Antipsychotic medications can have extremely negative side effects, including uncontrollable twitching of the face or limbs, blurred vision, and weight gain, among others. They also must be taken frequently, and at high doses, in order to be effective. While relatively little is known about the reasons for noncompliance, studies do suggest that in schizophrenia, age of schizophrenia diagnosis and medication compliance is positively correlated. Evidence also suggests that medication noncompliance is disproportionally prevalent in individuals of a low socioeconomic status (SES) due to issues such as homelessness, lack of insurance benefits, and lack of familial or social support.

2.5

Researchers were interested to see how drug education might affect compliance or noncompliance with psychotropic medications based on patient socioeconomic status. In a study of 1200 mentally ill individuals in the Los Angeles metro area, researchers measured baseline psychotropic medication compliance, then provided patients with a free educational seminar on drug therapy, and then measured psychotropic medication compliance six months later. The one-day, 8-hour seminar included information on positive effects of psychotropic medication, side effects of psychotropic medication, psychotropic medication interactions with other substances such as alcohol and non-prescribed drugs, and information on accessing Medicare benefits. Compliance was measured by the number of doses of prescribed psychotropic medication that the patients took in a week, over the course of 12 weeks, as compared to the number of doctor-recommended doses per week. Compliance was measured using a self-report questionnaire.

Results indicated that post-seminar, mentally ill patients from middle or upper class backgrounds (Upper and Middle SES) were significantly more compliant with their psychotropic medication regimens than prior to the seminar. However, no significant differences were found in patients at or below the poverty level (Lower SES). Table 1 displays psychotropic medication compliance by SES and disorder.

Table 1   Psychotropic Medication Compliance by Socioeconomic Status (SES) and Disorder

Disorder	SES	Pre-Seminar Compliance	Post-Seminar Compliance
Bipolar I	Upper	60%	73%
	Middle	57%	61%
	Lower	25%	27%
Schizophrenia	Upper	53%	65%
	Middle	51%	62%
	Lower	22%	26%

Analysis and Passage Map

This Experiment/Research Presentation passage follows a very common pattern for psychology/sociology passages. It starts off with an introduction of a topic and background information, provides a frame for the research, describes methodology, and presents results. The way this is presented varies, but in this example each point is given its own paragraph. The first paragraph starts with an introduction to the topic, psychotic disorders (specifically schizophrenia and bipolar disorder). This is primarily a background information paragraph and can be skimmed quickly, with a few specific words/phrases highlighted.

The second paragraph starts with "however," indicating a change in direction. This change in direction establishes the frame for the research. The first paragraph said that schizophrenia is easily managed with drugs and therapy, but the second paragraph indicates that that isn't the whole story; in fact, the main topic of the passage is presented—medication noncompliance, particularly in low socioeconomic (SES) individuals.

The third paragraph presents relevant information about the study conducted to determine the impact of drug education on medication noncompliance in various SES groups. This is essentially the methodology section. It is important to highlight the key features of the study here—what is it looking at, and how is data collected. You do not necessarily need to highlight every single detail, but understand the basic premise of the study.

The final paragraph describes the results of the study, and presents the data in Table 1. The paragraph provides you with the significant finding that is demonstrated by the data in the table—while upper and middle SES individuals demonstrated an increased medication compliance after the drug education seminar, low SES individuals did not.

Here is what your noteboard should look like:

> (Your heading would go above this list)
> *P1—psychotic disorders are manageable with medication and therapy*
> *P2—but medication compliance is a big problem, especially for low SES*
> *P3—STUDY: medication compliance by SES before and after a drug education seminar*
> *P4—RESULTS: medication compliance increases for upper and middle SES, no improvement for low SES*

One more thing about passages on the MCAT: you can do the passages in any order you want to. There are no bonus points for taking the test in order. Therefore, tackle the passages that you are most comfortable with first, and save the harder ones for last (see "General Strategy" in Chapter 1 for more information on how to move around efficiently in the test).

2.6 TACKLING THE QUESTIONS

Questions on the Psych/Soc section mimic the three typical science question types: Memory, Explicit, and Implicit.

Memory Questions in the Psych/Soc Section

Memory questions are exactly what they sound like: they test your knowledge of some specific fact or concept. While Memory questions are typically found as freestanding questions, they can also be tucked into a passage. The questions, aside from requiring memorization, do not generally cause problems for students because they are similar to the types of questions that would appear on a typical college psychology or sociology exam. Below are two examples of Memory questions, taken from the passage above:

1.   What is one "positive" symptom of schizophrenia?

A)   Catatonia
B)   Weight gain
C)   Flattened affect
D)   Auditory or visual hallucinations

2.   Bipolar disorder involves periods of mania and depression, and for some, episodes of hypomania. Hypomania, a state that is less severe than mania, is characterized by "feeling good/high" and increased well-being and productiveness. Which of the mechanisms is most likely involved with the hypomanic episodes experienced by individuals diagnosed with bipolar disorder?

A)   Increased dopamine in the brain
B)   Decreased stimulation of the enteric plexus
C)   Increased activation of the posterior pituitary
D)   Decreased serotonin in the central nervous system

These are Memory questions because, even though they are associated with the passage, you could have answered them (and should be able to answer them) without reading the passage. It is important that you recognize them as Memory questions so you don't go back to the passage and waste time looking for answers that are not there! There is no specific "trick" to answering Memory questions; either you know the correct answer or you don't.

If you find that you are missing a fair number of Memory questions, it is a sure sign that you do not know the content well enough. Go back and review.

Here are the answers for the questions above.

1. **D**   A "positive" symptom of schizophrenia is an addition to, excess of, or distortion of normal functions; auditory or visual hallucinations are positive symptoms of the illness (choice D is correct). A "negative" symptom of schizophrenia is a diminishment or absence of normal function; catatonia (lack or responsiveness to stimuli) and flattened affect (lack of emotion) are both negative symptoms (choices A and C are wrong). Weight gain is often a side effect of psychotropic medications, not a symptom of schizophrenia (choice B is wrong).

2. **A**   Dopamine is the primary neurotransmitter involved with the "reward centers" of the brain; since hypomania is characterized by "feeling good/high," it can reasonably be concluded that an increase of dopamine in the brain could produce this effect (choice A is correct). The enteric plexus or enteric nervous system is a portion of the autonomic nervous system that controls the gastrointestinal tract; decreased stimulation of the enteric nervous system would not produce any of the characteristics of hypomania described (choice B is wrong). The posterior pituitary is responsible for producing oxytocin, a hormone that controls lactation and uterine contractions, and vasopressin, a hormone that controls how much water the kidneys resorb; therefore, increased activation of the posterior pituitary would not produce any of the characteristics of hypomania described (choice C is wrong). Serotonin is a neurotransmitter with widespread effects in the brain; a decrease of serotonin in the brain has been shown to produce symptoms of depression, not hypomania (choice D is wrong).

Explicit Questions in the Psych/Soc section

True, pure Explicit questions are rare in the Psych/Soc section. A purely Explicit question can be answered with only information in the passage. Below is an example of a pure Explicit question from the passage above:

3. What is the incidence of psychotic disorders in the American population?

A)   1%
B)   2%
C)   4%
D)   Unknown

Referring back to the first paragraph of the passage, it clearly states that "Psychotic disorders—most notably schizophrenia and bipolar disorder with psychotic features—affect approximately 2% of Americans;" therefore, choice **B** is correct.

However, more often on the Psych/Soc section, Explicit questions are more of a blend of Explicit and Memory; they require not only retrieval of passage information, but also recall of some relevant information. They usually do not require in-depth analysis or connections. Here is an example of a common type of Explicit question:

4. Based on the design of the study described in the passage, what limits the researchers' abilities to draw conclusions about the causal relationship between socioeconomic status and psychotropic medication compliance?

A) Age at first diagnosis was not measured.
B) Participants were not randomly assigned to socioeconomic status.
C) The sample contained only Los Angeles metro area residents.
D) Severity of symptoms were not measured.

2.6

To answer this question, you first need to retrieve information from the passage about the study's experimental design (from paragraph 3). You also need to recall some information about experimental design, and what sort of factors limit a researcher's ability to infer a causal relationship.

Here is the solution to the question above:

4. **B** Causation is extremely difficult to determine when experimenting with humans, particularly because all of the variables in a given experiment must by controlled by the researcher, and subjects must be randomly assigned to experimental and control groups. Therefore, random assignment of subjects to a group (in this case, a socioeconomic status group) is one of the many variables that should have been controlled for in order to determine a causal relationship between socioeconomic status and psychotropic medication compliance (choice B is correct). While age at first diagnosis and symptom severity are important variables that could have been measured, neither specifically limits the researchers' ability to draw conclusions about the causal relationship between socioeconomic status and psychotropic medication compliance (choices A and D are wrong). The fact that the sample only contained participants from the Los Angeles metro area limits the researchers' ability to draw conclusions about how their results might apply to the general population, not about causality (choice C is wrong).

A final subgroup in the Explicit question category is graph or data interpretation questions. These questions will either ask you to take graphical information from the passage and convert it into a text answer, or they will ask you to take text from the passage and convert it into a graph. Below is an example from the passage above:

2.6

5. Which of the following graphs would best illustrate the relationship between age of schizophrenia diagnosis and medication compliance described in the passage?

A)

B)

C)

D)

The passage states, in the second paragraph, that "...studies do suggest that in schizophrenia, age of schizophrenia diagnosis and medication compliance is positively correlated." Therefore, as age of diagnosis increases, so does compliance. So, a graphical representation should look like the figure in choice **A**.

If you find you are missing Explicit questions, practice your passage mapping. Make sure you aren't missing the critical items in the passage that lead you to the right answer. Slow down a little; take an extra 15 to 30 seconds per passage to read or think about it more carefully.

Implicit Questions

Implicit questions require the most thought. These require recall not only of Psych/Soc content information but also information gleaned from the passage, and a more in-depth analysis of how the two relate. Implicit questions require more analysis and connections to be made than Explicit questions. Often they take the form "If...then...." Below is an example of a classic Implicit question, based on the passage above:

6. The experiment described in the passage was repeated, but instead of testing how drug education affects compliance, researchers measured how incentives affect compliance in low SES schizophrenics. The low SES schizophrenia group was broken into two groups. Group A received an incentive every time they took their medication for seven consecutive days, while Group B received an incentive every two weeks, regardless of compliance level. Based on operant conditioning principles, what results should the researchers see?

A) There should be no difference in compliance levels from the first study.
B) Group A's compliance should be higher than Group B's compliance.
C) Group B's compliance should be higher than Group A's compliance.
D) Both groups should demonstrate increased compliance from the first study but it is impossible to tell which group's compliance is expected to be higher.

To answer this question, conclusions have to be drawn about the experiment described in the passage, and the new experiment described in the question stem, and then applied to your content knowledge about reward schedules in operant conditioning. Many, many more connections need to be made than when answering an Explicit question. A detailed explanation for this question is below.

6. **B** According to the question, Group A is receiving an incentive on a fixed-ratio schedule (after every seven consecutive days of medication compliance) and Group B is receiving an incentive on a fixed-interval schedule (every two weeks, regardless of compliance). According to operant conditioning principles, a fixed-ratio schedule should produce a high rate of desired behavior (in this case, medication compliance), while a fixed-interval schedule produces

a steady rate of response that tends to increase closer to the reward, but is not nearly as frequent as what is expected from a fixed-ratio reward schedule (choice B is correct; choice C is wrong). Based on operant conditioning principles, rewarding desired behavior should increase behavior (choice A is wrong), and applying a fixed-ratio and fixed-interval reward schedule should increase behavior in predictable ways (choice D is wrong).

If you find that you are missing a lot of Implicit questions, first of all, make sure that you are using POE aggressively. Second, go back and review the explanations for the correct answers, and figure out where your logic went awry. Did you miss an important fact in the passage? Did you forget the relevant Psych/Soc content? Did you follow the logical train of thought to the right answer? Once you figure out where you made your mistake, you will know how to correct it.

2.7 SUMMARY OF THE APPROACH TO PSYCHOLOGY AND SOCIOLOGY

How to Map the Passage and Use Your Noteboard

1) The passage should be skimmed, NOT be read like textbook material. Do not try to learn something from every sentence (science majors especially will be tempted to read this way). Passages should be read to get a feel for the type of questions that will follow, and to get a general idea of the location of information within the passage.

2) Highlighting—Use this tool sparingly, or you will end up with a passage that is completely covered in yellow highlighter! Highlighting in a Psych/Soc passage should be used to draw attention to a few words that demonstrate one of the following:
   - the main theme of a paragraph
   - an unusual or unfamiliar term that is defined specifically for that passage (e.g., something that is italicized)
   - main points of the research: methods, participants, groups, hypotheses, results, conclusions

3) Pay brief attention to figures and experiments, noting only what information they deal with. Do not spend a lot of time analyzing at this point.

4) For each passage, start by noting the passage number, the general topic, and the range of questions on your noteboard. You can then work between your noteboard and the Review screen to easily get to the questions you want (see Chapter 1).

5) For each paragraph, note "P1," "P2," etc. on the noteboard and jot down a few notes about that paragraph. Try to translate psych/soc jargon into your own words using everyday language. Especially note down simple relationships (e.g., the relationship between two variables). Be brief here. Use annotations and symbols to represent main ideas and results.

6) The noteboard is only useful if it is kept organized! Make sure that your notes for each passage are clearly delineated and marked with the passage number and question range. This will allow you to easily read your notes when you come back to a review a flagged question. Resist the temptation to write in the first available blank space, as this makes it much more difficult to refer back to your work.

Psych/Soc Question Strategies

1) Remember that the content in Psychology and Sociology is broad, but not necessarily super deep, so don't panic if something seems completely unfamiliar. Understand the basic content well, find the basics in the unfamiliar topic, and apply them to the question.

2) Process of Elimination is paramount! The strikeout tool allows you to eliminate answer choices; this will improve your chances of guessing the correct answer if you are unable to narrow it down to one choice.

3) Answer the straightforward questions first (typically the memory questions). Leave questions that require analysis of experiments and graphs for later. Take the test in the order YOU want. Make sure to use your noteboard to indicate questions you skipped.

4) Make sure that the answer you choose actually answers the question, and isn't just a true statement.

5) Try to avoid answer choices with extreme words such as "always," "never," etc. In psych/soc, there is almost always an exception and answers are rarely black-and-white.

6) I-II-III questions: Whenever possible, start by evaluating the Roman numeral item that shows up in exactly two answer choices. This will allow you to quickly eliminate two wrong answer choices regardless of whether the item is true or false. Typically then, you will only have to assess one of the other Roman numeral items to determine the correct answer. Always work between the I-II-III statements and the answer choices. Once an item is found to be true (or false), strike out answer choices which do not contain (or do contain) that item number. Make sure to strike out the actual Roman numeral item as well, and highlight those items that are true.

7) LEAST/EXCEPT/NOT questions: Don't get tricked by these questions that ask you to pick the answer that doesn't fit (the incorrect or false statement). It's often good to use your noteboard and write a T or F next to answer choices A–D. The one that stands out as different is the correct answer!

8) Again, don't leave any question blank.

A Note About Flashcards

For most of the exams you've taken previously, flashcards were likely very helpful. This was because those exams mostly required you to regurgitate information, and flashcards are pretty good at helping you memorize facts. However, the most challenging aspect of the MCAT is not that it requires you to memorize the fine details of content knowledge, but that it requires you to apply your basic scientific knowledge to unfamiliar situations: flashcards alone may not help you there.

Flashcards can be beneficial if your basic content knowledge is deficient in some area. For example, if you don't know the stages of Erikson's psychosocial model of development, flashcards can certainly help you memorize these facts. Or, maybe you are unsure of the functions of the different brain regions. You might find that flashcards can help you memorize these. But unless you are trying to memorize basic facts in your personal weak areas, you are better off doing and analyzing practice passages than carrying around a stack of flashcards.

2.7

Chapter 3
Research Methods and Study Design

To understand human behavior and the complex interplay of human societies, researchers in the social sciences use a variety of methodologies to test hypotheses regarding behavior. Conducting social science research presents ethical and logistical complications that are unique from those faced by scientists in the physical and biological sciences. As a result, social scientists must be creative about how they combine methodologies, design research, and especially how they draw conclusions from the research they conduct. Determining causal relationships between variables is especially difficult when complex human behavior is considered. This chapter explores the types of problems researchers face, and the different tools at their disposal to assess human behavior and draw conclusions on why we do the things we do and what makes us who we are.

In addition to psychology and sociology content at the first-year undergraduate level, the MCAT Psychology and Sociology section will also feature many questions that incorporate research methods and study design (about 20-25% of the section). These questions will require knowledge of the elementary aspects of social research, such as types of study design, especially the experimental method, and what types of conclusions can be drawn from each. Almost all Psychology/Sociology passages will contain a study, and the majority of these passages will contain at least one question in which you are asked to evaluate the study or make a prediction about the implications of the research. Fortunately, the amount of content associated with these questions is manageable and is not heavy in statistics. What *is* required is knowledge of the common types of research conducted by social scientists, the strengths and weaknesses of each method, and the types of conclusions that can reasonably be drawn from each.

3.1 EXPERIMENTAL DESIGN

Because the word "experiment" is often used interchangeably with "research," it is easy to forget that "experimental design" is a technical term for a *specific type* of research. To emphasize this difference, let's examine an area of research in which social scientists might be interested. Many different types of studies have shown that a Mediterranean diet (one rich in seafood, legumes, nuts, olive oil, fruits, and vegetables) is associated with cardiovascular health and longevity. However, to show that consuming a Mediterranean diet helps *cause*, or helps *lead* to cardiovascular health and longevity, an experimental design is needed.

To see why this is the case, imagine a study in which a team of social scientists creates a scale to measure the extent to which an individual follows the Mediterranean diet: the subject would answer questions about how frequently she eats foods associated with that diet. Based on the responses on this food-frequency questionnaire, researchers assign a score for each individual from 1 (diet least resembles a traditional Mediterranean diet) to 12 (diet most resembles a traditional Mediterranean diet). Let's call this scale the Mediterranean Diet Index (MDI). Suppose researchers find that as individual MDI scores increase, so do measures of cardiovascular health. This finding does not show that adherence to the Mediterranean diet causes cardiovascular health to improve.

What the team has found is a positive correlation (discussed below) between the MDI and cardiovascular fitness, but correlation is not causation. For example, it is possible that people with a genetic predisposition toward good cardiovascular health produce a profile of digestive enzymes that leads to a natural preference for a Mediterranean-style diet. This implies that a predisposition to good cardiovascular health causes high MDI scores. This actually flips the causal direction! Another possible explanation is that some third factor, such as exercise or social support, leads to both greater cardiovascular health *and* a preference for Mediterranean foods (see Figure 1). A fourth possibility is that some third factor causes an increase in cardiovascular health, but does not actually lead to consuming a Mediterranean diet. This causal factor is merely positively correlated with Mediterranean-diet consumption. To rule out these other possible explanations and determine that a Mediterranean diet actually does cause improved cardiovascular health, the team must conduct a follow-up study with an experimental design.

A → B
A causes B

B → A
B causes A

C ⇄ B / A
C causes both
A and B

C ↗ B / A
C causes B, but is only
correlated with A

Figure 1   Possible causal relationships that could explain a correlation
that is found between two variables, A and B.

There are several steps to good experimental design. In this case, the researchers hope to show that adherence to a Mediterranean diet actually *causes* greater cardiovascular health.

1) <u>Select the population.</u> The first thing the researchers must agree on is the population of interest. Whom do they want to study? It may seem obvious that they would be interested in "all humans;" however, for various reasons, this may not be the best group to select. For example, many experiments in the social sciences are done by scholars at universities. Suppose our team of researchers were all tenured at a university—let's call it Healthy Living U. Then the easiest way for the researchers to get a large group of participants at low cost would be to use students at Healthy Living U as participants in the experiment.

Of course, our researchers would ideally like their findings to apply to everyone, but if they select the greater population as the population of interest, the researchers would have to find older (and younger) participants. Researchers would have to come up with ways to incentivize them to participate in the research and follow through to make sure they follow the experimental protocol correctly. Because this would be very taxing in terms of resources and logistics, the researchers are likely to decide that their population of interest will be healthy young adults in their early twenties. The research team now has access to thousands of willing participants that they can recruit by offering course credit or a small cash payment, and follow up on more easily since they are all located at the university.

Think about what this (very reasonable) decision about what population to study implies for later findings. If they *do* find that Mediterranean diet adherence leads to cardiovascular health, can they say that this result is also true for individuals in their 50s or 60s? It very well might, but this conclusion now lies outside the scope of the Healthy Living U experiment. Follow-up studies would be needed to say for sure whether the effect also applies to older adults. The researchers have compromised the reach and scope of their experiment, but they now have the advantage of a large pool of willing participants that they can sample for their experiment. In practice, social science researchers often make the (very dubious) assumption that the findings they made while studying a group of young adults in college apply to all adults in a society.

2) Operationalize the independent and dependent variables. The **independent variable** is the variable manipulated by the research team. The **dependent variable** is the variable that is measured. In the correlational study described earlier, researchers found that high MDI scores were associated with better cardiovascular health. In this follow-up experimental study, the *causal* relationship that researchers want to test experimentally is whether eating a Mediterranean diet *leads* to greater cardiovascular health. The researchers must specify exactly what they mean by this.

The independent variable in this experiment is adherence to a Mediterranean diet; to qualify as an experimental design, this variable must be *directly manipulated* by the researchers. Researchers want to have maximum control over the experimental environment so that they can be sure that differences between the groups actually led to the effect, assuming one is measured. Good experimental design requires experiments that can be reproduced by other researchers, an important quality of research design known as **reproducibility**. These other researchers may want to verify the results or adapt some aspect of the experiment. For this reason, precise definitions are key. A related concept to reproducibility, **replicability**, refers to obtaining consistent results across various studies attempting to answer the same scientific question but using different data and/or new statistical methods.

The researchers at Healthy Living U decide that they will work with the cafeteria on campus to serve a special diet to participants. They team up with a group of nutritionists to create a six-month-long diet plan of twenty-one meals per week that participants will be required to consume. Participants can also consume a set of preselected snacks and beverages for their dorm rooms, but outside foods are not allowed. The diet the team constructs is such that it would score a perfect 12 on the MDI scale.

The dependent variable in the experiment is cardiovascular health. This is the variable that the researchers will measure to see if their diet has an effect. To obtain rigorous results, the researchers must create an **operational definition**, a specification of precisely what they mean by each variable. The independent variable was operationalized as a very specific set of foods consumed over a 6-month period. The dependent variable must be equally well-defined and must also meet the criterion of being **quantitative**, or numerical, as opposed to **qualitative**, or descriptive. Quantitative data will be necessary later to conduct statistical analyses that will test the research hypothesis. The researchers decide that the dependent variables they will measure are heart rate, blood pressure, peak oxygen uptake, aerobic recovery rate, blood glucose levels, and ejection fraction. Each of these will produce a numerical value that they will measure before and after the 6-month period. The difference in these values will test the effect of the dietary regimen on health.

These are strong operational definitions. Both the independent and dependent variable definitions are specific and replicable, and the dependent variable is sufficiently quantitative to allow for statistical analyses. However, notice that the researchers have introduced new limitations to the experiment. Look first at the independent variable. What if the Mediterranean diet only starts to be effective after many years? Perhaps there is an adjustment period to the new dietary protocol and we only start to see benefits over time spans much longer than 6 months. If that were the case, the present experiment would not detect a result, and the research team might wrongly conclude that the diet is ineffective.

The operationalization of the dependent variable also introduced limitations. The variable is quantitative and rigorous; however, it only indirectly measures what we are really interested in: cardiovascular health (and ultimately increased longevity). The variables the researchers selected can only *indirectly* suggest that the quality-of-life variables we really care about are improving. Again, good experimental design often involves making compromises to meet conditions or to make conducting a study realistic.

It would be great if we could verify experimentally that eating a specific diet decreases the risk of heart attack and leads to increased longevity. However, let's reflect for a moment on how difficult that would be in practice. The Healthy Living U experiment we are developing is already shaping up to be *very* restrictive for participants, even though we have created a rather optimal scenario by defining variables so that many able participants who live in the research environment could be used. Imagine if we extended the dietary regimen for a lifetime, then measured average life expectancy and morbidity due to cardiovascular disease over the course of decades. This would be nearly impossible to accomplish in practice, but that is what we would need to do to conclusively show that the diet led to health benefits! To conduct experiments that are realistically feasible, the Healthy Living U researchers must compromise by narrowing the scope of their study and selecting measurable dependent variables like heart rate and blood pressure that *imply* cardiovascular health, rather than trying to measure cardiovascular morbidity and life expectancy directly.

3) <u>Carefully select control and experimental groups.</u> The group of participants that receives treatment is the **experimental** group. To draw conclusions about the effect of the treatment, researchers also need a **control** group, which acts as a point of reference and comparison.

Suppose the high-MDI six-month-long diet leads to improvements for participants with respect to each of the cardiovascular variables measured. This would seem to be a great success for the experiment, but it could not confirm the experimental hypothesis without a control group. For example, it is probable that being given *any* dietary regimen would offer some health benefits. The researchers need a point of comparison to rule this possibility out and conclude that it was actually the Mediterranean diet, and not following a dietary regimen that offered benefits, if any are found.

Having a control group is critical to this experimental design; otherwise the study would not qualify as experimental and no causal conclusions could be drawn. Researchers want to show that eating a Mediterranean diet causes cardiovascular health. To show this, they need a control group that is **homogenous**, the same throughout, and as similar as possible to the experimental group except for the variable of interest —the treatment.

The objective of having a similar control group is to rule out **extraneous (or confounding) variables**, variables other than the treatment that could potentially explain an experimental result. What sorts of variables could affect the current experiment? Gender, age, and socioeconomic status might play a role. Certainly exercise, BMI, and stress levels could play a role as well. If researchers agreed on this list of potential extraneous variables, they would carefully select experimental and control groups that were as similar as possible in age, gender, status, serum cortisol levels, and BMI. To control for exercise, they might create a regulated regimen for both groups to follow.

Remember that to optimize study design, the experimental and control groups must be *as similar as possible*. When evaluating research methodology in published articles, you might think the care that researchers take to maintain this quality can seem extreme. However, many studies have shown that unexpected and seemingly unrelated variables can lead to an effect. One of the many phenomena that complicate social research and can lead to erroneous results is the **placebo effect**, the well-known fact that just *believing* that treatment is being administered can lead to a measurable result.

It works like this. Tell a group of depressed subjects that they are getting a cutting-edge neurological treatment for depression, confirmed through years of double-blind clinical trials. Bring them into a state-of-the-art medical research center and test them through EEG, fMRI, and stress hormone exams to "establish a baseline measure of cortical activity." Then, give them each a sugar pill to take twice a day for six weeks. It is likely, if the environment and protocol seemed authentic, that depression would actually decrease. This would be especially likely if the doctors and medical aides administering the tests and giving the prescriptions also believed the pill was the real thing. That's right, if researchers know that they are administering a treatment, that can also lead to a placebo effect! To help counter the placebo effect, studies must be **double blind**: neither the person administering treatment nor the participants truly know if they are assigned to the treatment or control groups.

If we apply these considerations to the Healthy Living U experiment, then the control group subjects need their own special diet, with physiologists taking their readings, and special chefs to cook the meals in the cafeteria. Neither the physiologists taking the readings nor the chefs should be privy to the hypotheses of the experiment, and both the experimental and control groups should be operating under the belief that they will potentially receive health benefits from participating in the study. Now, finally, we are almost ready to recruit participants and begin the procedure.

But before we start recruiting participants and conduct the study, we must take one more thing into account. The study is designed to test for the *Mediterranean* diet, specifically. To appropriately isolate this variable (also for ethical reasons, see below), researchers had better give a healthy alternative diet to the control group. The researchers might select a diet that scores a 6 on the MDI so it is relatively average in "Mediterranean-ness," but is known to also be composed of fresh, healthy foods. Then later, if a difference were to be measured, researchers could be relatively sure that this result was due to the Mediterranean diet specifically, and not just the effect of eating a healthy diet designed by a team of professional nutritionists.

Researchers can never account for *every* potential extraneous variable. Firstly, *any* variable could theoretically be a potential confound, so researchers must focus on the most likely candidates. Beyond that, it may not be possible to control for a variable even if researchers would like to.

4) Randomly sample from the population. Finally, researchers can start recruiting participants for the study. The sampling should be random: it should be equally likely for any member of the population to be a participant in the study. This is an ideal that is almost never accomplished in practice. For the Healthy Living U study, any healthy young adult in their early 20s should have an equal chance of participating in the study. However, since the study is done at a specific university, only students at that school can be used. One of the most common flaws in social research is the fact that most studies are done on undergraduate students, and results are then applied to the greater population. This is often a dubious and highly precarious leap in logic. If it is not equally likely for all members of a population to be sampled, this is known as **sampling bias**.

    Selection bias is a more general category of systemic flaws in a design that can compromise results. Aside from sampling bias, another type of selection bias is purposefully selecting which studies to evaluate in a **meta-analysis**, a big-picture analysis of many studies to look for trends in the data. Attrition, discussed below, is also a type of selection bias.

    Usually, participants in a study are incentivized in some way, which could range from monetary compensation to access to new treatments and medication. The team at Healthy Living U might use extra points on an exam or nominal tuition rebates as an incentive for students to participate. This introduces another potential problem into the study—**attrition**, participants dropping out of the study. If the reason that participants are dropping out is non-random, this might introduce an extraneous variable.

5) Randomly assign individuals to groups. Once the individuals who will participate in the study have been incentivized and rounded up, it is time to assign them to the experimental and control groups. In a well-designed experiment, it should be equally likely that they are assigned to either group. In contrast to the previous step, this one is relatively easy to pull off. In this study, there are many extraneous variables that the researchers decided to account for, so they might use a **randomized block technique.** In this technique, researchers evaluate where participants fall along the variables they wish to equalize across experimental and control groups. Then they randomly assign individuals from these groups so that the treatment and control groups are similar along the variables of interest.

6) Measure the results. For this experiment, the dependent variable is a set of well-known physiological measurements with standardized collection procedures and error measures. In more general situations, they must check to make sure that their measurements are valid. The most important aspects of measurement for an experiment are that the dependent variable is quantitative (and therefore measurable) and that instruments used are **reliable** and **valid**. Reliability means that an instrument produces stable and consistent results; validity means that it actually measures what it's supposed to measure. For example, if every morning when you step on

your bathroom scale it indicates that you weigh three pounds, that scale is reliable but not valid. Replicability means that the experiment would produce similar findings if conducted by another researcher on different subjects. This requires clarity and precision in terms of the experimental procedure and measurements that are used. This is often a point of consideration for psychological studies that test dependent variables like mood, memory, and attitude. **Psychometrics** is the study of how to measure psychological variables through testing. Another concern with surveys is **response bias**, the tendency for respondents to not have perfect insight into their state and provide inaccurate responses.

There are many ways that researchers could choose to compare groups and measure results. In the Healthy Living U study, researchers are comparing two different groups: one experimental group that receives a high-MDI diet, and a control group with an alternative dietary regimen. This is known as a **between-subjects** design; the comparisons are made between subjects, from one group to another. An alternative approach is to use a **within-subjects** design and compare the same group at different time points. For example, the research team could also choose to measure cardiovascular fitness before and after the dietary regimen, thereby making the comparisons within subjects. If researchers were to use both techniques, and make both within-subjects and between-subjects comparisons, this would be a type of **mixed methods** research. Mixed methods are any combination of different research techniques, such as within-subjects and between subjects, or qualitative and quantitative.

7) <u>Test the Hypothesis.</u> Scientists and philosophers of science over the years have generally agreed that it is better to incorrectly conclude that there is no effect (**type 2 error**, or false negative) than to falsely suppose the veracity of a result that does not actually exist (**type 1 error**, or false positive). In fact, a way to remember this distinction is to think of type 1 error as predominant, because it is a graver problem in hypothesis-testing. Much like the legal concept of "innocent until proven guilty," it is better to reason from a point of skepticism. For this reason, scientists generally start with the **null hypothesis**: they assume that there is no causal relationship between the variables and any effect that they measure, if there is one, is due to chance. Then, they see whether evidence from the experiment suggests that the null hypothesis is true or false. Taking this position and reasoning in this way places the "burden of proof" on the **experimental hypothesis,** the proposition that variations in the independent variable cause changes in the dependent variables.

To reject the null hypothesis, it is not satisfactory simply to observe a difference between two groups. After all, the observed difference may simply be due to chance. Even two identical groups or identical measures are subject to randomness and can therefore produce different measures even if there is no fundamental difference. To see why, and to get an idea of how social scientists and statisticians conduct hypothesis-testing, consider the following example.

Imagine you and a friend roll two dice (each a cube with six faces labeled from "1" to "6"). Suppose you roll a 3, and your friend rolls a 5. Should you conclude that your friend cheated, and is using an unfair die? Of course not. Chances are, the difference in that individual roll is simply due to chance. If the dice are in fact fair, after many rolls, you will find that both your averages start to converge to the natural average, 3.5[1]. If, for example, you each roll 1,000 times, and your average score is 3.497 while your friend's average score is 3.501, you will conclude that the dice were fair and the slight difference measured is simply due to chance.

---

[1] The sum of the possible scores divided by the number of possibilities (1 + 2 + 3 + 4 + 5 + 6).

Likewise, if the Healthy Living U researchers find slight differences between the experimental and control groups in cardiovascular fitness, they will not rush to conclude that the difference was *significant*. In statistics and hypothesis-testing, a **significant difference** is a measured difference between two groups that is large enough that it is probably not due to chance. The vagueness of this definition is intentional. It is up to the researchers to determine when the difference is big enough.

To see how this works in practice, let's return to the example of rolling dice. Suppose that this time around, when you and your friend roll 1,000 times, your average is 3.506 and your friend's average is 3.813. Did your friend cheat? It is not immediately obvious what you should conclude. Maybe they just got lucky. Although you can never be absolutely sure, using statistics it is possible to calculate the probability that your friend obtained this value using a fair die. The mathematics used to compute this probability are briefly covered in the statistics chapter and generally are beyond the scope of Psychology/Sociology questions on the MCAT.

Now, suppose that you ran the necessary statistical tests and they show that the chance of the measured difference in dice scores was 17%. What would you conclude? Using the legal analogy from above, you would not want to wrongfully incriminate your friend. But what if the probability you found was 6%? 3%? 0.04%? At what point would you accuse your friend of cheating? It is not an easy decision to make, since whatever value you choose as the threshold point will inherently be arbitrary.

Scientists evaluating data from experiments have the same problem. They can never be certain that a difference measured in an experiment actually reflects a fundamental difference between the groups. They must arbitrarily pick a cutoff point at which it is reasonable to conclude "beyond reasonable doubt" that there was a difference. Conventionally, social scientists have decided that if the probability of an observed difference is found to be 5% (or 0.05) or less, this constitutes a significant difference. A **p-value** is a number from 0 to 1 that represents the probability that a difference observed in an experiment is due to chance. By convention, if (and only if) $p < 0.05$, scientists reject the null hypothesis. Other p-values such as 0.01 or 0.001 are also used as the threshold for significance in some cases. To make sure that the experiment picks up an effect, it is necessary to have a large enough **sample size**, or number of participants. Usually 30 or more participants are necessary to meet the mathematical criteria needed to conduct statistical tests. A larger sample size is usually preferred. This increases the **power** of the experiment, or the ability to pick up an effect if one is actually present.

Whatever researchers decide to do, they must select the significance threshold in advance, or they might be extremely tempted to change the number so that their data reach significance. For the MCAT, make sure you know what p-values represent, and that a lower value suggests a stronger relationship.

Table 1 Summary of Good Experimental Design

Step:	Objective:	Common Flaws in Design:
1. Select the population	• Determine the population of interest • Consider what group will be pragmatic to sample	• Population is too restrictive • Sampling all individuals of interest is not practical
2. Operationalize variables	• Determine the independent and dependent variables • Specify exactly what is meant by each • Make sure the dependent variable can be measured quantitatively within the parameters of the study	• Insufficient rigor in description • Manipulation of the independent variable presents practical problems
3. Divide into groups	• Carefully select experimental and control groups • Homogenize the two groups • Isolate the treatment by controlling for potential extraneous variables	• Control group does not resemble treatment group along important variables • Experiment is not double-blind • Participants can guess the hypothesis, purpose of the study, and ways in which they're expected to behave
4. Random sampling	• Make sure all subsets of the population are represented • Ideally each member has an equal chance of being selected • Meeting these criteria is often not possible for practical reasons	• Sampling is not truly random • Sample does not represent the population of interest
5. Random assignment	• Individuals who have been sampled are equally likely to be assigned to treatment or control groups • Consider matching along potential extraneous variables which have been pre-selected	• Groups are not properly matched • Assignment is not perfectly random
6. Measurement	• Make sure measurements are standardized • Make sure instruments are reliable and valid	• Tools are not precise enough to detect a result • Instruments used for measurement are not reliable and valid
7. Test the hypothesis	• Use statistics to check for a significant difference • Assign a pre-established threshold at which the null hypothesis will be rejected	• Small sample size leads to insufficient power • Researchers do not set thresholds in advance and make after-the-fact conclusions that are suspect

3.2 EXPERIMENTAL DESIGN CONSIDERATIONS

Validity

As we took a step-by-step look at experimental design, we looked at some of the potential flaws that come up in experiments, and how they might compromise our ability to draw conclusions about the real world from our study. These flaws can be placed into two categories. In one case, the flaw or limitation might make it difficult to apply our conclusion to the real world. This is known as a flaw in **external validity**. For example, the fact that only students of Healthy Living U can participate in the study is a threat to external validity. We cannot be absolutely sure that a result that rejects the null hypothesis applies to all healthy young adults in their twenties.

Another threat to external validity is that the subjects in this experiment ate a special diet, constructed by professional researchers, cooked by culinary professionals at a university, and monitored by a team of scientists. Can we really expect an average person trying to eat an experimental diet to match this rigor? An affirmative finding that a high-MDI diet leads to healthier outcomes might not apply to conditions outside the conditions of the study.

On the other hand, a limitation of the study might be such that the experiment is not "well done," leaving doubts about the conclusion because of some inherent flaw in the design. This is known as **internal validity**. Internal validity is high if confounding variables have been considered and minimized, and the causal relationship between the independent and dependent variable can be established by the way the experiment was set up. Another important component of a well-done study is construct validity, or the extend to which a psychometric instrument measure what it purports to. If the researchers forgot to control for sex differences, used a diet that was not actually Mediterranean, or gave the control group unhealthy foods, for example, internal validity could be threatened. **Demand characteristics**, or subtle cues (usually subconscious or inadvertent) that let subjects know how they are expected to behave, can also threaten internal validity.

Another consideration, especially when psychometric evaluations are used, is **predictive validity**. For example, consider the MCAT. Does the test predict performance after the exam-taker enters school (or becomes a doctor)? This is a question about predictive validity: does the test tell us about the variable of interest? Below is a summary of the frequently-tested common threats to validity in social science experiments.

Table 2 Threats to Internal Validity

Impression Management	Participants adapt their responses based on social norms or perceived researcher expectations; self-fulfilling prophecy; methodology is not double-blind; Hawthorne Effect
Confounding Variables	Extraneous variables not accounted for in the study; another variable offers an alternative explanation for results; lack of a useful control
Lack of Validity/Reliability	Measurement tools do not measure what they purport to, lack consistency
Sampling Bias	Selection criteria are not random; population used for sample does not meet conditions for statistical test (e.g., population is not normally distributed)
Attrition Effects	Participant fatigue; participants drop out of study
Demand Characteristics	Researchers inadvertently give subtle cues about the hypothesis and how subjects are expected to behave

Table 3 Threats to External Validity

Experiment doesn't reflect real world	Laboratory setups that don't translate to the real world; lack of generalizability
Selection Criteria	Too restrictive of inclusion/exclusion criteria for participants (i.e., sample is not representative)
Situational Effects	Presence of laboratory conditions changes outcome (e.g., pre-test and post-test, presence of experimenter, claustrophobia in an MRI machine)
Lack of Statistical Power	Sample groups have high variability; sample size is too small

Ethical Considerations

Finally, all researchers should consider the ethical implications of the procedures they employ. Ethical problems tend to arise more frequently in experimental designs because researchers are directly manipulating variables, not just observing what they see in nature. Ethical controversies arose regarding many social science experiments of the early 20th century as researchers, institutions, and society gradually came to an agreement as to the correct protocol for running experiments. Some studies became infamous for their egregious breach of ethical protocols. One such experiment was the Tuskegee syphilis experiment. In this study, African-American males in Alabama who had contracted syphilis were not told they had the disease after they tested positive, and were not treated for the disease, even though treatments were available. The participants were recruited under false pretexts and treated with an inhumane disregard for their health and well-being. This experiment and others have become classic examples of ethical breaches that researchers must avoid. Any procedures that could lead to detrimental health consequences must be ruled out. If researchers become aware that patients have a condition or disease they must be immediately notified and given treatment options. Over time, ethical standards for human experiments have strengthened to include the emotional health of participants and potentially traumatic experimental procedures must include protocols for dealing with the harm they might cause, such as counseling or other clinical treatment.

To be sure that these ethical standards are met, modern experiments must be cleared by an independent internal commission. They must also contain some type of **disclosure**, an outline given to participants before the experiment begins that clarifies incentives and expectations while reminding them of their right to terminate the experiment at any time. Finally, experimental protocol should include **debriefing**, in which participants are told after the experiment exactly what was done and why the experiment was conducted. In some cases, particularly if the experiment may have triggered psychological vulnerability, participants may be offered access to treatment or counseling services as part of debriefing.

3.3 NON-EXPERIMENTAL DESIGNS

We have seen that experiments are difficult to conduct, sometimes prohibitively, and introduce many possible problems concerning validity and ethics. However, they are often worth the trouble. Experimental design offers the only way to confidently establish a causal relationship between two variables. When, however, experiments are not feasible for practical or ethical reasons, researchers in the social sciences have many other types of design at their disposal. Each offers its own benefits and potential drawbacks. In general, non-experimental designs tend to offer the benefit of observing phenomena in a more naturalistic setting, often improving external validity. The trade-off is reduced control of the variables of interest, which tends to reduce the internal validity. Below are the most frequently tested non-experimental research designs that appear on the MCAT.

1) **Correlational studies** explore the relationship between two quantitative variables. The most commonly used type of correlation is the **Pearson correlation**. A Pearson correlation assigns a number from −1 to +1 to a pair of variables. If the value is negative, the two variables are negatively correlated. This means that if one increases, the other will decrease, and vice versa. On the other hand, a positive value represents a positive correlation, which means that as one variable increases, the other also increases, and if one variable decreases the other will also decrease. A value of zero indicates no correlation, that there is no *linear* relationship between the two variables, although a nonlinear relationship is still plausible. Significance testing can be combined with Pearson correlations to see if the computed correlation is likely to have occurred by chance or not.

   For example, many studies have shown that size and mass of the amygdala, a brain area associated with fear and primal emotions, is positively correlated with subjective reports of anxiety. We expect that as reported anxiety increases, so too will measures of amygdala size. Note that this does not imply that one variable *causes* the other. As we mentioned earlier, the causal relationship could go in either direction, or some third variable (say, childhood abandonment) could be responsible for both.

   An example of a negative correlation is the relationship between social support and introversion. Some studies have shown that as social support increases, measures of introversion tend to decrease, and vice versa. Correlational studies offer the advantage of showing a numerical relationship between two variables, and are usually easier to conduct than experiments. Researchers can take the measurements of a population as it exists and do not need to directly manipulate the variables. The main disadvantage, as we've discussed, is that causality cannot be inferred.

2) **Ethnographic studies** are a qualitative method in which researchers immerse themselves completely in the lives, culture, or way of life of the people they are studying. These studies tend to be lengthy and thorough and involve as little interference or intervention by the researchers as possible. The culture studied is often unique or remote in some way, or offers a special insight into a scientific question. A researcher interested in the effects of the Mediterranean diet on health might go to a remote Sicilian village and study the lives of the participants, scrutinizing their everyday lives and recording everything they possibly can over the span of several years.

   Many of the early ethnographic studies were anthropological in nature: they often explored the lives and habits of remote cultures with little outside contact. Over time, ethnographic methods came to be used throughout the social sciences.

Nowadays, a lot of ethnographic research is conducted through online tools and technology. By utilizing social media, researchers can explore the habits, lifestyles, and social interactions of millions of individuals, then use data analytics to analyze the research and draw conclusions. There are many web tools that now make this type of research relatively easy to conduct, and it can be less resource intensive and time consuming than traditional forms of ethnographic research.

In general, perhaps the greatest strength of the ethnographic method is depth of analysis. Researchers can get a thorough understanding of a culture and the factors that influence it over many years. There are also many potential weaknesses. The researcher in an ethnographic study is often working alone, so there is no one to critique the methodology. Also, the mere presence of the researcher can affect the findings. It is likely that the members of the group will probably want to present themselves and their group/culture in a good light. This also makes replication of the study difficult, and deep immersion in a culture can result in feelings of association and attachment with the culture by the researchers, which threatens objectivity.

3) **Twin studies** are often run to test the relationship between nature and nurture. They are the best way to measure **heritability**, the extent to which an observed trait is due to genetics versus the environment. For example, twin studies interested in the heritability of intelligence might look at correlations in IQ scores between monozygotic (identical) twins and dizygotic (fraternal) twins. It is reasonable to conclude that any differences between these two correlations are due to genetics, since both types of twins share an environment. Similarly, an intelligence study might look at the difference in correlations between IQs of identical twins reared together versus reared apart. These differences would likely be due to the environment, since both sets of twins would share the same percentage of genes, namely 100.

4) **Longitudinal studies** can be run when researchers may be interested in how individuals develop over time along some research variable. While some longitudinal research is experimental, most longitudinal studies do not involve independent-variable manipulation. The New York longitudinal study is a classic example of the **longitudinal method**, which involves intervallic measurements of a dependent variable over long time frames. The New York longitudinal study asked a simple research question: what effect does our disposition at birth have on the life we lead? Researchers categorized newborns according to their dispositions: agreeable or irritable, healthy or sickly, regular or irregular in biological functions. Then they checked in on subjects over periodic intervals to see if temperament at birth was consistent throughout life. These types of research are costly, difficult to execute, time-and-resource intensive, and likely to have high attrition rates. The benefit is the ability to detail how an effect or factor can develop over time. This allows researchers to have high accuracy when observing for change. A related (but slightly different) methodology is known as a **cross-sectional study**, data collection or survey of a population or sample at a specific time.

5) **Case studies** involve in-depth exploration of individual, small group, entity, event, or phenomenon. Suppose that a researcher from Healthy Living U met a native Sicilian in her late 90s with extraordinary health and fitness. The researcher might want to know everything possible about this person's diet and lifestyle to understand how she was able to obtain such a high level of fitness, including dietary habits over time, exercise frequency, interaction with family, and sleep patterns. They would then compile this data and offer a report for critique by the scientific community. This would offer an excellent way to thoroughly explore the potential causes that

lead to a phenomenon, but of course the limitation is that there is no isolation of variables or control over the conditions. It is also difficult to determine how the different variables involved in a phenomenon interact.

6) **Phenomenological studies** are interested in describing phenomena, using the introspective method to explore research questions. All the studies we have discussed so far have involved researchers studying another individual or group of individuals. Another type of study could involve researchers studying themselves, or researchers recording what individuals report about their own personal experiences. Hermann Ebbinghaus made many groundbreaking discoveries in learning and forgetting by taking detailed data and notes on his own learning and memory performance. These investigations were phenomenological; Ebbinghaus attempted to understand his own perceptions and understandings, rather than make a comparison between variables or draw a causal conclusion.

Not all phenomenological studies are confined to self-observation. A phenomenological study attempts to understand people's perceptions, perspectives, and understandings of a situation (or phenomenon). Although the sample size may be greater than one, it is almost always small. Phenomenological studies offer the advantage of detail and in-depth understanding, but the data is subjective, potentially affecting validity. It is also difficult to generalize data, and the small sample sizes reduce external validity.

7) The **survey** is a method for collecting information or data as reported by individuals. Participants answer a series of questions and self-report the information. Surveys are used to ascertain the beliefs and attitudes of a particular group about issues such as politics and religion, as well as their opinions about, for example, the quality of new businesses, academic classes, consumer products, etc. Additionally, surveys can be a way for people to measure how often or how little people engage in different behaviors, such as smoking or drinking alcohol. The benefits of surveys are that they are easy to administer and tend to be cost effective. Nowadays, they can be administered online, which further boosts the reach and facility of conducting survey studies. Potential flaws are that respondents may not feel encouraged to provide honest and accurate answers and that validity can be adversely affected by an unrepresentative sample or poor survey questions. Surveys must be assessed for reliability and validity to make sure they are consistently measuring what they're supposed to measure.

8) A few other types of studies are worth mentioning briefly since they may appear on the MCAT Psychology/Sociology section. **Archival studies** analyze already collected data from historical records and authentic original documents. **Biographical studies** are exhaustive accounts of an individual's life experience. Finally, many of the study types we've looked at fall under the category of **Observational Studies**. An observational study is any study in which individuals are observed and outcomes measured with no attempt to control the outcome. Table 4 provides a summary of the non-experimental designs that are likely to show up on the MCAT.

Table 4   Summary of Non-Experimental Designs

Type of Study:	Description	Strengths	Weaknesses
Correlational	• Measures the quantitative relationship between two variables	• Great preliminary technique • Usually easy to conduct	• Does not establish causality • May not pick up nonlinear relationship
Ethnographic	• Deep, lengthy qualitative analysis of a culture and its characteristics	• Provides detailed analysis and comprehensive evaluation	• Researcher's presence may affect individuals' behavior • Heavily dependent on the researcher conducting the study, difficult to replicate, and objectivity may be compromised
Twin	• Analysis of heritability through measuring characteristics of twins	• Offers insight into how nature and nurture might interact to lead to various characteristics	• Difficult to find participants who meet criteria • Difficult to analyze the complex variables involved and how they interact
Longitudinal	• Long-term analysis that intermittently measures the evolution of some behavior or characteristic; usually nonexperimental	• Scientists can understand how trait of interest changes over time	• Logistically demanding, expensive and difficult to implement • High attrition rate
Case	• Deep analysis of a single case or example	• Offers comprehensive details about the single case	• Results may not be generalizable • Does not offer points of reference or comparison
Phenomenological	• Self-observation of a phenomenon by researcher or small group of participants	• Introspection can provide insight into behaviors and occurrences that are difficult to measure	• Lacks objectivity due to results coming from self-analysis • Difficult to generalize results to other circumstances or individuals
Survey	• Use of a series of questions to allow participants to self-report behaviors or tendencies	• Easy to administer • Can provide quantitative data that can be compared to large participant pools	• Self reporting creates limitations in objectivity

Archival	• Analysis of historical records for insight into a phenomenon	• Provide insight into events from the past that are different from everyday behavior	• Quality of analysis subject to the quality and integrity of records • Difficult to conduct follow-ups • Data are unlikely to be comprehensive, leaving ambiguity and unanswered questions
Biographical	• Exploration of all the events and circumstances of an individual's life	• Comprehensive knowledge of all the details of an individual's life	• Limitations in objectivity • Difficult to generalize observations
Observational	• Broad category that includes any research in which experimenters do not manipulate the situation or results	• Naturalistic observation of circumstances as they are	• Difficult to tease out the complex interplay of many variables

Chapter 3 Summary

- The experimental method is the primary method used by researchers to establish causality.

- Several steps must be scrupulously followed in order to meet the rigorous requirements of experimental research: selecting the population, operationalizing variables, creating the different groups and the protocols for each, randomly sampling from the population, and randomly assigning subjects to groups.

- The independent variable is the variable manipulated by the researcher.

- The dependent variable, or measurement variable, is the variable that is measured to test for an effect.

- An operational definition is a precise and concrete definition of a research variable.

- Quantitative indicates numerical, whereas qualitative indicates descriptive or categorical.

- A control group is the group researchers use as a point of comparison; it does not receive the treatment.

- An experimental group is the group that does receive the treatment in a study.

- Extraneous (or confounding) variables are variables other than the research variable that could potentially explain a result in an experiment.

- A research sample should reflect the population from which it is drawn.

- Individuals who are sampled from the population should be randomly assigned to the control and experimental groups.

- In hypothesis testing, researchers assign the null hypothesis: the hypothesis that any effects are due to chance and there is no experimental result.

- Type 1 error is known as a false positive, rejecting the null hypothesis: any observed effects are not systematic and are simply due to chance.

- Internal validity is how well done a study is, or how well it allows researchers to draw conclusions from measured effects. External validity is how well a research result applies to the population at large and real-life scenarios.

- Non-experimental methodologies, which do not allow researchers to draw conclusions about causality, include the correlational method, the observational method, the longitudinal method, ethnographic studies, and case studies.

CHAPTER 3 FREESTANDING PRACTICE QUESTIONS

1. A team of researchers measures a negative correlation between income and length of labor time in a group of pregnant women. It is expected that as income increases, labor time:

   A) decreases.
   B) increases.
   C) stays the same.
   D) The change in labor time cannot be determined.

2. Due to scheduling and logistical limitations, researchers conducting a study could only conduct the study on Tuesdays and Thursdays between 7 P.M. and 9 P.M. They were therefore limited to individuals who were available at this time to participate in the study. This set up would have created issues in:

   A) external validity, due to the selection criteria.
   B) internal validity, due to a potential Hawthorne effect.
   C) external validity, due to the lack of a control group.
   D. internal validity, due to impression management.

3. Researchers want to explore the experience of subjects as they engage in the Stroop task, a task in selective attention that measures the ability to distinguish between discordant stimuli. The researchers are not merely interested in response time but want to know qualitative details about the subjects' internal experiences. Which of the following methodologies should the researchers implement?

   A) Correlational method
   B) Observational method
   C) Survey method
   D) Phenomenological method

4. Which of the following is a limitation of the ethnographic method?

   A) Cultural validity is low, since the observer is not a member of the society of interest
   B) External validity is low, because the conditions under which the research is conducted do not match the real world
   C) External validity is low, because only one culture is sampled
   D) Construct validity is low, since the instruments have not been checked for reliability

5. A team of researchers finds that there is a complex relationship between IQ and sociability. Measures of sociability were found to be high for individuals within one standard deviation of the mean for intelligence, and gradually decreased for individuals with both very high and very low IQ scores. Which of the following correlations would be measured in this instance?

   A) A strong positive correlation
   B) A weak negative correlation
   C) No correlation
   D) A moderate negative correlation

6. In a study of the impact of personality type on the interpretation of a social symbol, which of the following is a possible operational definition of the independent variable?

   A) Personality type is the independent variable, so it can be defined as results on a questionnaire designed to measure five-factor model personality traits.
   B) Personality type is the independent variable, so it can be defined as degree of sympathetic arousal and amygdala activation when seeing a symbol.
   C) Symbol interpretation is the independent variable, so it can be defined as average ranking, from positive to negative, of a series of neutral symbols.
   D) Symbol interpretation is the independent variable, so it can be defined as degree of sympathetic arousal and amygdala activation when seeing a symbol.

7. Attrition, or subjects dropping out of a study before its completion, is a threat to:

   A) internal validity, because it introduces a potential confounding variable.
   B) internal validity, because the group may no longer be representative.
   C) external validity, because it introduces a potential confounding variable.
   D) external validity, because the group may no longer be representative.

8. Which of the following research methodologies would best explore the development of human memory over time?

   A) Case study
   B) Longitudinal study
   C) Observational study
   D) Archival study

CHAPTER 3 PRACTICE PASSAGE

Recent adaptations in technology, such as smartphones and the Internet, have been found to have potentially negative effects on physical and psychological well-being. Sociologists refer to the time it takes to catch up to technology as cultural lag. Researchers have been interested in studying the effects of cultural lag on attention, cognition, and psychopathology.

A study was conducted by recruiting 347 students from first year introductory psychology courses at a four-year state university in the Midwest, where a large majority of students were in-state residents. They were incentivized with extra credit in their course, and of the 347 that were invited, 62 participants that chose to participate were first asked to respond on a Likert scale from 1 to 5 on how often they used their cell phones, social media, and the Internet. Based on the results, participants were divided into 2 groups of 31 students each. Both groups contained more females, 21 and 23 in the low usage and high usage groups, respectively. Researchers also considered GPA, and found that the cumulative GPAs for both groups were similar, 3.16 and 3.32, respectively, a difference that was not found to be significant. It was hypothesized that the group that used various types of digital media more would manifest detrimental effects along a range of variables, measured by a battery of exams on reaction time, working memory, and ability to conduct tasks while ignoring a distractor. Participants were given a questionnaire designed to measure depression and a second questionnaire designed to measure anxiety.

Results supported the research hypotheses. Based on the results, researchers determined that the stress response may have been the link between technology use and the measurement variables, since various studies showed that stress was known to have detrimental effects on each of these areas. The group suggested to campus health experts that they should recommend students limit their use of digital media to mitigate the effects of cultural lag.

1. If the researchers are correct in their conclusion, what is likely to happen in a second study of elderly adults who are known to be more sensitive in their response to stress?

A) They will have difficulty attending to stimuli.
B) They will score higher on depression.
C) The low digital usage group will have slower reaction times.
D) The high digital usage group will demonstrate increased anxiety.

2. Which of the following conclusions can be most reasonably drawn from the study in passage?

A) Stress plays a critical role in the relationship between technology and cognitive effects, because it provides the most plausible mediating variable.
B) There was a relationship between technology use and psychopathology because the research utilized various psychometrics.
C) Cultural lag regarding digital media is an ongoing problem on college campuses because the research conducted used random assignment and random sampling to test the hypotheses.
D) Use of social media caused detrimental effects on cognition because of the strain placed on the attentional mechanism, as demonstrated by comparison with the control group.

3. A likely confounding variable created by the experimental design was:

A) school performance.
B) gender.
C) extraversion.
D) academic major.

4. The methodology described in the passage created threats to external validity due to each of the following considerations EXCEPT:

A) geographic location.
B) lack of a control group.
C) student availability.
D) age.

5. Which of the following pairs represents a qualitative and quantitative variable, respectively?

A) Reaction time and coping ability
B) Reaction time and depression score
C) Type of coping response and level of depression
D) Attending fluidity ability and reaction time

6. Each of the following could be an operational definition of the dependent variable EXCEPT:

A) depression inventory score.
B) sympathetic nervous system arousal.
C) size of social media network.
D) time attending to distracting variables.

SOLUTIONS TO CHAPTER 3 FREESTANDING PRACTICE QUESTIONS

1. **A**   A negative correlation suggests that as the value measured for one variable increases, the other decreases, and vice versa. Therefore, as income increases, labor time is expected to decrease (choice A is correct). Labor time would increase if the correlation were positive (choice B is wrong). There was a result measured, so the measurement would not stay the same (choice C is wrong), and the direction of change is known because the type of correlation is given in the question stem (choice D is wrong).

2. **A**   This question can be attacked more quickly with the observation that the second part of the answer choices cuts the set of choices in half. The first step is to determine if the situation described in the question stem is a threat to internal or external validity. The recruitment method is problematic because the experiment will not sample individuals who have different schedules and are not available at that time. A sample that is not representative of the population is a threat to external validity (choices B and D are wrong). Selection criteria are the processes used to select participants for an experiment. This describes the scheduling issue presented in the question stem (choice A is correct). A lack of control group is a threat to internal (not external) validity, as this factor is related to how well-designed the study is and to what extent researchers can draw conclusions based on findings (choice C is wrong).

3. **D**   The phenomenological method is a technique used to evaluate the experience of some phenomenon and often obtains more introspective details about an event than is possible with other methods. This method is also usually qualitative, or descriptive, as the question stem suggests (choice D is correct). The correlational method is a quantitative measure of the relationship between two variables (choice A is wrong). The observational method involves observation and minimal interference by the researcher. It would be very difficult to know about subjects' internal experiences by simply observing them (choice B is wrong). The survey method tends to reveal only general aspects of an event or experience, since it contains general questions that are tested on numerous individuals. This characteristic would make it difficult to know about subjects' unique internal experiences. The survey method is also quantitative in most cases, since subjects often provide a numerical assessment of their self-reported beliefs or feelings (choice C is wrong).

4. **C**   External validity is an issue in ethnographic studies, mainly because the methodology involves deep exploration of a single culture or subculture, so it provides limited information on how the results might apply to other cultures (choice C is correct). Cultural validity is not a type of validity checked for by researchers (choice A is wrong). Conditions in ethnographic research are usually very close to the real world, since the researcher makes every attempt to not disrupt the environment. The goal of ethnographic research is to observe the culture in a naturalistic setting (choice B is wrong). Ethnographic researchers do not usually use surveys, but deep analysis, in their evaluations of the cultures they study, so construct validity is very unlikely to be a consideration. Construct validity usually applies to psychometric instruments such as surveys (choice D is wrong).

5. **C** The results described in the question are curvilinear in nature. They do not represent a linear relationship and would show up as a bell on a graph. Correlational research does not pick up nonlinear trends (choice C is correct; choices A, B, and D are wrong).

6. **A** This question can be resolved more quickly by noticing that the first part of the answer choices is divided in half. The first step is to determine whether personality type or symbolic interpretation is the independent variable. The study described is designed to measure how personality affects symbolic interpretation. Therefore, the independent variable—the variable manipulated by the researcher—is personality type (choices C and D are wrong). The five-factor model is a common measure of personality (choice A is correct). Sympathetic arousal and amygdala activation do not define personality type (choice B is wrong).

7. **A** Attrition is primarily a threat to internal validity, because there may be some non-trivial reason that subjects are dropping out. This would present a confounding variable, because if the reason for attrition were related to the hypothesis, it could provide an alternative explanation for the results (choice A is correct). Non-representative samples are a threat to external, not internal, validity (choice B is wrong). Confounding variables are a threat to internal, not external, validity (choice C is wrong). It is less likely that enough subjects drop out to threaten the external validity of the study. Also, if participants began to drop out, internal validity would be threatened first, such that it would be difficult to draw a conclusion that would then be applied to the external population (choice D is wrong).

8. **B** Longitudinal studies are best for exploring how variables develop over time. They involve conducting periodic measurements of the same individuals over many years to see how certain variables change. This is the ideal methodology for exploring the question presented in the stem (choice B is correct). Case studies are best for understanding individuals in a comprehensive way. This would be an ideal methodology for understanding one person's memory development, but would not allow for generalization to human memory (choice A is wrong). An observational study could meet the criteria, but observational studies do not specifically deal with the development of variables over a long period of time. This study methodology usually involves observing events in a naturalistic setting, and although this could be done over time intervals, this is not usually a feature of observational research (choice C is wrong). Archival studies would be best for exploring how a phenomenon was different many years ago, to use as a comparison with other epochs. However, archival research would not be ideal for understanding how memory evolved for groups of individuals, since it is impossible to control for variables with data taken many years ago, and there are often gaps in the data available (choice D is wrong).

SOLUTIONS TO CHAPTER 3 PRACTICE PASSAGE

1. **D** The researchers concluded that stress was a potential mediating result because of its known relationship with the cognitive variables. Stress and anxiety are known to be related to each other, so high digital usage would be associated with increased anxiety (choice D is correct). The research described showed a relationship between digital usage and attention, not stress response and attention. Note that stress response does not necessarily mean that the group will actually experience more stress, but that they will respond with greater sensitivity if stress occurs. Therefore, the known relationships between stress and attention and stress and depression do not necessarily apply (choices A and B are wrong). Slower reaction time was associated with the high digital use group, not the low digital use group (choice C is wrong).

2. **B** Psychopathology refers to mental disorders or abnormal behavior. The research described found a relationship between time spent using various forms of technology and slowed cognitive function. The psychometrics used were the battery of exams on cognitive functions (reaction time, working memory, and multitasking) as well as the Likert scale that was used to assess technology use (choice B is correct). The researchers proposed stress as a possible mediator in paragraph 3, however, the actual research to establish this relationship was not actually conducted. A mediating variable is a variable that provides a link in a causal relationship and helps to show why that relationship exists. The researchers did not conduct any tests on stress and how stress relates to technology use (choice A is wrong). The research did suggest that cultural lag was a point of concern since new technologies seemed to be related to cognitive problems. However, the study did not contain random sampling from the population described in the answer choice, namely college campuses. The study only sampled from one university, and without follow-up research, we cannot be sure that the results apply to students on other campuses (choice C is wrong). The researchers cannot be sure that social media caused the detrimental effects because the independent variable is not manipulated directly by the researchers in this case. Instead, it is measured and the subjects are placed into groups. Also, there was no control group. There was only a high technology and low technology group (choice D is wrong).

3. **C** Extraversion is a characteristic related to how energizing individuals find social interactions which others. Individuals who are high in extraversion tend to be more sociable, garrulous, and spend more time interacting with others. It may therefore be more likely that they engage more with social media and technology, spending more time on their phones. This could make high extraversion individuals more susceptible to the effects of the study (choice C is correct). School performance and gender were both measured in the study, and the researchers did not find large differences between the two groups in either variable (choices A and B are wrong). Academic major is unlikely to be a confounding variable since there is not a clear link between major and digital media usage. Also, there are many academic majors, and variables with many groups are less likely to confound, since any effect will be distributed across a spectrum (choice D is wrong).

4. **B**   For except/not/least questions, evaluate each answer choice and eliminate the answer choices that are true. Only using subjects from one geographic location (a Midwestern university) is a threat to external validity because these individuals may not be representative of the larger population (choice A is true and can be eliminated). The study did lack a control group, but this is a threat to internal validity, not external validity, because it is a flaw in the way the research is designed that affects the ability to draw conclusions from the variables (choice B is false and the correct answer choice). Student availability is a threat to external validity, because only some students participated in the study, so the research results may not apply as well to the entire student population, which includes students who may be too busy to participate in the research (choice C is true and can be eliminated). Age is a threat to external validity since most students will be in their early 20s. This means the results may not apply to older adults (choice D is true and can be eliminated).

5. **C**   The correct answer choice will pair a qualitative variable with a quantitative variable. Type of coping response suggests that coping responses will be broken into categories, a sign that it is a qualitative variable, since it would not involve a numerical continuum but rather placement into one of several different coping styles. Depression level can be measured quantitatively, since "level" suggests a score along a scale (choice C is correct). Reaction time is a quantitative variable (choices A and B are wrong). Attending fluidity ability suggests a measure along a continuum. Most variables along a continuum tend to be quantitative in nature, whereas most categorical variables tend to be qualitative. Since attending fluidity ability suggests a range of abilities along a single variable, attending fluidity, this suggests a quantitative variable (choice D is wrong).

6. **C**   For except/not/least questions, evaluate each answer choice and eliminate the answer choices that are "true" or work for this question (i.e., could be an operational definition of the dependent variable). A dependent variable is an outcome variable measured by the researchers to test the extent of effect of the manipulation in the study. Depression is one of the dependent, or measurement, variables (choice A works for this question and can be eliminated). Sympathetic nervous arousal is related to anxiety, one of the dependent variables (choice B works for this question and can be eliminated). Size of social media network is related to how much time an individual spends using digital media, which is an independent, not dependent, variable in the study (choice C does not work for this question and is therefore the correct answer choice). Attention and ability to tune out distracting variables is a dependent variable in the study (choice D works for this question and can be eliminated).

Chapter 4
Sociological Theories and Social Institutions

Sociologists employ various theoretical lenses to provide a framework for how individuals and social structures interact with each other. Each theory provides a perspective for understanding social phenomena and guides the type of research conducted by social scientists. Theories can focus on society as a whole and other big-picture issues, or individual interactions, or both. One of the primary large scale issues sociologists explore is the nature of social institutions: how they organize, evolve, and impact the lives of individuals within the society.

4.1 SOCIOLOGY: THEORETICAL APPROACHES

A **society** can be defined as a group of people who share a culture and live/interact with each other within a definable area. **Sociology** is the study of how individuals interact with, shape, and are subsequently shaped by the society in which they live. Because culture influences individuals and individuals influence their culture, sociologists consider both individual actions and the patterns of behavior of groups.

There are four major sociological theories that explain society: functionalism, conflict theory, symbolic interactionism, and social constructionism. The first two, functionalism and conflict theory, are macro-level theories which focus on the effects of large scale social structures. Macro-level theories try to answer fundamental questions such as why societies form, why societies change, and why their social structures function in the manner that they function.

The third major perspective is **symbolic interactionism**, which analyzes society on a **micro-level**. Micro-sociologists are interested in small-scale individual considerations, most prominently one-on-one and small group interactions. From the micro-sociological perspective, societies are best understood as emergent properties of individual human social interactions and best understood by analyzing very specific relationships among individuals and small groups. The fourth theory, **social constructionism**, can be either macro or micro, depending on the context.

Presented in this section are these four major theories along with the **feminist**, and **rational choice/ social exchange theories**.

Functionalism (also known as Structural Functionalism)

The oldest of the three major theories of sociology, **functionalism** is a paradigm that conceptualizes society as a living organism with many different interrelated and interdependent parts, each of which has a distinct and necessary purpose. Functionalism can trace its genesis to the philosopher **Herbert Spencer** (1820–1903). Spencer postulated that just as the various organs and systems in a human body work together to keep the body functioning and regulated, the various structures and institutions of a society work together to keep that entire society functioning and regulated. Spencer also contended that societies were subject to evolutionary pressures and could evolve in response to these pressures just as organisms do.

The functionalist perspective focuses on the social functions of different social structures by asking what these structures contribute to society at large. For example, the contribution of our lungs to the body is to orchestrate the exchange of air. Similarly, we can think about the function of schools, churches, hospitals, and other social structures. Just as organs function interdependently to help the organism survive, social structures work together to sustain society. According to the functionalist perspective, societies can thrive and grow or become disease-addled and die, like living organisms.

Émile Durkheim (1858–1917) was a pioneer in modern social research and a major proponent of functionalism. Durkheim established sociology as an academic field of study separate and distinct from psychology and political philosophy. Through the influential scientific journal he edited and his groundbreaking scientific work, Durkheim is considered by many to be the founder of sociology. Durkheim extended Spencer's analogy to explain how societies form, grow, persist, and function. To Durkheim, a society's capacity to maintain social order and stability is paramount to its functional success.

Durkheim believed that modern societies were more complex than primitive societies. In primitive societies, people are held together because they are all quite similar, sharing a common language as well as common tasks, values, and symbols. In modern societies, Durkheim argued, people rely upon each other to make the society function as a whole. According to functionalist theory, all the interrelated parts of modern societies, including all major social structures such as the government, the police force, the educational system, and the medical system have interdependent roles to play. For society to thrive, all of these complex, interdependent parts must work together to keep society ordered, balanced, and stable. When a healthy society faces an imbalance or crisis, functionalist theory proposes that the major structures of society will work together to return to a state of **dynamic equilibrium**. Healthy societies can successfully achieve and maintain this dynamic equilibrium; unhealthy ones cannot.

Durkheim further believed that society should always be viewed holistically—as a collective of social facts, rather than individuals. **Social facts** are the elements that serve some function in society, such as the laws, morals, values, religions, customs, rituals, and rules that make up a society. Durkheim felt that such cultural links create societal "solidarity." He proposed the existence of a "collective conscience," his name for how people of a shared culture come to think in the same manner due to their shared beliefs, ideas, and moral attitudes, all which operate to unify society.

There is an important distinction in the functionalist framework made between manifest and latent functions. **Manifest functions** are the official, intended, and anticipated consequences of a structure. Manifest functions are at least arguably beneficial. For example, the manifest functions of a police department include enforcing laws against violent crime and property crime. In contrast, **latent functions** are consequences of a structure that are not officially sought or sanctioned. Latent functions can be beneficial, neutral, or harmful. For example, the latent functions of a police department can include providing employment to community residents, raising government revenue by issuing traffic tickets, or even promoting social inequality through selective law enforcement.

Functionalism recognizes that not all of the effects of social structures are beneficial. A **social dysfunction** is a process that has undesirable consequences and may actually reduce the stability of society. For example, a dysfunctional police department could routinely commit police brutality. However, functionalist theory predicts that in a healthy society other social structures such as a free press and a responsive government will, over time, work together to mitigate such dysfunctions.

While functionalism was the prevailing theory in sociology in the 1950s, many sociologists began to argue that functionalism's focus on the structures of healthy society working together to maintain societal order, balance, and stability could not accurately account for the many rapid sociological advances taking place in the 1960s and 1970s. Though functionalism is still considered useful in many respects, other sociological theories have become more popular in recent decades.

Conflict Theory

Like functionalism, **conflict theory** is also a macro-level theory that focuses primarily on large-scale social structures and their effects on individuals. However, conflict theory views society as a never-ending competition for limited resources, and at least in some respects, conflict theory is diametrically opposed to the functionalist perspective. According to conflict theory, all past and current societies have had unequally distributed resources; therefore, individual members of these societies must compete for social, political, and material resources such as money, land, power, and leisure. Furthermore, social structures and institutions will reflect this competition in their degree of inherent inequality. Those with the most resources, power, and influence will use their relative advantages to amass more resources, power, and influence by suppressing the advancement of others.

Karl Marx (1818–1883), who is closely identified with conflict theory, looked at the economic conflict between different social classes. According to Marx, every society is divided into two major classes based upon the ownership of the means of production (such as tools, factories, and land). In the economic system of **capitalism**, which encourages competition and private ownership, the bourgeoisie, or ruling class, owns the means of production, while the proletariat, or working class, provides labor. The working class is oppressed and exploited by the capitalist bourgeois class that pays the members of the working class only a fraction of the production value of their labor. These differences result in an inherent conflict of interests between the two groups. Those who already have want to use their advantages to maintain their position at the top of society, while the interests of the have-nots is to overthrow the haves in order to create an egalitarian society.

According to conflict theorists, this unequal social order is maintained through ideological coercion that creates societal consensus, or **hegemony**—a coerced acceptance of the values, expectations, and conditions as determined by the capitalist class. Conflict theorists maintain that societal "consensus" is imposed by the "superstructure" of society, comprised of social institutions, political structures, and culture. This coerced consensus justifies the social, political, and economic status quo as natural, inevitable, and perpetual, as well as beneficial for everyone in society rather than only for the capitalist class that engenders this cultural hegemony.

Marx believed that revolution was inevitable in any capitalist society because of the inherent instability of the extreme class inequality that capitalism promotes. To maximize profits, members of the capitalist class pay the lowest possible wages while providing the worst possible working conditions. Such exploitation will eventually result in the development of **class consciousness**, which Marx defined as exploited workers' awareness of the reasons for their oppression. This in turn would inevitably lead the more numerous workers to revolt against less numerous capitalists, overthrow their oppressors, and replace capitalism with an extreme form of **socialism**, that Marx called **communism** in which all means of production are owned by all workers equally.

Max Weber (1864–1920), who is best known for refining and critiquing many of Marx's tenets of conflict theory, agreed with Marx that inequalities in a capitalist system would lead to conflict, but Weber did not believe that the collapse of capitalism was inevitable. Instead, Weber believed that Marx's focus on economic inequality alone was too narrow and extreme. Weber also believed that Marx did not pay enough attention to the power of values and beliefs to influence, transform, and stabilize societies. Weber theorized that the **Protestant/Puritan work ethic**, a widely held religious belief that lauded the morality of hard work for the sake of godliness, was a critical factor in the success of the capitalist system in replacing the feudalist system that preceded it in Western Europe. Weber contended that the fundamental trend of modern society was the increasing **rationalization of society**, which he defined as our increasing concern with efficiency (achieving the maximum result with the minimum amount of effort). Weber also argued that several factors moderate people's reaction to inequality, such agreement with authority figures, high rates of social mobility, and low rates of class difference.

Like functionalism, conflict theory strongly emphasizes the effects of large-scale structures of society over individuals, making it a macro-sociological theory. Although the perspectives of Karl Marx and Max Weber fundamentally differ from the perspective of Émile Durkheim, these three men are generally considered the founders of sociology.

The major criticism of conflict theory is that it focuses too much on competition and does not recognize the role of stability within society. Critics of conflict theory contend that conflict theorists focus too myopically on economic factors, view society only from the perspective of those who lack power, and ignore the cooperative ways in which people and groups can reach pragmatic agreements for the good of society as a whole.

Symbolic Interactionism

While the first two sociological perspectives look at society from a macro (top-down and zoomed-out) perspective, **symbolic interactionism** starts at the micro (bottom-up and zoomed-in) level and views society as built up from typical everyday interactions. Rather than considering individuals as entities who are acted upon by the large-scale structures of their society, symbolic interactionism emphasizes the ways by which individuals actively shape their world through their understanding and subsequent behavioral responses to the meanings they attribute to the societal symbols through which individuals define their reality.

While symbolic interactionism's focus was presaged by Max Weber's assertion that individuals act according to their respective interpretations of the meaning of their world, the term "symbolic interactionism" was not officially coined until 1969 (by Herbert Blumer, a proponent of the theory). However, the works of **George Herbert Mead** (1863–1931) are considered most important in the initial development of the paradigm.

Symbolic interactionism examines the relationships between individuals and society by focusing on the exchange of information through language and symbols in one-on-one and small-group communication. According to symbolic interactionism, individuals can make sense of the world around them by ascribing meaning to the symbols and language of their shared culture, and these meanings depend on both individual interpretations and social context.

Symbolic interactionism analyzes society by addressing the subjective meanings that people impose upon objects, events, and behaviors. Subjective meaning is important because people behave based on what they believe to be true, whether or not their beliefs are actually true. Therefore, society is constructed through human interpretation; people must continually interpret their own behaviors as well as those of others around them, and these interpretations form a social bond.

Symbolic interactionism holds the principle of meaning to be the central aspect of human behavior: (1) humans ascribe meaning to things and act toward those things based on their ascribed meaning; (2) language allows humans to generate meaning through social interaction with each other and society; (3) humans modify meanings through an interpretive thought process that observes and considers the reactions of others as well as the social context of these interactions.

Mead and other interactionists have also been interested in identity and the development of the self. For interactionists, the self is developed through three important activities: language, games, and play. Language is probably the most prominent system of symbols in all human interactions and incorporates not only what we say and hear, but all modes of communication including body language and interpretation of meaning. The distinction between play and games is also worth noting. These are words that often suggest interactions among children and are sometimes used interchangeably. However, Mead meant for them to apply to all humans and established a clear distinction between them. Social play is characterized by spontaneity and freedom, with minimal social rules and limited stakes. Two children playing in a sandbox and building castles with the sand would be an example of play, as would two adults meeting for coffee. Social games, on the other hand, have a much stricter set of rules and have greater stakes. Classic board games like monopoly are clearly a type of social game, but so is taking the MCAT: the rules are clearly defined and there are spoils that go to the winner. Language, play, and games are the primary ways that we interact with each other and interpret the role of the self, and each plays a critical role in the formation of identity.

Another important distinction Mead proposed was the difference between the "I" and the "me." Mead thought there were two important components to identity: the individualistic self, which sought to establish its own unique identity through social interactions in the face of social pressures and expectations, and the social self, which internalized the characteristics of the social environment. The "I" represents the individualistic self. There is a connection with grammar and linguistics. I, as a subject pronoun, represents the part of the self that is the active agent, the part that acts on other people and things and has its own autonomy and will. On the other hand, the object pronoun "me" is used to represent the social self. This governs when others are acting and interpreting our behavior and we are the object of their actions and interpretations. Both the "I" and "me" are in constant dialogue with each other, sometimes agreeing, sometimes in conflict; and thinking itself, Mead believed, represents the internal dialogue between the individualistic and social self.

People interpret one another's behavior, and it is these interpretations that form our social bonds. These interpretations are called the "definition of the situation." An example of this phenomenon is called the **Thomas theorem**, the theory that interpretation of a situation affects the response to that situation.

A specific type of interactionist philosophy is called the **dramaturgical approach**, which was developed by **Erving Goffman** (1922–1982), a prominent proponent of symbolic interactionism. As the name suggests, this paradigm views people as theatrical performers and everyday life as a stage. Just as actors project a certain on-screen image, people in society choose what kind of image they want to communicate to those they interact with. For example, a college student who lands a coveted internship downtown will project a different image while at her internship than she will in class, and an even different image still when hanging out with her friends at a bar, or visiting her family in her childhood home.

Critics of symbolic interactionism contend that the theory neglects the macro-level of social interpretation and may miss the larger issues of society by focusing too closely on individual interactions.

Social Constructionism

Like symbolic interactionism, **social constructionism** asserts that people actively shape their reality through social interactions; reality is therefore something that is socially constructed rather than inherent. Both social constructionism and symbolic interactionism share the **belief** that society is subject to cultural "meaning-making" and collective definition-building and that the primary way that societies evolve is through changes in collective meaning-making. This similarity is not coincidental and derives from the fact that most social constructionists have been greatly influenced by the tenets of symbolic interactionism. Both of these theories challenge the scientific viewpoint that there is one objective reality shared by all humans.

Social constructionists focus on **social constructs** (mechanisms or practices created and sustained by society) that change across cultures and within a single culture over time. Social constructionism claims that social attributes such as race, gender, sexuality, and class are constructs of society, and that the same is true of our concepts of occupational status, power, and mental health/illness. Even concepts we typically think of as completely measurable physical characteristics, such as money, wealth, age and even time itself, are only social constructs. Whether the phenomenon in question is depression or higher education, social constructionists argue that the "reality" people see when they consider such phenomena is actually socially constructed, or an "artifice of society."

A major difference between symbolic interactionism and social constructionism is that while symbolic interactionists focus almost exclusively on one-on-one and small group interactions, social constructionists examine the constructs of society from both macro- and micro-sociological perspectives.

Other interests of social constructionists include our individual **stocks of knowledge** that allow us to classify objects and actions we observe quickly and to routinely structure our own actions in immediate response through a process called **typification**. Frequently repeated actions evolve into patterns that we learn to reproduce without much effort. As these actions become routines, they form a general store of knowledge that can be institutionalized by society. Once knowledge becomes institutionalized, we experience it as objective, unquestionable reality, the truth of which is continuously affirmed by others around us as well as concretized by the language we use to describe as "real" what was previously only a routine.

Social constructionism also analyzes the effects of mass media and contends that mass media corporations have become the main mechanisms by which our social institutions transmit culture to preserve power and authority. Echoing conflict theorists, these social constructionists feel that disempowering societal constructs are derived from, or at least bound up with, larger social structures and institutional practices.

Feminist Theory

Feminist theory is concerned with the social experiences of both men and women and the differences between these experiences (for example, manhood versus womanhood and masculine versus feminine). Feminist sociologists strive to understand both the social structures that contribute to gender differences (macro-level questions) and the effects of gender differences on individual interactions (micro-level questions). Feminist theory is related to the concept of feminism, but feminism is better described as a collection of social movements with the purpose of establishing men and women as equals in terms of social rights, roles, statuses, etc.

The feminist perspective sometimes extends to the idea of active oppression in which both individuals and structures maintain inequalities. Micro-level oppression can occur as the result of authoritative principles that allow men to restrict women. Domestic violence is an example of this. Macro-level oppression can occur when economic, political, and other social structures permit the domination of women. The driving ban for women in Saudi Arabia is a high-profile modern example of this.

Feminist theory can also extend to questions of **intersectionality**. Intersectionality posits that various human aspects subject to societal oppression (such as class, race, sexual orientation, and gender) do not exist isolated and separated from each other, but instead have complex, influential, and interwoven relationships.

Rational Choice and Social Exchange Theories

Economic considerations also have a place in the sociological tradition. Economics is a social science concerned with resources, whether goods or services, and their production, distribution, and consumption by both individuals and groups (for example, corporations). Capitalist societies, in particular, are built on competition, and thus economics influences social behavior. Under the broad heading of **rational choice theory** can be included **social exchange theory**, **game theory**, and **rational actor theory**. No matter what name is used, the rational choice paradigm brings a decidedly economic approach to the analysis of why, when, and how people interact.

In all rational choice theories, individuals seek to maximize the benefits they gain and minimize the disadvantages they sustain in all of their social interactions. If an individual decides that the benefits of an interaction outweigh its disadvantages, this individual will initiate the interaction (or continue it if it has already begun). If an individual instead decides that an interaction's disadvantages outweigh its benefits, this individual will decline interacting (or stop the interaction if it has already started). Social order is possible because individuals realize that their best interests are often served through cooperation and compromises with others.

All rational choice paradigms share the fundamental premise that human behaviors are utilitarian. **Utilitarianism** is based on two assumptions: (1) that individual humans are rational in their actions, and (2) that in every human interaction, individuals will seek to maximize their own self-interest. Since utilitarianism focuses on the individual social choices that individuals make, rational choice theory and all of its related theories, such as social exchange theory, are often **micro-sociological theories**. However, because they can also look at the tendencies and behaviors of large groups of people, they are also capable of being **macro-sociological theories**.

Rational choice theorists tend to treat society as a kind of market or game in which each person is constantly making choices among available options, based on a cost-benefit or risk-reward analysis and according to his or her own set of value preferences. The players in the game may not have perfect information about exactly what their options are or about the rewards, costs, and risks of each option. Rational choice theorists examine the relative power of interacting individuals and analyze how differing parameters of an exchange relationship can shape an individual's ability to get favorable returns from that exchange.

Rational choice theory is widely criticized for assuming the inherent rationality of human actions and minimizing the role of culture and subjective meaning in individual and group behavior. Advocates claim that rational choice theory provides an integrated theoretical analysis of human behavior that has the potential to unify many branches of social science.

4.2 SOCIAL INSTITUTIONS

Social institutions are complexes of roles, norms, and values organized into a relatively stable form that contribute to social order by governing the behavior of people. Social institutions provide predictability and organization for individuals within a society and mediate social behavior between people. Social institutions provide harmony and allow for specialization and differentiation of skills. Examples of social institutions in the United States include our educational systems, family, religions, government, and health care systems.

Family

The family, in all of its many different forms, is part of all human cultures. A family may be defined as a set of people related by blood, marriage, adoption, or some other agreed-upon relationship that signifies some responsibility to one another. Throughout history families have tended to serve five functions:

1) Reproduction and the monitoring of sexual behavior
2) Protection
3) Socialization—passing down norms and values of society
4) Affection and companionship
5) Social status—social position is often based on family background and reputation

One way of conceptualizing family is to distinguish **nuclear family**, consisting of direct blood relations, and **extended** family, in which grandparents, aunts, uncles, and others are included. Across cultures and even within a culture, the members of the family that typically live together may vary.

The extension of a family through marriage can occur in many different ways. **Monogamy** refers to a form of marriage in which two individuals are married only to each other. **Polygamy** allows an individual to have multiple wives or husbands simultaneously. Throughout world history, polygamy has actually been more common than the monogamous relationships currently considered the norm in the United States. There are two subtypes of polygamy. **Polygyny** refers to a man married to more than one woman, while **polyandry** refers to a woman married to more than one man. In choosing a mate, **endogamy** refers to the practice of marrying within a particular group. **Exogamy** refers to a requirement to marry outside a particular group, with it being the norm in almost all cultures to prohibit sexual relationships between certain relatives.

How we think about who we are related to is referred to as **kinship**. Kin do not have to live together, and kin is considered a cultural group rather than a biological one. Kinship groups may include extended family and members of the community or friends (like godparents and close family friends that are referred to as "aunts" and "uncles"). If kin groups involve both the maternal and paternal relations, this is called **bilateral descent**. Preference for paternal and maternal relations is called **patrilineal** and **matrilineal** descent, respectively.

Families may differ in terms of who has the power and authority to make decisions. In some families, each individual is given power over certain tasks, such as cooking, shopping, working, cleaning, and finances. There are three types of authority patterns based on gender. In a **patriarchy**, men have more authority than women, and in a **matriarchy**, women have more authority than men. In an **egalitarian family**, spouses are treated as equals and may be involved in more negotiation when making decisions.

There are many alternatives to the traditional family. A few of the differences seen in the United States are described as follows:

1) *Cultural differences:* many cultures emphasize the importance of extended family, often living with grandparents, cousins, and the like. In some cases, "kin" who are non-blood related members of the community may be considered part of the family.
2) *Divorce:* The divorce rate has generally risen in the United States due to several factors. First, there is a growing social and religious acceptance of divorce. Second, more and more opportunities are becoming available for women to succeed autonomously, making divorce a realistic possibility. Third, the financial and legal barriers to divorce have lessened over time as it has become more common.
3) *Cohabitation:* there has been a large increase, especially among couples in their 20s and 30s in living together without getting married. Sometimes these couples will have children and do many of the same things "traditionally" married couples do (like buy property and have a joint checking account) but remain legally unmarried.
4) *Lesbian and gay marriage/relationships:* Lesbian and gay couples often engage in all of the same behaviors that a "traditionally" married couple might, including property ownership and raising children.

Both individual and group experiences can threaten the strength of families. **Family violence** is a dramatic example in which one member of the family is directly responsible for the threat through their mistreatment of another person, often in an attempt to gain power, leaving the target fearful and powerless. **Child abuse** involves abusive behavior directed toward a child target. There are four categories of child abuse: physical abuse, emotional abuse, sexual abuse, and neglect. **Domestic abuse**, also referred to as dating abuse or spousal abuse, involves abuse directed toward one partner of an intimate relationship, where the abuser is the second partner. **Elder abuse** involves abuse directed toward an older target. The added element in elder abuse is that there is an expectation of trust from the older person, which is violated in the course of violence or other mistreatment. Abuse has been linked to alcohol consumption, mental illness, and certain social conditions.

Education

Educational institutions have both manifest and latent functions. Their manifest functions are to systematically pass down knowledge and to give status to those who have been educated. For example, patients trust doctors mainly because of the conferral of an awarded degree and subsequent licensure. This degree and licensure represents an agreed-upon amount of information, skills, and training acquired in order to practice medicine. Latent functions include socialization, serving as agents of change, and maintaining social control.

As a social institution, schools transmit aspects of the dominant culture. School plays a role in teaching the dominant language and literature, holidays and traditions, historical figures and events, and exposes people to existing beliefs. This involves a significant degree of interpretation. Schooling also helps maintain social norms by disciplining students and otherwise teaching them socially acceptable behavior.

While many forms of student socialization are intentional (manners, learning to talk only when called on, learning to work independently), there are other lessons learned in school known as the **hidden curriculum**. The hidden curriculum often conflicts with the manifest curriculum. For example, medical educators know that medical students experience a conflict between the stated values of their curriculum and the lived reality of hospital work they encounter during their third and fourth years. While students may have learned about the sanctity of patient care during their lectures, they often encounter hospital staff whose actions inadvertently teach them that patients are nuisances.

Within schools, benefits such as small class size, excellent teachers, and the availability of the latest technology and resources, are based on the socioeconomic status of the school district for public schools. The option of private school is only really an option for those in the higher income brackets. Access to higher education, a key factor in getting a good job, is also highly dependent on family income, as well as other factors. Level of education then continues to be influential in terms of power, respect, and social standing. Therefore, the education system has often been criticized as one that serves to maintain or widen socioeconomic and privilege gaps. This is accomplished through the processes of educational segregation and stratification.

These processes lead to an informal type of **educational segregation**, the widening disparity between children from high-income neighborhoods and those from low-income neighborhoods. In wealthier neighborhoods, parents have the time and resources to be more involved, and would potentially intervene in the event of poor teacher performance. On the other hand, children in poorer neighborhoods have public schools that are poorly funded, and teachers that may not get enough resources to do their job well. Consequently, research has found that poorer schools may be more likely to have higher teacher turnover, lower quality instruction, and provide a lower quality of education to students.

- tend to attend poorer schools and receive poorer educations
- are far less likely than children from wealthier neighborhoods to pursue a four-year college degree, and even more unlikely to pursue education beyond college, like a graduate or medical degree
- are more likely to end up with lower-paying jobs, and perpetuate the cycle of poverty for themselves

Additionally, teachers can greatly affect students' achievement. Research has shown that teachers tend to quickly form expectations of individual students, and once they have formed these expectations, they tend to act toward the student with these expectations in mind. If the student accepts the teacher's expectations as reasonable, the student will begin to perform in accordance with them as well. This is known as **teacher expectancy theory**.

While education has long been touted as the path to upward mobility in the United States, it can also reinforce and perpetuate social inequalities. This is known as **educational stratification**.

Religion

Organized religion is a social institution involving beliefs and practices. These practices are based on objects and ideas that are recognized as sacred and worthy of reverence. The MCAT may include information regarding the forms of religious organizations, common information on the five major world religions, and the social functions of religion. The forms of religious organizations include the following:

1) **Ecclesia:** a dominant religious organization that includes most members of society, is recognized as the national or official religion, and tolerates no other religions. It is often integrated into political institutions, and people do not choose to participate but are born into the social institution. Examples of countries with this social structure are Sweden (Lutheranism is the official state religion) and Iran (Islam is the official state religion).

2) **Church:** a type of religious organization that is well-integrated into the larger society. Church membership tends to occur by birth, but most churches allow people to join. Congregations are typically concerned both with the sacred and ordinary aspects of life and have well-stipulated rules and regulations. An example in the United States is the Catholic Church.

3) **Sect:** a religious organization that is distinct from that of the larger society. Sects are often formed from breaking away from larger religious institutions. Over time, some sects may develop into churches. Membership may be by birth or through conversion. Examples of sects in the United States include the Mormon community and the Amish community.

4) **Cult/New religious movement:** a religious organization that is far outside society's norms and often involves a very different lifestyle. Examples of cults in the United States include the Branch Davidians and Heaven's Gate.

From a functionalist standpoint, religion can create social cohesion (as well as dissent), social change (as well as control), and provide believers with meaning and purpose. Social cohesion is often experienced by members of religious groups due to the system of shared beliefs and values that they provide. Religious communities can be a source of emotional, spiritual, and material support in difficult times. However, religion can also be a source of social dissent, as a history of violence between religious factions indicates. Religion can be a vehicle for social change. Teachings such as the Protestant work ethic can have a profound impact on how members live their lives. Liberation theology refers to the use of the church in a political effort against various social issues, such as poverty and injustice.

Religion can prompt social change as mentioned above, but there are also cases wherein it must respond to social change. The classical sociologists predicted that as societies became more modern, there would be a decline in religious practice in favor of more rational thought. **Secularization** is the process through which religion loses its social significance in modern societies. However, evidence of secularization is contested, and even in the United States, religious factors continue to influence economics and politics. **Fundamentalism** is a second response to modernist societies in which there is strong attachment to traditional religious beliefs and practices and a strict adherence to basic religious doctrines resulting from a literalist interpretation of these texts.

A very brief overview of the five major world religions is as follows:

1) **Christianity** is the largest single faith in the world, with about 30% of the population across the globe identifying as Christian, though there are multiple denominations. About two-thirds of people in the United States identify as Christian, and although church and state are legally separate, many social and political matters reference God. Christianity is monotheistic (one God), and its followers also believe in prophets (Jesus as the Son of God), an afterlife, and a judgment day.

2) **Islam** is the second largest religion in the world. Its followers are known as Muslims, and it is estimated that between 20–25% of the world's population is Muslim. It is also monotheistic (Allah), and its followers believe in prophets (with the final one being Mohammad), an afterlife, and a judgment day. Muslim governments often do not separate religion and state, and religion frequently dictates law in Muslim countries. Muslim cultures vary in their norms, with issues such as the hijab worn by women being cultural rather than religious.

3) **Hinduism** developed in India and is a polytheistic religion (many gods) practiced by about 14% of the world's population, although there are major deities such as Shiva and Vishnu. Hinduism also includes a belief in reincarnation, or rebirth after death.

4) **Buddhism**, a religion that recognizes no deity, also originated in India. Based on the teachings of Siddhartha Gautama (the Buddha), Buddhism centers on the goal of achieving enlightenment. Buddhism teaches overcoming cravings for physical or material pleasures primarily through meditative practices.

5) **Judaism** is monotheistic and formed the historical basis for Christianity and Islam. Jews believe that God formed a covenant with Abraham and Sarah, and that if certain rules were followed (the Ten Commandments), God would bring paradise to Earth. Jews make up about 0.2% of the world's population.

There are many individual differences among people who consider themselves members of a particular religion. **Religiosity** refers to the extent that religion influences a person's life. Some may be very devout, with the extreme form being **fundamentalists**, who adhere strictly to religious beliefs. Others may adhere more to the beliefs of the religion without the rituals or to the rituals without the beliefs. Still others may define themselves by some sort of religion but do not practice their religion actively or attend any formal religious events.

Government and Economy

Our political and economic structures both influence and are influenced by social structure. Power structures are a fundamental part of both politics and economics. Governments across the world derive their power from different places. The United States government is one based on **rational-legal authority**, legal rules and regulations are stipulated in a document like the Constitution. Many corporations, including health care organizations, work within this structure and are often organized in a similar way. Other governments around the world may derive power from **traditional authority**, from custom, tradition, or accepted practice. Still other leaders may be powerful due to **charismatic authority**, the power of their persuasion.

Political sociologists are interested in the relationship between the government and the people; these scholars are concerned with the organization of governments in terms of the distribution of power and the effects of this distribution on social control. **Aristarchic governments** are controlled by a small group of people, selected based on specific qualifications, with decision-making power; the public is not involved in most political decisions. Aristarchies include **aristocracies** (those ruled by elite citizens, like those of noble birth) and **meritocracies** (those ruled by the meritorious, like those with a record of meaningful social contributions). **Autocratic governments** are controlled by a single person, or a selective small group, with absolute decision-making power. Autocracies include **dictatorships** (those ruled by one person) and **fascist governments** (those ruled by a small group of leaders). **Monarchic governments** are controlled by a single person, or by a select small group who inherited the leadership role, like kings and queens. In addition to absolute monarchies, there are constitutional monarchies, in which leaders are limited through formal constitutions.

There are also concerns of how the leadership is elected. **Authoritarian governments** consist of unelected leaders; the public might have some individual freedoms but have no control over representation. Authoritarianisms include **totalitarianism** (those in which unelected leaders regulate both public and private life through coercive means of control). **Democratic governments** consist of elected leaders; the public has some degree of political decision-making power through either direct decisions or representation. Democracies include **direct democracies** (governments in which there is direct public participation) and **representative democracies** (governments in which there is indirect public participation through the election of representatives). Democratic structures are common in the Western world, such as in the United States, where most of the population is granted the right to vote through public elections, although there might not be an equal distribution of this decision-making power (for example, minorities have been denied the right to vote in the past). This often results in the formation of **political parties**, formal groups of people that share the same principal political beliefs and organize with a common purpose of ensuring governance that supports these principles through appropriate policies. **Oligarchic governments** are less clear as leaders can be elected or unelected; the public might have the power to elect representation, but people have little influence in directing decisions and social change. Oligarchies are controlled by a small group of people with shared interests; for example, theocracies are governments ruled by the religious elite.

Finally, the structure of governments can be studied. **Republican governments** consider their countries to be public concerns and are thus democratic in nature, meaning that the people have the supreme power in these societies. **Federalist governments** include a governing representative head that shares power with constituent groups. There is the division between the central government, or the federal government, and the constituent governments, or the state, provincial, and local governments. **Parliamentary governments** include both executive and legislative branches that are interconnected; members of the executive branch (ministers) are accountable to members of the legislature. **Presidential governments** also include organizing branches, as well as a head of state. Other political concepts include **anarchy**, which refers to societies without a public government; here, there is a common implication of "lawlessness."

Economics is concerned with the production, distribution, and consumption of resources, both goods and services. Most economic structures fit into one of four categories: command, market, mixed, or traditional. In **command economies**, also known as **planned economies**, economic decisions are based on a plan of production and the means of production are often public (state-owned); these include socialism and communism. In **market economies**, economic decisions are based on the market ("supply and demand") and the means of production are often private; these include laissez-faire and free market economies. **Mixed economies** blend elements of command and market economies with both public and private ownership. There are various forms of mixed economics; for example, in some societies, there is public oversight, and even funding, of private production, such as in the United States. **Traditional**

economies consider social customs in economic decisions; this practice is most common in rural areas and often involves bartering and trading.

In addition to deriving power from rational-legal authority (i.e., governmental power is legitimized by laws and rules), our political and economic system is influenced greatly by capitalist ideals, although the United States is not purely capitalist. **Capitalism** is an economic system in which resources and production are mainly privately owned, and goods/services are produced for a profit. The driving force in capitalist societies is the pursuit of personal profit. It is thought that the advantages of capitalism are that it benefits the consumer by allowing for competition, which theoretically promotes higher quality and lower price of goods and services. Capitalism is also thought to emphasize personal freedom, by limiting government restrictions and regulations.

On the other hand, **socialism** is an economic system where resources and production are collectively owned. Socialism includes a system of production and distribution designed to satisfy human needs (good/services are produced for direct use instead of for profit). Private property is limited and government intervenes to share property amongst all. The driving force in socialist societies is collective goals; everyone is given a job and everyone is provided with what they need to survive. In socialist societies, the economy is usually centrally controlled and run by the government. **Communism** is a specific socialist structure in which there is common ownership of the means of production, as well as the absence of currencies, classes, and states, based on shared economic, political, and social ideologies.

Most nations incorporate both capitalist and socialist ideas. **Welfare capitalism** is a system in which most of the economy is private with the exception of extensive social welfare programs to serve certain needs within society. Most countries in Western Europe demonstrate welfare capitalism because most of their economies are based on capitalist principles, but universal health care is provided by the state. **State capitalism** is a system in which companies are privately run, but work closely with the government in forming laws and regulations. In the United States, most businesses are privately owned, but the government runs many operations, such as schools, the postal service, and the military. However, most hospitals and other health care providers, as well as insurance companies, remain privately run in the United States.

Numerous trends have led to the economic system that currently exists. Notably, the Information Revolution has been followed by a deindustrialization. Instead of focusing on tangible products, the emphasis has shifted to intangible products, such as information technology and services. This has changed the focus from factory work to work that can be done almost anywhere, and emphasizes literacy over mechanical skills. This shift has led to a focus on **professions**, highly esteemed white-collar occupations that require a great deal of education.

The **division of labor** occurs as societies become so complex that it is not possible for an individual to meet all of his or her needs alone, such as happened with the rise of capitalism. Different occupations emerge as a response; these occupations are specialized to serve a specific social need (for example, doctors can treat medical problems and mechanics can address our automobile issues). Because individuals no longer participate in all of the activities required for survival, there is an increase in interdependence. The division of labor has had both positive and negative consequences for social order; for example, it has increased the rate of production but it has also decreased the similarities in social experience among individuals, contributing to class differences. Thus, the division of labor is about more than economic interests.

Durkheim contributed to our current understanding of the division of labor and differentiated between two forms of social solidarity in relation to economic approaches. **Mechanical solidarity** allows society to remain integrated because individuals have common beliefs that lead to each person having the same fundamental experience. **Organic solidarity** allows society to integrate through a division of labor, which leads to each person having a different personal experience; thus, each movement is distinguishable and separate.

Health and Medicine

Medicine is the social institution that governs health and illness, particularly with respect to diagnosis, treatment, and prevention of illness. The **delivery of health care** in the United States is accomplished by teams of health-care providers with different training backgrounds and specialty areas, such as physicians and nurses of all specialties, physical and occupational therapists, dentists, hospitalists, social workers, community health workers, caregivers, pharmacists, alternative medicine providers, and rehabilitative therapists—to name only a few! The delivery of health care is organized into different levels: primary, secondary, and tertiary care. Primary care describes the care provider responsible for ongoing preventative care or disease management, or community-based care (such as an urgent care center). Secondary care includes acute care (emergency department), as well as specialty care, which is often received following a referral from a primary care provider. Tertiary care is a very specialized form of health care. It is based on consultations with specialist care providers and often occurs in hospitals or care facilities designed just for the purpose of caring for patients with a limited set of conditions. Examples of tertiary care include cancer hospitals, burn centers, and palliative care (end-of-life care) facilities. It is also important to remember that community centers and agencies can provide para-medical care, such as patient education, in-home care work, and public health outreach.

Society plays a large role in defining health/illness and acceptable health care practices. For example, societies differ in the degree of emphasis that they put on physical health versus mental health. In many nations, ADHD and depression are not considered illnesses and are not treated. The United States has experienced the spread of the **medical model of disease**, which emphasizes physical or medical factors as being the cause of all illness. Because the medical model characterizes all illness as having a physiological or pathological basis, the medical profession has been able to reframe many conditions as disease states based on the success of empirical treatment or the hope that scientific research will eventually expose the underlying cause of disease. The process by which a condition comes to be reconceptualized as a disease with a medical diagnosis and a medical treatment is known as **medicalization**. When medicalization results in medical explanations for social problems, the physician can act as the expert on a variety of issues including child development, criminality, drug addiction, and depression. However, the medical model is only one way of understanding illness, and it does not always describe illness from the patient's point of view.

An alternate way of understanding illness is known as the **social model of disease**. The social model of disease emphasizes the effect one's social class, employment status, neighborhood, exposure to environmental toxins, diet, and many other factors can have on a person's health. While someone working from the perspective of the medical model might look for the *ultimate* cause of a person's illness, someone working from the social model would be attuned to a more *proximate* cause—something about the patient's life circumstances that put him/her at greater risk of exposure.

The social model of disease, as discussed above, postulates that social pressures create the conditions for health and illness. The field that studies how social organization contributes to the prevalence, incidence, and distribution of disease across and within populations is known as **social epidemiology**. Being low-income can predispose individuals to conditions that limit individuals' ability to eat healthy food, exercise, get enough sleep, and avoid the long-term effects of severe stressors. Low-income individuals often work multiple jobs, which may cause sleep deprivation and leave little time for the exercise needed to maintain a healthy weight. Very low-income neighborhoods are often food deserts. A **food desert** is an area where healthy, fresh food is difficult to find because there are no proper grocery stores, making people more likely to eat high-calorie foods that have low nutritional value. Also, living paycheck-to-paycheck is extremely stressful. The effects of chronic stress on the body take their toll as poor health: low infant birth weight, high blood pressure, obesity, and cognitive deficits, to name only a few.

Being ill impacts not only the patient, but also the patient's social networks. Two main sociological concepts describe what illness can be like for a patient. One concept, the sick role, describes society's response to illness. The second concept, illness experience, explains the patient's subjective experience of illness.

The **sick role** is a concept developed by American sociologist Talcott Parsons. According to this concept, when a person is ill, he or she is not able to be a contributing member of society. Being ill, from Parsons' point of view, is a type of deviance. For others to take up the extra work in this person's absence they must consider the person's illness to be legitimate—they must sanction this person's deviance by exempting him/her from normal social roles and by not blaming the person for his or her illness. In return, the person must fulfill the role obligations of an ill person: the person should seek medical care and the person should make a sincere attempt to get well.

However, the sick role concept does not always hold up empirically. Other sociologists have pointed out the limitations of this role for those with chronic disease, stigmatized diseases, and "lifestyle" diseases. For example, if a person is suffering from a condition about which little is known, such as fibromyalgia, others may not accept that the person is actually ill and not confer the legitimation of the sick role. Second, the sick role concept was developed to describe acute illness and cannot explain chronic illness, where a person has good days and bad days, and often must carry on with normal life despite poor health.

Other research has examined the type of doctor-patient relationship the concept of the sick role implies. The sick role implies a passive patient and an authoritative physician. Research on **illness experience** takes the patient's subjective experience of illness as its main concern. When studying illness experience, sociologists are not just interested in the meanings people give to their illness, but also how the experience of being ill affects patients' daily lives—their ability to work, spend time with friends and family, and cultivate their identities. With a chronic disease a patient can have no reasonable expectation of getting better; thus, she or he must adjust normal daily life to fit the constraints of the illness.

Chapter 4 Summary

- A society is defined as the group of people who share a culture and live/interact with each other within a definable area.

- Functionalism is a sociological theory that conceptualizes society as a living organism with many different parts and organs, each of which has a distinct purpose; Émile Durkheim was a major proponent of functionalism.

- Manifest functions are the intended and obvious consequences of a structure; latent functions are unintended or less recognizable consequences of a structure.

- Conflict theory views society as a place where there will be inequality in resources, therefore individuals will compete for social, political, and material resources like money, land, power, and leisure; Karl Marx, a proponent of conflict theory, advocated for socialism.

- Symbolic interactionism examines the relationship between individuals and society by focusing on communication, the exchange of information through language and symbols.

- The dramaturgical approach suggests that people in society choose what kind of image they want to communicate verbally and nonverbally to others.

- Social constructionism argues that people actively shape their reality through social interactions; it is therefore something that is constructed, not inherent.

- Social institutions are a complex of roles, norms, and values organized into a relatively stable form that contributes to social order by governing the behavior of people. They provide predictability and organization for individuals within a society and mediate social behavior between people.

- Social institutions include family, education, organized religion, government and economy, and medicine.

CHAPTER 4 FREESTANDING PRACTICE QUESTIONS

1. Social institutions include all of the following, EXCEPT:

A) social networks.
B) families.
C) schools.
D) churches.

2. Joy lives in a neighborhood where 40% of the population is obese. Almost half of the adults in her neighborhood are unemployed and rely on food stamps. There are no grocery stores within a ten block radius of where Joy lives, but there are many fast-food chains. The economic and social situation in Joy's neighborhood could be described as:

   I. a food desert.
  II. absolute poverty.
 III. relative poverty.

A) I only
B) II only
C) I and II
D) I and III

3. A country where the economy is profit-driven and privately-owned, but public services like health care and education are state-funded, would be considered:

A) socialist.
B) capitalist.
C) collectivist.
D) welfare capitalist.

4. A study finds that lower-income Hispanic women from a specific urban community located near a factory are more than twice as likely to develop a rare form of cancer than women in the general population. This finding could be potentially attributed to all of the following, EXCEPT:

A) class-dependent health care disparities.
B) environmental injustice.
C) gender-dependent health care disparities.
D) ethnicity-dependent health care disparities.

5. Which of the following is NOT a macro theory of sociology?

A) Functionalism
B) Conflict theory
C) Feminist theory
D) Symbolic interactionism

6. Which of the following is NOT true regarding the sociology theory structural functionalism?

A) Functionalism is less concerned about the interactions of small groups.
B) Functionalism involves the idea that society is like an organism.
C) Functionalism encourages people to actively change the status quo of society for their own benefit.
D) Functionalism believes that once one part of an institution changes, it will always affect the other parts of the institution.

7. An adolescent gets into a fight with her parents over curfew rules. Her parents tell her that she is often irresponsible and gets distracted from her school work when her friends invite her out, so she must respect their rules. The girl responds that she knows how to manage her time and when she can spend more time with her friends without sacrificing her grades. When the girl returns to her room she is likely to experience a conflict between:

A) the "I" and "me."
B) the "I" and the individualistic self.
C) the "me" and the social self.
D) her real self and her ideal self.

8. Religion has been famously described as "the opiate of the masses" since it keeps poorer members of societies from attaining class consciousness. This concept is most consistent with:

A) exchange-rational theory.
B) structural functionalism.
C) conflict theory.
D) symbolic interactionism.

CHAPTER 4 PRACTICE PASSAGE

The term *arbovirus* is used to describe the hundreds of predominantly RNA viruses that are transmitted by mosquitoes and other arthropods. One of these, Zika virus, was first discovered in Uganda in 1947. For many years, the virus was found predominantly in primates and was restricted to a thin, equatorial belt running from Africa through Asia. Only in the second decade of the 21st century did a Zika pandemic spread to the West.

The symptoms of Zika, which is related to dengue but displays milder symptoms, include eye pain, fever, maculopapular rash, muscle aches, and prostration. Zika is also believed to sometimes carry complications. In Brazil, the incidence of microcephaly increased about 20-fold from 2014 to 2015; many public health officials believe the condition is linked to a significantly increased incidence of Zika among pregnant mothers in the region. Although a causal relationship between Zika in pregnant women and microcephaly was not definitively established, pregnant women and women planning to become pregnant were advised to refrain from traveling to areas in which the virus is apparent.

Some of the best preventive measures include applying insect repellent as well as wearing long pants and shirts. Other precautions that may be taken are using screens, mosquito nets, and air-conditioning as well as eliminating debris and still water that provide conditions for mosquito- breeding. Access to these items can be limited in developing regions, and this partially explains the prevalence of the disease in countries with less robust economies. Also, Zika is classified as a disease of poverty, meaning it is a disease that is endemic to poor regions with underdeveloped public health systems that can allow diseases to spread unchecked. Confronting these diseases in regions where the capacity of public health officials to respond in a systematic and orchestrated way is limited is an ongoing challenge for health policy officials and governments, due to limited availability and accessibility of preventative measures in lower income regions. Historically, studies have found that the most effective preventative measures are much more available and accessible in higher income regions.

Adapted from A.S. Fauci & D.M. Morens. "Zika virus in the Americas—Yet another arbovirus threat." The New England Journal of Medicine. © 2016 Massachusetts Medical Society.

1. Ana lives in a small village in Latin America. Her parents, like many other parents in the area, have always struggled to provide food and clean water for their five children. When Anna becomes sick with Zika, she does not have access to healthcare and must suffer the symptoms with no reprieve or definitive diagnosis. This situation demonstrates:

A) absolute poverty.
B) cyclical poverty.
C) relative poverty.
D) situational poverty.

2. Which type of research design would be most appropriate to determine the hypothesized relationship between Zika and pregnant women mentioned in paragraph 2?

A) A correlational study
B) An experimental design
C) A phenomenological study
D) A case study design

3. A team of researchers is testing an intravenous vaccine to prevent the spread of Zika. One hundred participants are divided into two groups. Members of the first group are given glucose fluid intravenously, while members of the second group are given the vaccine. Which of the following is true in this study?

A) The independent variable is vaccine efficacy, and the dependent variable is health outcomes.
B) The independent variable is type of fluid, and the dependent variable is health outcomes.
C) The independent variable is the type of fluid, and the dependent variable is the vaccine.
D) The independent variable is the vaccine, and the dependent variable is vaccine efficacy.

4. Which sociological theory would be most consistent with the findings regarding the availability and accessibility of Zika virus preventative measures mentioned in the final paragraph?

A) Structural functionalism
B) Symbolic interactionism
C) Social constructionism
D) Conflict theory

SOLUTIONS TO CHAPTER 4 FREESTANDING PRACTICE QUESTIONS

1. **A** Social institutions are complexes of roles, norms, and values organized into a relatively stable form that contribute to social order by governing the behavior of people. Families, schools, and churches are all examples of social institutions (choices B, C, and D can be eliminated), while social networks are not (choice A is not a social institution and is the correct answer choice).

2. **D** Item I is true: a food desert refers to an area, typically in a highly populated lower-income urban environment, where healthy, fresh food is difficult to find. Joy's neighborhood does not have a nearby grocery store but does have a plethora of fast-food restaurants, therefore, it would arguably qualify as a food desert (choice B can be eliminated). Item II is false: absolute poverty is the inability to meet a bare minimum of basic necessities, including clean drinking water, food, safe housing, and reliable access to health care; the scenario described is not absolute poverty (choice C can be eliminated). Item III is true: relative poverty is defined as an inability to meet the average standard of living within a society. The fact that so many people in Joy's neighborhood are unemployed suggests that she is living in relative poverty (choice A can be eliminated, and choice D is correct).

3. **D** Welfare capitalism refers to a system of government where most of the economy is private with the exception of extensive social welfare programs to serve certain social needs within society (such as health care and education; choice D is correct). Socialism is an economic system where resources and production are collectively owned. Socialism includes a system of production and distribution designed to satisfy human needs; good/services are produced for direct use instead of for profit (choice A is wrong). Capitalism is an economic system in which resources and production are mainly privately owned, and goods/services are produced for a profit; strict capitalism does not include state-funded public services (choice B is wrong). Collectivism is an economic or social outlook that emphasizes interdependence between people; a profit-driven economy would not be a part of a collectivist country (choice C is wrong).

4. **C** Gender-dependent health care disparities highlight differences in the treatment and outcomes between men and women; because this question relates lower-income Hispanic women to women in the general population, there is no evidence that the disparity is based on gender because no comparison is made to men (this finding is not attributable to choice C, so it is the correct answer choice). Class-dependent health care disparities are based on socioeconomic differences between classes and ethnicity-dependent health care disparities are based on ethnic differences between groups; because this question relates lower-income Hispanic women to women in the general population, it is possible that this disparity exists due to either class and/or ethnicity (the finding could be attributable to either choices A or D, so both choices can be eliminated). Environmental injustice refers to the fact that people in poorer communities are more likely to be subjected to negative environmental impacts on their health and well-being; because these women live near a factory, this health care disparity could be the result of environmental injustice (the finding could be attributable to choice B, so it can be eliminated).

5. **D** Macro theories are concerned with interactions between groups of people, while micro-level theories are concerned with interactions between individuals. Symbolic interactionism, which is concerned with the way individuals use symbols to communicate in society, is the only micro-level theory listed (choice D is not a macro-level theory and is the correct answer choice). Functionalism explains how social processes work on a broad scale. It considers the function and purpose of large groups within society, e.g., churches, schools, hospitals, and the like, and is considered a macro-level theory (choice A can be eliminated). Conflict theory explains society based on constant competition between groups for limited resources and is considered a macro-level theory (choice B can be eliminated). Feminist theory is concerned with inequality between the genders (whole groups of people) rather than inequalities between particular individuals (choice C is a macro-level theory and can be eliminated).

6. **C** Functionalism discourages people from changing the norm because it emphasizes the idea of stability through the universal agreement to abide by the norms of society (choice C is false and therefore the correct answer). Functionalism focuses on society as a whole rather than the individual aspects of society (choice A is true and can be eliminated). Organic solidarity is an idea within functionalism that compares society to an organism (choice B is true and can be eliminated). Functionalists believe that if one part of the system changes, then the rest of the system will have to adjust to the dysfunction until social stability can be restored (choice D is true and can be eliminated).

7. **A** The adolescent in the question stem has just received an interpretation of her identity from her parents that she is at odds with. Her individualistic belief of her own character is different from the feedback she is getting from her social environment. This is exactly the difference between the "I" and the "me," the individualistic self and the social self (choice A is correct). The I and the individualistic self are one and the same, so would not cause a conflict (choice B is wrong). This is also true for the me and the social self (choice C is wrong). Real versus ideal self is a gap between who one is in the real world and who one wishes to be. This is a concept in Humanistic psychology and client-centered therapy that does not apply to the situation (choice D is wrong).

8. **C** Karl Marx, one of the founders of modern sociology, said that religion was "the opiate of the masses." This statement is most consistent with conflict theory, as he saw the state's use of religion to ensure the continued inequality of the system (choice C is correct). Exchange-rational theory asserts that people use cost-benefit analyses to choose which action will be most beneficial to them (choice A can be eliminated). Structural functionalism says that there are individual structures in society that all work together for the good of the whole—for dynamic equilibrium. Religion is one of these structures (choice B can be eliminated). Symbolic interactionism is a micro-level theory that says that people use language express what objects mean individually to them. While Marx might be expressing his own symbolic understanding of religion, the quote itself refers not to an individual interpretation on the micro-level, but rather to how the larger society uses religion as a tool (choice D can be eliminated).

SOLUTIONS TO CHAPTER 4 PRACTICE PASSAGE

1. **A** Absolute poverty is when individuals do not have access to basic necessities such as clean water, food, and healthcare (choice A is correct). Cyclical poverty usually lasts for a transient period and is related to the overall state of the economy (choice B is wrong). Relative poverty refers to the idea that some persons may not be able to attain the average standard of living within a given society, but it does not indicate absence of the basic necessities (choice C is wrong). Situational poverty arises because of a change in circumstances, which may be related to health, environmental, or personal issues, among others. The question stem does not indicate a change in circumstances, and it emphasizes that the family has always struggled to make ends meet (choice D is wrong).

2. **B** Paragraph 2 mentions that "a causal relationship between Zika in pregnant women and microcephaly was not definitively established...". To determine causality, an experimental design must be used (choice B is correct). Choices A, C, and D may give insight to a relationship between two variables but would not allow researchers to infer any cause-and-effect relationship (choices A, C, and D are incorrect).

3. **B** In this scenario, the independent variable (the one that can be manipulated or controlled) is whether or not the subject receives the vaccine. Thus, there are two conditions for the independent variable: vaccine and placebo (glucose fluid), and the independent variable is best described as the type of fluid given, not one of the two conditions (choices A and D can be eliminated). The dependent variable is the type of health outcome observed (choice C can be eliminated, and choice B is correct). Note that vaccine and vaccine efficacy are both conditions, not variables.

4. **D** The final paragraph discusses both limited access and availability of the Zika virus preventative measures, as well as economic disparities in terms of the availability and accessibility. The sociological theory that would be most concerned with limited resources and economic discrepancies would be conflict theory (choice D is correct). Structural functionalism is more concerned with the institutions and groups of society functioning together to maintain social stability, which does not clearly apply (choice A is incorrect). Symbolic interactionism is a micro-level theory, and the final paragraph is discussing macro-level trends (choice B is incorrect). Social constructionism is concerned with socialization and the construction of social realities, neither of which clearly apply to this scenario (choice C is incorrect).

Chapter 5
Culture, Demographics, and Social Inequality

Human beings live within societies, so in order to best understand human behavior, we must consider both the impact of the individual on the collective and that of the collective on the individual. By understanding social structures we can better understand the individual. Moreover, these social structures, along with cultural and demographic factors, play a key role in determining a person's health. Social stratification and inequality affect all societies across the globe, and afford power and privilege to some while denying it to others.

5.1 CULTURE AND DEMOGRAPHICS

Culture

Culture simply refers to a shared way of life, including the beliefs and practices that a social group shares. Although cultures can vary a great deal, they are composed of some common elements. **Symbolic culture** consists of symbols that are recognized by people of the same culture. Symbols convey agreed-upon meaning, can communicate the values and norms of the culture, and include rituals, gestures, signs, and words that help people within a society communicate and understand each other.

Symbols and rituals can differ between cultures, for example, some cultures celebrate the life of a deceased relative with a party, while others mourn at a more somber funeral. While symbolic elements of culture involve values and norms, **material culture** involves physical objects or artifacts. This includes clothing, hairstyles, food, and the design of homes. The importance placed on material objects can reflect the culture's values; for example, the American dream often includes a car, a symbol of mobility and independence. In contrast, **non-material culture** is specific to social thoughts and ideas, such as values.

Popular culture is a phrase used to describe features of culture that appeal to the masses, often those communicated through mass media such as radio and television. This is distinguished from **high culture**, which describes those features often limited to the elite, like the ballet or opera.

While comparing different cultures is useful for noticing differences, some anthropologists assert that there are also some **cultural universals**—patterns or traits that are common to all people. Cultural universals tend to pertain to basic human survival and needs, such as securing food and shelter, and also pertain to events that every human experiences, including birth, death, and illness. Despite these very important similarities that unite us all, cultural differences are far more common than cultural universals.

Two of the most crucial elements of culture are its values and beliefs, which people within a given culture tend to share. **Values** can be defined as a culture's standard for evaluating what is good or bad, while **beliefs** are the convictions or principles that people hold. Values often define how people in a society should behave, but they may not actually reflect how people do behave. For example, in the United States, open-mindedness and tolerance are considered to be values, yet examples of racism and homophobia abound. In order to promote societal values, laws, sanctions, or rewards may be in place to encourage behavior in line with social values and discourage behavior counter to social values. For example, it is against the law to discriminate based on race, color, religion, gender, or national origin when making employment decisions. **Norms** are the visible and invisible rules of social conduct within a society.

Culture and Social Groups

Sociobiology is a study of how biology and evolution have affected human social behavior. Primarily, it applies Darwin's principle of natural selection to social behavior, suggesting there is a biological basis for many behaviors. That is, particular social behaviors persist over generations because they are adaptive for survival. Sociobiologists would argue that biological predisposition is influenced by social factors; an aggressive individual may learn to channel these tendencies away from socially unacceptable acts (for example, assault) and toward socially accepted activities (for example, cage-fighting).

Scientists also believe that the origins of culture lie in human evolution. Through time, humans in various societies evolved the ability to categorize and communicate human experience through the use of symbols (as discussed above). As these codified systems for communication were learned and taught to future generations, they began to develop independently of human evolution. While people living in different areas will likely develop their own unique cultures, culture can still be taught and learned. Therefore, anthropologists consider culture to be not just a product of human evolution, but a complement to it; it is a means of social adaptation to the natural world.

Cultural Construction and Transformation

Cultural diffusion is the transfer of elements of culture from one social group to another. This contributes to cultural similarities between different societies. Diffusion can be direct or indirect, or sometimes even forced, as with cultural imperialism. The rate of diffusion has increased as a result of cross-cultural communication, like modern media and transportation. This is important for **cultural competence** or effective interactions between people from different cultures. For example, in medicine, the diffusion of cultural understanding—which leads to effective communication—is an important element in reducing disparities in health and health care. **Cultural transmission** is the process through which this information is passed down to successive generations.

Elements of culture are not static. In some cases, **social change** occurs, in which societies experience a change in state. This can be subtle, like with the development of new linguistic phrases, or radical, like with **revolutions**. Transformative social changes, such as technological innovations, often challenge our understanding of the world because there is no social consensus about the new innovation; the creation of new social rules "lags" behind. This is described as **cultural lag**. The foundational work on cultural lag explains that material culture changes much faster than non-material culture, which often resists change.

When individuals experience changes that necessitate a period of adjustment, there is often **transition shock**. When this disorientation is the result of an individual being subjected to alternative cultures and foreign environments, such as through leisure travel or permanent relocation, it is called **culture shock**. This is a real experience that involves deeper emotions than homesickness; it challenges an individual's assumptions about their social surroundings. Different cultures have different cuisines, fashions, languages, gestures, etc., and individuals must grow accustomed to all of these changes. For example, the transition to medical school causes a definite reaction for most students; there is a feeling of "information overload" as the result of exposure to unfamiliar content and the disruption of established schedules. **Reverse culture shock** involves the same experiences but upon an individual's return to their initial environment.

Sociocultural evolution is a set of theories describing the processes through which societies and cultures have progressed over time. Both individuals and social structures experience continuous transformation in response to their complex needs. Sociologists argue that these changes are the result of social factors, such as social interactions, rather than biological factors. Thus, sociocultural evolution is less concerned with the evolution of human bodies, but instead questions how human minds have evolved for us to succeed as beings with natural social tendencies. While myriad societies have existed throughout the centuries, as revealed by historical research, most of these have declined naturally and only a couple hundred remain today. Two modern theories of sociocultural evolution, *modernization* and *sociobiology*, are discussed previously.

POPULATION STUDIES

Human **population** is the collection of people in a defined geographical area, and also refers to the number of people in the area. Population studies are interested in demographic shifts and can be quite complex. There is periodic population growth and population decline as a result of birth rates, death rates, and migration rates. The world as a whole is experiencing a period of population growth that is predicted to continue for many decades. Much of this growth is attributed to advances in agricultural production and innovations in medicine that have contributed to changes in birth and death rates. In contrast, studies of population decline are often concerned with great reductions in population as a result of catastrophes, such as epidemics and massacres, or widespread social changes (such as rural flight). Population growth and decline are measured using the **population growth rate**: the rate of population change in a specified time period, reported as a percent of the initial population.

In societies experiencing population growth, there is concern of reaching **overpopulation**, at which point there are more people than can be sustained; in societies experiencing decline, there are concerns about maintaining economic success. The total possible population that can be supported with needed resources and without significant negative effects in a given area is referred to as the **carrying capacity**. Populations tend to increase and decrease until **population equilibrium** is met at this maximum load.

Population projections are estimates of future populations made from mathematical extrapolations of previous data. Traditional projections are based on birth rates, death rates, and migration rates, and thus do not consider unpredicted effects on population, like the chance of catastrophes. The global population reached 7.9 billion in 2021. Experts project an increase in this population until at least 2050 with upper estimates ranging from 9 to 11 billion despite decreases in worldwide fertility rates. The projections suggest that the greatest contributions will be made in less-developed regions. In fact, nine countries are expected to contribute to more than half of the world's population; these countries are underdeveloped regions, including China and India, with the exception of the United States where international migration rates are an important consideration. In contrast, in some developed regions the death rate exceeds the birth rate which, coupled with increasing life expectancies, suggests population decline. In the United States, national population growth rates have been in decline since the turn of the century.

Population distributions—in particular, age and sex distributions—are sometimes represented through graphical illustrations called **population pyramids** (Figure 1). These representations create age- and sex-specific groups (cohorts) using either total population or percentages. The *x*-axis represents the population and the *y*-axis separates men and women with the tradition positioning males on the left and females on the right. This creates a clear and distinct shape that describes the social structure. For example, an expansive population pyramid is wide at the base, representing a high birth rate and a high death rate. Thus, population pyramids can help predict population trends and determine the social needs for dependents, such as children and people of retirement age.

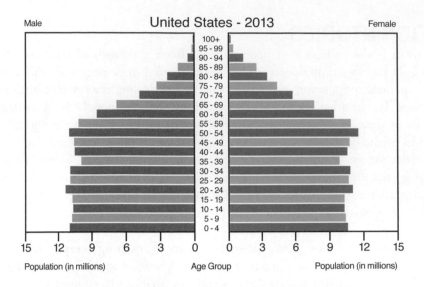

Figure 1 Population pyramid: birth rates, death rates, and migration rates are the main determinants of changes in population

Fertility and Mortality

Birth rates and death rates are often reported through statistical measures. The **crude birth rate** (CBR) is the annual number of births per 1,000 people in a population. Experts consider crude birth rates of 10–20 to be low and those of 40–50 to be high. The **crude death rate** (CDR) is the annual number of deaths per 1,000 people in a population. Experts consider crude death rates below 10 to be low and those above 20 to be high. The **rate of population change** is the difference between the crude birth rate and crude death rate. There are also **age-specific birth rates** and **age-specific death rates**, which are the annual number of births or deaths per 1,000 persons in an age group.

In broad terms, **fertility** is the ability of a woman to reproduce. The **general fertility rate** is the annual number of births per 1,000 women in a population. The more complicated measure of **total fertility rate** predicts the total number births per single woman in a population with the assumption that the woman experiences the current recorded age-specific fertility rates and reaches the end of her reproductive life. Most women are capable of reproduction between the ages of 15 and 45 ("childbearing years"). The **replacement fertility rate** is the fertility rate at which the population will remain balanced, and **sub-replacement fertility** indicates that the birth rate is less than the death rate, thus the population size will not be sustained. The **population-lag effect** refers to the fact that changes in total fertility rates are often not reflected in the birth rate for several generations. This is the result of **population momentum**, in which the children produced during periods of higher fertility rates reproduce; there are more women of reproductive age and thus more births overall, regardless of the number of births per woman. Because crude birth rates do not consider age or sex differences, fertility rates offer a clearer idea of demographic trends.

Regarding decreases in population, **mortality** refers to the death rate in a population, and this also includes both general and specific measures. This is distinguished from **morbidity**, which refers to the nature and extent of disease in a population; the **prevalence rate** measures the number of individuals experiencing a disease and the **incidence rate** measures the number of new cases of a disease. Reference to death rates in medicine often concern the **case fatality rate**, which measures deaths as the result of a set diagnosis or procedure, sometimes specific to the beginning or late stages. The current leading cause of death worldwide is ischemic heart disease, but there are also variations in causes of death by location; for example, age-related issues are a major cause of death in developed countries, while malnutrition is a major cause of death in developing countries. There is an inverse correlation between a nation's crude death rate and its gross domestic product (GDP). There are two additional common and reliable indicators of important qualities of life: the infant mortality rate and life expectancy. The **infant mortality rate** is the annual number of deaths per 1,000 infants under one year of age. This rate is lowest in European countries, such as Iceland, at a low of 5 and highest in the sub-Saharan regions of Africa, such as Sierra Leone, at a high of 170. **Life expectancy** is the number of years that individual can expect to live based on year of birth and other demographic factors. Estimates of global life expectancies range from 36 to 79 years.

Developed regions tend to have lower birth rates and death rates. Factors contributing to decreasing crude birth rates include access to contraception, costs associated with raising a child, and other social changes. For example, teenage births are at a historic low in the United States and an increasing number of older couples are choosing to postpone reproduction, or to not reproduce at all. Factors contributing to decreasing crude death rates include improvements in agriculture, medicine, and sanitation.

Migration

In addition to birth rates and death rates, population is also determined through rates of **migration**, the geographical movement of individuals, families, or other small or large groups of people. Migration is distinct from non-permanent movement. For example, non-permanent travel for leisure, pilgrimage, or seasonal reasons and **nomadism**, which is a traditional method of continuous travel in search of natural resources as a method of sustenance ("hunting and gathering"), are not considered migration because there is no intention to settle. **External migration**, also referred to as cross-border or international migration, involves migration to another nation. Motivations for external migration are often economic or political in nature. **Internal migration** involves migration to another region of the same nation. Motivations for internal migration are often more economic in nature as individuals pursue better opportunities, such as education. **Voluntary migration** is the result of internal factors (a personal decision). **Involuntary migration**, or forced migration, is the result of external factors that pose a threat to the individual in their initial environment and are often a form of social control, such as ethnic cleansing. Those who migrate to unsettled areas are **settlers** and those who migrate to settled areas as a result of displacement are **refugees**. More complicated is **colonization**, which involves migration to settled areas in which dominance is exerted over the foreign state. **Immigration** involves entering a new area and these people are called immigrants (and can be either legal or illegal residents); **emigration** involves leaving an area and those who do so are called emigrants. For example, there is a high rate of emigration from Mexico and a high rate of immigration to the United States. There is also a high rate of illegal immigration, which has disadvantages for both the migrant individual and their new home. **Reverse migration**, or return migration, is the return of individuals to their former homes.

There are numerous historical theories describing the reasons for migration and its effects. Everett Lee, a popular theorist, differentiated between push and pull factors in migration. **Push factors** are those features that are unattractive about an area and "push" people to leave. Push factors are often economic, political, or religious (e.g., housing **discrimination** or insufficient access to social resources). There are also more extreme examples, such as destructive violence or natural disasters, and **genocide**, or mass execution with the intention of eliminating a specific social group. **Pull factors** are those features that are attractive about an area and "pull" people there. These often include opportunities for economic, political, or religious freedom and success. The interaction between push and pull factors contributes to the rates of migration.

Urban Growth, Decline, and Renewal

Internal migration includes the movement between rural and urban areas. The spatial distribution of individuals and social groups is an interest of **social geography**. **Urbanization** refers to the growth of urban areas (as people move from rural to urban areas) as the result of global change. Urbanization is tied to **industrialization**, the process through which societies transform from agrarian to industrial, and industrialized countries have more people living in urban areas than non-industrialized countries do. The global urbanization rate is roughly 55%, and approximately 80% of the U.S. population lives in urban areas (including cities and suburbs). People move to urban areas predominantly for the economic advancement that cities provide. Furthermore, people can access more social services in cities. This is related to **rural flight**, the migration from rural areas to urban areas. Emigration from rural areas is often related to a decreasing emphasis on agricultural processes.

In contrast to urban growth, suburbanization leads to urban decline. **Suburbanization** refers to population growth on the fringes of urban areas (as people move from urban areas to suburban areas). The **suburbs** are residential satellite communities located in the peripheral regions of major urban centers that are often connected to the cities in some fashion. In the United States more people live in the suburbs (which are considered "urban" for statistical purposes) than in the cities themselves. **White flight** is a historical example of suburbanization that involved the migration of whites from cities to more racially homogenous suburbs. Migration to such areas that are adjacent to the cities is an example of **urban sprawl**, or the migration of people from urban areas to otherwise remote areas. The negative effects of urban sprawl include **urban blight**, which occurs when less functioning areas of large cities degrade as a result of urban decline. These forms of migration can thus lead to desolate properties, such as condemned houses, and the resulting dangerous conditions can contribute to an increase in crime levels in blighted areas. Those who remain in the blighted areas are often poor and have less access to social amenities and opportunities.

Gentrification refers to the renovation of urban areas in a process of urban renewal. Gentrification is often specific to the introduction of wealthier residents to the cities who then help to restore the existing infrastructure, which alters the region's demographics and economics. Gentrification is a form of **urban renewal**, or the redevelopment of urban areas. This causes much social change with both positive and negative effects; for example, it can increase the tax base, but it can also lead to the displacement of the original local people. Urban renewal can be a mechanism for reform or a mechanism for control (for example, eminent domain).

Theories of Population Change

There are multiple theories of population change. **Demographic transition** (DT) is the transition from overall higher to overall lower birth and death rates as a result of a country's development from a pre-industrial to industrial framework due to both economic and social changes; thus, both fertility and mortality rates decrease as in the transition from an agricultural to a manufacturing society. This has long-term effects, such as a stable population. The model includes specific stages of transition and, in general, developed countries are further along in this transition than developing countries but most countries have started to experience changes in crude birth rate and crude death rate. However, the model is limited; for example, it does not consider additional social factors that affect birth rates, like religious influences.

Thomas Robert Malthus argued that population is the result of available resources for sustenance, such as productive farmland. Humans are inclined to reproduce and thus population growth is often exponential, especially during times of excess. However, **Malthusianism** states that the possible rate of population increase exceeds the possible rate of resource increase. Malthus described two forms of checks on population growth: **positive checks** that raise the death rate, like disease, disasters, hunger, and wars, and **preventative checks** that lower the birth rate, like abstinence, birth control, late marriage, and same-sex relationships. A **Malthusian Catastrophe** occurs when the means of sustenance are not enough to support the population, resulting in population reduction through famine or predicted famine (i.e., people have fewer children because they fear serious food shortages in the future). **Neo-Malthusianism** is a movement based on these principles that advocates for population control in order to reduce the negative effects of population strain.

Demographics in U.S. Society

Demography is the study of human population dynamics, including the size, structure, and distribution of a population, and changes in the population over time due to birth, death, and migration. An analysis of the demographics of a given society can provide powerful information about many sociological phenomena. Demographic data are largely derived from censuses.

As of 2020, the population of the United States was approximately 331,449,000, roughly 50.8% of whom were female. Approximately 22.3% of the population were eighteen years old or younger, while approximately 16.5% were sixty-five or older.

In 2020, approximately 13.6% of the population was foreign-born, including approximately 11 million noncitizens. Latin America accounts for just over half of all of the people who are foreign-born in the United States, so is thus the largest source of both legal and illegal immigration to the United States.

In regards to population studies, there has been a rapid decline in the total global fertility rate; this is of particular concern in the United States where the average woman has fewer than two children, which is below the population replacement level. The infant mortality rate has decreased in recent years and is now approximately 6 deaths per 1,000 live births. The current life expectancy at birth is approximately 79 years (76 for males and 81 for females). The current migration rates (external migration) have caused increases in population despite low birth rates and death rates (although population growth is nonetheless near a historical low). There are also examples of internal migration. There have been historic migrations from the eastern states to the western states (expansion), as well as the migration of African Americans from the rural south to the urban north after abolition of slavery, called the Great Migration. The **New Great Migration** is an example of a domestic reverse migration. During this period, there was an increase in Black migration to the now urban South as racial relations improved.

Researchers often use aggregate statistics to provide a demographic profile of a specific population (based on region or time). **Minorities** are those demographic groups that receive differential treatment through processes of prejudice and discrimination due to their shared characteristics. These groups have lower statuses than other groups, and may be viewed as inferior. It is important to note that despite the title, these groups are termed minorities not for their size but instead for their disparate social experiences and the description holds regardless of population size. Thus, despite the gender and sex distributions being near equal in most societies, women are sometimes considered minorities because of their perceived status as inferior and subordinate to men. The **dominant groups** are those with the social power to assign these labels.

Demographic measures discussed on the next pages include age, gender, race and ethnicity, sexual orientation, and immigration status.

Age

People's temporal position between birth and death is measured through **age**. In Western societies, the most common use is numerical age, a chronological measurement that begins at birth (thus babies are age 0 at birth). This is distinguished from measures of prenatal development, such as gestational age, although some societies do consider this period (thus babies are age 9 months at birth if full-term). Years are the most common units of measurement for age, but months or even weeks are also used in certain situations, such as with infants.

Age cohorts are an example of statistical cohorts in which a group of subjects share the characteristic of age. Generational cohorts, or **generations**, are groups of people born in the same period. Demographic age profiles describe populations in terms of age groups. Populations with a proportionate distribution are the most stable. **Population aging** occurs when there is a disproportionate percentage of older people in a population. This raises concerns such as health-care demands and provider shortages. **Ageism** is prejudice or discrimination against a person based on age, often against older people.

The concept of aging has both biological and social components. *Social aging* reflects the biological changes in a multidimensional process in which individuals experience complex emotional and social changes. There are serious social implications of an aging population. Economic consequences of a rising median age include increased requirements for pension liabilities, retirement packages, and worker's compensation. In contrast, an increase in children leads to greater demands for social resources such as education. Furthermore, younger people are more likely to contribute to social changes, such as the creation of new technologies or the push for political changes.

There are theories that explain the social construction of age. These perspectives assert that perceptions of age are not inherent but instead social creations based on cultural customs, traditions, and values. Eastern cultures tend to respect older people for their experience and wisdom. Western cultures, however, tend to see aging as undesirable. It is thus common to take measures to control appearances and impressions, such as cosmetic surgeries. The response to aging parents exemplifies these cultural differences. Retirement homes are more popular in developed societies and public perceptions of these resources are accepting; in less modern societies, it is expected that children will care for their parents and assisted living options might be seen as disrespectful.

Gender

Sex is a biological characteristic that is assigned at birth and permanent in most cases; it is based on chromosomes, external genitalia, gonads, and hormones. Thus, categories of sex are male (XY) and female (XX). The third sex, albeit rare, is intersex. This classification is applicable when a single sex cannot be identified. **Gender** is a social characteristic that is based on behavioral role expectations. Thus, categories of gender are masculine and feminine. Developed societies often discuss gender in dichotomous terms, where masculine and feminine are opposites, but in some societies, there are third genders, such as the Native American two-spirit: individuals who are neither male nor female, and are held in high regard in some traditional Native American tribes.

Gender is thought to be influenced by both nature and nurture. In terms of nature, biological measures can have behavioral effects (for examples, hormones influence emotions). The natural sciences are interested in the consequences of biological differences between men and women on gender. In some cases, genetic abnormalities (such as the XXY chromosomal abnormality in Klinefelter's syndrome) might cause unexpected presentations in light of one's biological sex. In terms of nurture, our social surroundings have a profound effect on the development of our gender identities. Gender identification occurs through multiple agents of socialization and **gender roles** (the socialization of gender roles is also known as **gender conditioning**) describe the social and behavioral expectations for men and women. These expectations are internalized and become connected to our self-identities (how we think about ourselves) and thus influence our behaviors. **Gender expression** is the external manifestation of these roles. **Gender schema theory** is the study of how gender beliefs become socialized in society. A similar theory states that individuals learn sexual behavior through gender scripts, a series of predictable patterns that are internalized through socialization.

Sexism is prejudice or discrimination against a person based on gender or sex, often against women. Despite revolutionary social changes, there continues to be a flawed perception in which men are viewed as dominant and women are viewed as subordinate; men are the reference group and women are the "other" group in continuous reference to men. Men and women are different and unequal in the social resources afforded to them; women are marginalized and given less power at birth and fewer opportunities throughout their lifetime to gain power. A classic example of gender inequality concerns the institution of marriage. Upon entering into a marriage, women often gain many more responsibilities. The division of labor further limits the representation of women in the public sphere, which also limits the opportunities women have to develop the intellectual reasoning skills that society values. These disparate experiences are an interest of the previously discussed Feminist Theory.

Gender roles are those behaviors that are considered appropriate or proper for men and women. Gendered behaviors that follow social conventions are approved while those that do not are disapproved; thus, deviation from gender roles tends to create social disorder. **Transgender** individuals have gender identities that are inconsistent with their biological sex. Some transgender individuals decide to make permanent changes to their bodies through hormone therapy, surgery, or some other means. There is much prejudice and discrimination against transgender communities.

Race and Ethnicity

Race and ethnicity are related concepts that are of much interest to sociologists because of their importance in human interactions. **Race** is a description of a distinct social group based on certain shared characteristics. These shared characteristics are often inherited biological traits or genetic differences (and thus manifest in physical appearances). According to the U.S. Census Bureau, the currently accepted race categories include Black/African American, white, Asian, American Indian/Alaska Native, Native Hawaiian/Other Pacific Islander, and "Other." **Ethnicity** is cultural and ethnicities are distinct from nationalities. For example, Arab populations originate in the Arabian Peninsula, which includes several modern nations including (1) Egypt, (2) Algeria, (3) Iraq, (4) Sudan, and (5) Morocco. In addition to Arab populations, Egypt also includes ethnic minorities, such as the Beja, Berber, Dom, and Nubian peoples. **Ethnogenesis** is a social process that results in the creation of separate ethnicities. Historical examples of this include the development of small sub-ethnic groups, **tribes**, into independent ethnic groups.

Members of the same racial or ethnic group do not develop a common identity based on shared characteristics alone; such identities are also formed on the basis of shared historical and social experiences. It is not the common origin that forms the group but the shared consciousness of the common origin, and the meanings ascribed to that specific origin. Prejudices and actions that discriminate based on race, or hold that one race is inferior to another, are called **racism**. While the exact definitions of "race," "ethnicity," and "racism" have been subject to much debate over the years, racism tends to be seen when the dominant or majority group holds a prejudice or engages in discrimination, whether intentional or not, against non-dominant or minority groups. Sometimes racism is used to describe discrimination on an ethnic or cultural basis, independent of whether these differences are described as racial. The ambiguity largely stems from confusion about the definitions of the terms "race" and "ethnicity." Ethnocentrism is a related concept that describes biases that result when people look at issues from the perspective of a particular cultural background. It is often whites who are said to be ethnocentric in sociological studies, but this is not absolute.

Michael Omi and Howard Winat's **racial formation perspective** was created with the purpose of deconstructing race in its modern form. Race is seen as a complex and fluid social construct, enforced through both micro- and macro-level social processes. In contrast to other theories that do not present race exclusively as a social construct, the racial formation perspective asserts that without these processes, the differences in biological features are meaningless.

Racialization, or **ethnicization**, is the social process by which the dominant group ascribes racial or ethnic identities, perceived or real, to groups that do not otherwise relate to the labels. These processes are used as forms of social control, often as a part of imperialism or nationalism. Historical examples of racialization and ethnicization have resulted in the eventual self-identification of these groups with the ascribed race or ethnicity.

Sexual Orientation

Sexual orientation concerns the target of a person's romantic or sexual attraction or behavior. There are three main sexual orientations:

- **Heterosexual**: the orientation toward the opposite gender or sex
- **Homosexual**: the orientation toward the same gender or sex
- **Bisexual**: the orientation toward both genders or sexes

Bisexual identities do not necessitate an equal attraction toward both genders or sexes; in some cases, there is a distinct, but not exclusive, sexual preference toward one gender or sex. Bisexual communities include those who are **pansexual** and attracted to people irrespective of gender or sex. **Asexuality** involves the lack of sexual attraction. This is different from the decision to be abstinent or celibate for personal reasons, such as religious beliefs. In fact, those with little or no sexual attraction sometimes participate in sexual behavior nonetheless for reasons like reproduction. Sexual orientation exists along a continuum, with the extremes being exclusive attraction to the opposite gender or sex (heterosexual) and exclusive attraction to the same gender or sex (homosexual). The Kinsey Scale, also called the Heterosexual-Homosexual Rating Scale assigns a number from 0 (exclusively heterosexual) to 6 (exclusively homosexual) that places each individual along this continuum.

Heterosexism is prejudice or discrimination against a person based on their sexual orientation toward the same sex (for example, homophobic attitudes). **Heteronormative beliefs** often enforce strict gender roles and involve prejudice and discrimination against non-heterosexual individuals. There are sometimes public sanctions, such as formal policies, reinforcing these beliefs. This has led to modern social movements for the recognition of legal rights, such as adoption rights, marriage rights, and health-care rights for same-sex couples.

There is much debate about the causes of sexual orientation, including both biological theories that consider factors like genetics and hormones and environmental theories that consider factors like parenting. Some argue that non-heterosexual behavior is unnatural for certain reasons (for example, it does not permit reproduction). However, research suggests that sexual orientation is a human characteristic that is generally resistant to change, leading to the argument that non-heterosexual behavior can be natural. Furthermore, there is no substantive scientific evidence to support the argument that sexual orientation can be changed through interventions.

Immigration Status

Immigration was introduced above as the migration of people to a new area. Immigration status is another common demographic measure. In the past, the United Nations estimated the international migrant population to be near 3 percent of the total world population. Most of these migrants moved to developed countries. European countries host the most immigrants worldwide (around 70 million); North American countries host the second most (around 45 million). Recent research recorded that the highest percentage of respondents (23%) in a study who identified as being interested in migration named the United States as their preferred destination. This can be attributed in part to the **American Dream**, an ideological construct that offers individuals the opportunities for happiness and success with the proper amount of determination. This central promise has contributed to the rise in migration to the United States in the search of a better life with enhanced personal freedoms.

The United States has had four main periods of immigration, based on the social context, as well as the distinct demographics (ethnicities, nationalities, and races) of the migrants.

1) **The seventeenth and eighteenth centuries**: During this period, English colonists migrated to the United States (the colonial period). Indentured servants also migrated through this process, accounting for more than half of all immigrants from Europe during the period.

2) **The mid-nineteenth century**: During this period, the most migrants came from northern Europe.

3) **The early twentieth century**: During this period, the most migrants came from southern and Eastern Europe. The peak of European migration was 1907, after which the social context of the United States made conditions less suitable for immigration. The Great Depression, for example, led to a period of higher national emigration rates than immigration rates (this occurred in the early 1930s).

4) **The late twentieth century (post-1965) to the present**: During this period, the majority of migrants have been from Asia and Latin America. The rates of immigration during this period have been unprecedented. For example, the decade with the historically highest rate of immigration was from 1990 to 2000; between 10 and 11 million legal and illegal immigrants entered the United States during this phase. There are now more than 44 million immigrants living in the United States; approximately 10.5 million of those are undocumented, according to 2017 estimates.

The United States has restrictive legal limits on immigration. There are current quotas based on origin, and these limits do not consider populations (thus, the maximum number of visas offered is the same for all countries). **Immigration controls** are formal policies that define and regulate who has the right to settle in an area. Today, most legal immigration is granted on the basis of family reunification (this accounts for two-thirds of all cases), employment skills, and humanitarian reasons. Historically, immigration decisions have been made for other reasons, such as ethnic selection. In some cases, the U.S. government has granted amnesties for undocumented immigrants. The presence of illegal immigrants presents definite challenges in describing the complex demographics of the United States.

The shared experiences of immigrants are of concern to sociologists. These individuals are often mistreated, and in some cases their rights are violated, in the immigration process. Immigrants are also a common target of prejudice and discrimination. Public attitudes, in general, are more positive toward established migrants (such as the Polish and Italian communities) and more negative toward recent migrants (such as Hispanic communities). For these reasons, there are often intersections between immigration status and race and ethnicity, as well as social class. There is also a distinction in the public opinion of legal and illegal immigrants, often fueled by media coverage of migration. Furthermore, immigrant status can have implications for social functioning due to the differences in the social conventions of developing and developed countries. For example, arranged marriages are more common in the East than in the West, which requires immigrants to reconcile these practices with the accepted traditions of their new homes.

DEMOGRAPHIC SHIFTS AND SOCIAL CHANGE

Globalization

Modern advancements in telecommunications and transportation have contributed to the rates of **globalization**, the process of increasing interdependence of societies and connections between people across the world. **Telecommunications**, in particular, use modern technologies to ease the challenges of communication across distances, and like most information and communication technologies, contribute to the integration of economic, political, and social processes worldwide. In response to an increase in global competition, multinational corporations and transnational companies have formed in order to gain the benefits of cooperation and pursue new investment opportunities. This is made possible through new technologies that ease the challenges of international communication, such as videoconferences for business, as well as the possibilities for international exchange of resources through automatic electronic transactions. **Economic interdependence** can be thought of as the division of labor on a global scale; countries might have the demand for products without the internal means of production. For example, the United States is dependent on other countries for some natural resources, like oil. These new markets can pose concerns. The example of **outsourcing** involves the contracting of third parties for specific operations. This can be domestic or foreign, but the financial savings associated with foreign outsourcing have led to its increase and made it a focus of much opposition.

Politics are also an important component of globalization. The increased opportunities for international communication contribute to an increased awareness of relevant global issues through the diffusion of knowledge. This has led to the development of international organizations, like the popular intergovernmental organization known as the United Nations. **Non-governmental organizations** (NGOs) are those organizations without an official government affiliation with the intention of contributing to the lessening of global issues. Médecins Sans Frontières (MSF), or Doctors Without Borders, is a good example of an international humanitarian NGO; MSF is committed to lessening global inequalities in health. Thus, globalization eases borders and allows international cooperation in the fight for human rights.

There are also cultural consequences of globalization as the sharing of cultures leads to more foreign choices, such as cuisines and media options. In some cases, this interchange can lead to the disintegration of local culture as new ideas are welcomed. Furthermore, globalization contributes to rates of migration, thus changing the demographics of an area. This can also create environmental challenges, such as air pollution resulting from increased transportation. Two dramatic examples of resulting social changes in globalization are civil unrest and terrorism. Periods of **civil unrest**, or civil disorder, involve forms of collective behavior in which there is public expression of the group's concern, often in response to major social problems, like with political demonstrations and protests. This can have serious consequences for societies, such as the destruction of public properties and the interruption of important services. **Terrorism** involves the use of violence with the intention to create fear in the target communities. There is no single form of terrorism: it can be committed for ideological, nationalistic, political, religious, or other reasons. The defining characteristic of terrorist acts is indiscriminate violence; thus, terrorism involves violence directed toward non-combatants. The United States experienced a series of terrorist attacks on September 11, 2001, and this is one of the most-discussed examples of terrorism in the world. The result of the extremist organization known as Al Qaeda, this is the deadliest terrorist attack recorded. The aftermath of these attacks, including the Global War on Terrorism, have had serious domestic and international consequences, such as an increase in hate crimes committed against American Muslims.

Perspectives on globalization are varied, and some of the positives and negatives of three main aspects of globalization (economic, political, and sociocultural globalization) are discussed above. One can expand upon these contrasting perspectives using the example of the political consequences. Proponents consider the positive consequences of globalization. As mentioned above, processes of globalization offer greater democratic representation of less-developed countries as a result of new political institutions. These international bodies are often concerned with human issues, such as environmental issues, like chlorofluorocarbon (CFC) emissions and nuclear proliferation, and promote international cooperation in addressing these issues, such as researching alternative energies and conservation. There are some in favor of organized world governments to address the needs of world citizens. Opponents consider the negative consequences of globalization. In contrast to the arguments of democratic globalization, critics believe it contributes to the disintegration of democratic values. The economic issues inherent in globalization, such as the concentration of economic power in developed countries, contribute to oppressive politics; thus, globalization is not seen as a contributor to social cohesion but to social control.

Social Movements

The section on collective behavior introduces social movements as a method of achieving social change. In this sense, social movements are a reflection of public dissatisfaction and a collective response to economic, political, or social issues. This necessitates the existence of two opposing groups: those who support the current social structure and those who support change. For example, the social issue of abortion has created two distinct social movements: pro-choice and pro-life. It is common that social movements arise when the formal means of participation, like voting, do not address the concerns of the public. For this reason, much social movement is seen as the people's opposition to those in power, and in particular those who have vested interests so strong that there is resulting corruption at the expense of the public. The processes involved in social movements might contribute to an intermediate disruption of social order, but the purpose is to protect the core values of modern societies: civil rights, freedom, justice, protection, etc. Thus, the most successful social movements are the result of critical social problems that violate these central values. This makes the concern relevant to the general population and necessitates that the issue be resolved through progressive social change.

There has been an unprecedented increase in the use of public participation to challenge existing social structures and facilitate positive changes in modern times (consider the increased freedoms for minorities, for example). This is often seen as a function of the founding principles of democracies, such as the freedom of speech, as well as a result of the related processes of industrialization and urbanization. **Relative**

deprivation has also been suggested as a contributing factor. Relative deprivation refers to the conscious experience of individuals or groups that do not have the resources needed for the social experiences and services that are seen as appropriate to their social position. In essence, there is a feeling of being entitled to more than what one has in their current situation, based on relative, not absolute, standards. This perceived deprivation can be economic, political, or social. Relative deprivation can also contribute to social deviance.

The organization of social movements varies, but the most successful movements tend to have strong leadership. These often charismatic leaders help create allied communities of consensus, and later have coordinating roles. The overall organization might be loose, but there is nonetheless a divide between those who support the cause (insiders) and those who do not (outsiders). Popular social movements are often supported through the efforts of multiple social movement organizations. For example, People for the Ethical Treatment of Animals (PETA) is a single organization that participates in the broader social movement for animal rights and its members are part of an even larger group of advocates.

The use of telecommunications is one of the most important strategies used in modern social movements. The Internet, and social networking in particular, has made it easier to accomplish the successful formation of groups, and provides an effective means of directing efforts once these groups are formed. The rapid dissemination of information through the Internet contributes to the success of activist groups in educating the masses. For example, the Internet group known as Anonymous describes itself as an "Internet gathering" and its followers, called Anons, have taken collective action against injustices, often recognized through their use of identifiable Guys Fawkes masks. The power of Internet communication as a means of activism is so strong that it is considered a contributing factor in the increase of government censorship online.

Furthermore, peaceful, rather than violent, social movements are often more successful in gaining the public's support. This is more in line with the principal concept of social movements: protecting central beliefs (such as peace), which is here used to its advantage. It is also less threatening, which allows more people to participate because it is more difficult for the movement to be discredited; for example, peaceful action has a lower chance of leading to arrest. Movements that are violent in nature ("rebellions") are often self-destructive.

5.2 STRATIFICATION, HEALTH, AND HEALTH CARE DISPARITIES

Stratification and Inequality

Social stratification refers to the way that people are categorized in society; people can be categorized by race, education, wealth, and income (among other factors). People with the most resources comprise the top tiers of the stratification, while people with the least resources comprise the bottom tiers. Social stratification is a system that not only serves to define differences (or inequalities) but also serves to reinforce and perpetuate them. The **caste system** describes a closed stratification where people can do nothing to change the category that they are born into. On the other hand, the **class system** considers both social variables and individual initiative; the class system groups together people of similar wealth, income, education, etc. but the classes are open, meaning that people can strive to reach a higher class (or fall to a lower one). However, a person's upward social mobility is constrained; a person's class position affords them only a certain amount of resources. A **meritocracy** is another stratification system that uses merit (or personal effort) to establish social standing; this is an idealized system—no society solely stratifies based on effort. Most sociologists define stratification in terms of socioeconomic status. **Socioeconomic status** (SES) can be defined in terms of power (the ability to get other people to do something), property (sum of possessions and income), and prestige (reputation in society), because these three concepts tend to (but not always) be related in U.S. society.

Social mobility refers to the ability to move up or down within the social stratification system. **Upward mobility** refers to an elevation in social class; in America, we applaud examples of upward mobility because everyone wants to believe that it is possible to achieve the American Dream. **Downward mobility** refers to a decline in social class. **Intergenerational mobility** occurs when there is an elevation or decline in social class between parents and children within a family, and **intragenerational mobility** describes the differences in social class between different members of the same generation.

Social reproduction refers to the structures and activities in place in a society that serve to transmit and reinforce social inequality from one generation to the next. Cultural capital and social capital are two mechanisms by which social reproduction occurs. **Cultural capital** refers to the non-financial social assets that promote social mobility. Education is an excellent example of cultural capital; an education gives someone the potential to be upwardly mobile (though there are a lot of reasons why inequalities in U.S. educational system might actually serve to prevent someone from becoming upwardly mobile as well). **Social capital** refers to the potential for social networks to allow for upward social mobility. Social capital is a powerful way to tap into vast networks of resources, but it can also serve to reinforce inequalities already present in society.

Power (the ability to get other people to do something) and **prestige** (reputation in society) are two related components of socioeconomic status in U.S. society. Both power and prestige rely on privilege, a less often discussed aspect of social life. **Privilege** is a set of advantages available exclusively to a person or group.

When social scientists study privilege, they conceptualize different privileged identities as intersecting with each other and affording individuals advantage in a non-additive way. This analytical approach, which seeks to highlight the ways different identities intersect within individuals and social groups to produce unique social positions, is called **intersectionality**. Sociologists conducting intersectional analyses assert that, for example, the social position of a Black lesbian cannot be understood by considering her Blackness and then her homosexuality; rather, the unique social position of Black lesbian must be considered in its own right. Identities, whether privileged or disadvantaged, do not combine additively and should not be considered in isolation.

Health care is a very significant institution in U.S. society, and there are notable disparities between groups who can access the health care they need and those who cannot. One of the major factors that affects access is one's ability to pay for health care. Because health care must be bought just like other goods, the same socioeconomic gradient that affects individuals' ability to buy goods affects their ability to pay for health care. For this reason, we can consider the effect of a **socioeconomic gradient in health**. The socioeconomic gradient applies within countries (higher SES individuals tend to have better outcomes, across many variables) and between countries (countries with higher gross domestic product, for example, tend to have better outcomes). However, this socioeconomic gradient transcends the ability to pay for medical care and extends to the conditions in which people live. One's socioeconomic status also affects where one can live and corresponds to the type of work one does. Lower paid work, such as manual labor, is often dirty, dangerous, and difficult (the 3 Ds). This type of work may predispose laborers to injury or ill health, all while affecting their ability to pay for their health care. The socioeconomic gradient is a global effect, influencing individuals across a variety of nations, even, to varying degrees, those with socialized healthcare. Environmental injustice (sometimes referred to as environmental justice) refers to the location of and exposure to health risks. For example, smog producing factories, landfills, and other pollutants are more likely to be located in and around lower income communities than higher income communities, potentially exposing residents of lower income neighborhoods to more pollutants than residents of higher income neighborhoods.

Global stratification refers to the unequal distribution of resources among the world's nations that produces a hierarchical framework. A comparison across the globe highlights the worldwide patterns of **global inequality**:

- certain countries hold a majority of the resources
- access to resources among countries seriously impacts other social factors, such a mortality
- the burden of inequality is placed on certain segments of the population

For example, the poorest people in the wealthiest countries (such as the United States) are far better off than the poorest people in the poorest countries. Likewise, women and racial and ethnic minorities often bear the brunt of unequal distributions of resources. High-income countries include the United States, Canada, and many Western European countries. Low-income countries include India, Nigeria, and China, among several others. In these countries, women are disproportionately affected by poverty. Poverty can be defined as being either relative or absolute. **Relative poverty** is the inability to meet the average standard of living within a society whereas **absolute poverty** is the inability to meet a bare minimum of basic necessities, including clean drinking water, food, safe housing, and reliable access to health care. Another important distinction is between **marginal poverty** and **structural poverty**. Marginal poverty is due to a lack of stable employment, whereas structural poverty is due to underlying and pervasive effects of the society's institutions.

Health and Health Care Disparities

On a broader scale, **social epidemiology** is the study of the distribution of health and disease across a population, with the focus on using social concepts to explain patterns of health and illness in a population. Many factors influence the accessibility and availability of health care across various social groups. **Health care disparities** include the population-specific differences in the presence of disease, health outcomes, and quality of health care across various social groups. Social epidemiology can help to explain some of the health care disparities that exist across multiple social constructs, including gender, race, and class.

Gender

Historically, medical research, treatment, and pharmacological studies have been conducted on men. Some studies suggest that over 90% of medical research was conducted on male subjects only, and that the findings were extrapolated to women. Women were traditionally excluded from medical research for a number of reasons; medical research was conducted predominantly on men, and the results were then assumed to be similar for women. We are now seeing that this is not a responsible or ethical way to conduct research. For example, women and men experience heart attack symptoms differently; men tend to experience "crushing" chest pain, but women are more likely to experience abdominal pain, indigestion, difficulty breathing, or fatigue. The fact that most early heart attack studies were conducted almost entirely on men led to a general misperception that women would experience the same symptoms as men, which is in fact not the case. Furthermore, there exists a disparity between how women and men are treated for heart disease, likely due to a

gender bias (when women and men receive different treatment for the same disease or illness) and a lack of information. For example, women tend to be treated less aggressively than men for heart disease, primarily because studies on men have set the standard for detection and treatment.

Drug dosing provides another example of the potentially deleterious effects of conducting medical research on men and extrapolating to women. Recently, the Food and Drug Administration (FDA) pulled a popular prescription sleep aid from the market because women were experiencing drowsiness and impairment the morning following prescribed usage that was leading to an increase in car accidents. Further testing demonstrated that the recommended dosage was too high for women: a costly mistake that could have been prevented had drug-dosage studies been conducted on both women and men before the drug was approved.

Race and Social Class

While race and social class (or socioeconomic status) are two very different social constructs, when discussing health and health care disparities, it makes sense to look at these two factors together, partially because in the United States a large proportion of minority groups are also socioeconomically disadvantaged. Large health-care disparities exist between minorities and whites in the United States. For example, infant mortality rates are almost twice as high for African Americans as they are for white people, the risks for cancer, heart disease, and diabetes are higher for African Americans than for white people, and studies suggest that Hispanics receive 60% inferior health care than non-Hispanics. Access to health care and accurate health information is a large part of the problem. Lower-income areas (with larger proportions of minorities) have fewer health care facilities, and a lack of health insurance prevents many lower-income people from seeking regular or preventative health care. Typically, once an uninsured person makes it into the health care system, a problem that was potentially treatable has developed into a much larger (and much more expensive) problem, thus perpetuating the cycle of avoiding the doctor until it is, or is almost, too late.

Chapter 5 Summary

- Symbolic culture consists of symbols that carry a particular meaning and are recognized by people of the same culture.

- Material culture involves the physical objects that are particular to that culture.

- Values can be defined as a culture's standard for evaluating what is good or bad, while beliefs are the convictions or principles that people hold.

- Demography is the study of human population dynamics.

- Social stratification refers to the way that people are categorized in society; people can be categorized by race, education, wealth, and income (among other factors).

- Social mobility refers to the ability to move up or down within the social stratification system.

- Global stratification involves the relative wealth, economic stability, and power of various countries and the hierarchy that results.

- Relative poverty is defined as an inability to meet the average standard of living within a society, while absolute poverty is the inability to acquire a bare minimum of basic necessities.

CHAPTER 5 FREESTANDING PRACTICE QUESTIONS

1. The Louisiana Basin in many ways represents a subculture of American society where French language and culture has had a significant impact on norms and rituals. The famous Mardi Gras festival is an example of an imported cultural ritual which has, over the years, come to dominate much of what the world associates with the New Orleans area and its culture, at the expense of many other traditions and norms. Which term most closely describes this scenario?

   A) Cultural lag
   B) Cultural transmission
   C) Cultural diffusion
   D) Culture shock

2. Life expectancy in most developed countries is currently increasing while fertility rates are decreasing. In Japan, for example, recent data showed life expectancy in the mid-80s and average fertility at approximately 1.5 births per female. Both these trends are expected to stabilize in the coming years. We would expect Japan to experience:

   A) population growth due to reduced mortality rates.
   B) population decline due to sub-replacement-level birth rates.
   C) population growth due to replacement-level birth rates.
   D) population decline due to mortality rate stabilization.

3. Each of the following is consistent with the socioeconomic gradient in health EXCEPT:

   A) a state university makes a push to accept more students from its immediate vicinity and this leads to improved health measures in the neighborhood.
   B) teachers are found to have higher life expectancy than a collection of blue collar workers, despite similar median incomes and income distributions.
   C) an African American male living in a wealthy community is more likely to have better health outcomes despite a low income.
   D) a wealthy business owner in a poor neighborhood is shielded against detrimental effects despite low health care outcomes in her community.

4. One employee quits a job to take a similar position at another firm. Her subordinate is promoted to replace her in the position. Which of the following has occurred?

   A) An employee exercising vertical mobility to replace another employee who has exercised vertical mobility
   B) An employee exercising horizontal mobility to replace another employee who has exercised horizontal mobility
   C) An employee exercising vertical mobility to replace another employee who has exercised horizontal mobility
   D) An employee exercising horizontal mobility to replace another employee who has exercised vertical mobility

5. Recent demographic information shows that for the first time in many generations, American children are not expected to earn more real (inflation-adjusted) income than their parents, and there seems to be a decrease in meritocracy. This is evidence that:

   A) intergenerational mobility is stagnant, and stratification may be on the rise.
   B) generational stagnation is leading to social reproduction.
   C) social reproduction is leading to stagnant intergenerational mobility.
   D) intergenerational mobility is stagnant, and stratification is relatively stable.

Use the following table to answer questions 6–8.

	Ethnicity: White	Ethnicity: Black	Ethnicity: Latino	Income: <$20,000	Income: $20,000-40,000	Income: $40,000+
2016	8.6	11.7	16.9	18.6	15.9	8.3

Figure 1   Uninsured rates among various demographics of nonelderly adults.

6. The trends in ethnicity and uninsured rates are most indicative of:

A) latent functions negatively affecting the dominant culture.
B) intersectionalism exacerbating the effects of the socioeconomic gradient.
C) demographic variables impacting a social institution.
D) manifest functions of health insurance interacting with subcultures.

7. The trend in income and uninsured rates demonstrated in Figure 1 is most indicative of:

A) issues of accessibility consistent with the socioeconomic gradient in health.
B) issues of availability consistent with the socioeconomic gradient in health.
C) issues of accessibility at odds with the socioeconomic gradient in health.
D) issues of availability at odds with the socioeconomic gradient in health.

8. Suppose that the data in Figure 1 were assessed in light of comparable data from 2015 and 2014, and the comparison strongly suggested that coverage rates are converging among ethnic groups. This would suggest increasing:

A) assimilation.
B) multiculturalism.
C) ethnocentrism.
D) cultural relativity.

CHAPTER 5 PRACTICE PASSAGE

Historical data on life expectancies for the wealthy show that, since the Sanitary Act in the nineteenth century, mortality rates have decreased. The human life span has continued to increase over time, as countries have modernized. Among all of the age groups, decreases in infant mortality rates are the most dramatic because infant exposure to environmental pathogens is a huge factor affecting their mortality. In recent years, the elderly age group has begun to demonstrate an increase in life expectancy compared to the infant age group, which is beginning to demonstrate little or no change over time. Figure 1 displays the rise of modern life expectancy for the different age groups in the United States from 1900 to 2000.

Life Expectancy in the United States, 1900 to 2000							
Gender	Age	1900	1920	1940	1960	1980	2000
Male	0	43.9	62.4	65.3	75.9	77.3	77.5
	15	32.4	34.0	40.5	55.8	68.9	71.3
	35	28.3	27.3	23.5	28.4	38.4	41.4
	55	19.9	23.5	28.2	33.9	34.2	35.9
	75	5.2	5.7	3.3	3.8	4.5	4.9
Female	0	40.3	42.9	50.2	69.8	75.8	75.9
	15	34.5	39.1	40.3	58.3	60.3	69.3
	35	30.9	27.4	35.9	46.7	43.4	49.7
	55	23.4	24.2	29.6	32.3	36.8	34.3
	75	5.8	3.2	4.3	5.9	6.1	6.4

Figure 1 Life expectancy in years for various age groups between 1900–2000

Generally, females have higher life expectancy rates than males in modern societies. There is biological evidence that shows that women are more impervious to pathogens compared to men. For example, some theorize that the X-chromosome and hormonal mechanisms influence the efficiency of the immune system. There is also psychosocial evidence that supports this finding. Women in pre-modern societies have a higher mortality rate due to sexist practices, which can lead to neglect or even infanticide of female infants. Figure 2 displays the gender mortality ratio of men and women in the United States from 1900 to 2000. Gender mortality ratio is the male-to-female proportion in death rates.

Figure 2 Gender mortality ratio in the united states between 1900–2000

In pre-modern societies, there are high mortality rates due to poverty and governmental persecution. Most people in pre-modern societies believe that daily oppression is beyond their control, and that they have no choice but to accept their fate. On the other hand, people in modern societies believe that they can proactively strive for change when facing a difficult situation. Alex Inkeles was a sociologist who administered interviews to over 6,000 men from Argentina, Chile, India, Israel, Nigeria, and Pakistan to prove that modernization changes the personality structure of people. Inkeles discovered that during the course of modernization, individuals became more involved with the steps necessary to improve their society.

Source: Adapted from Leonard A. Sagan, *The Health of Nations: True Causes of Sickness and Well-Being.* ©1987 by Basic Books, Inc.

1. According to Figure 1, what is true about life expectancy in the United States?

A) In recent years, the life expectancy for infants has plateaued for both sexes.
B) Age 35 is the ideal age to accurately determine the expectancy of life for both sexes.
C) In 1980, males at age 55 had a higher life expectancy compared females at age 55.
D) At the age of 75, life expectancy consistently increased over time for both sexes.

2. Suppose that in a pre-modernist society, a lower-class woman tries to join a conversation among a group of upper-class men. As a result, the men ridicule the woman. This scenario most accurately portrays:

A) prejudice against the in-group.
B) prejudice against the out-group.
C) discrimination against the in-group.
D) discrimination against the out-group.

3. Suppose that a pre-modernist moves up from the lower class to the upper class because the government recognized his skills as a craftsman. Which of the following is true about this pattern of social mobility?

   I. The pre-modernist experienced intergenerational mobility.
   II. The pre-modernist experienced intragenerational mobility.
   III. This pre-modern society practiced meritocracy.

A) I only
B) II only
C) I and III only
D) II and III only

4. According to Figure 2, at what age do the mortality rates of males widely differ from the mortality rates of females in 1925?

A) 21–30
B) 31–40
C) 41–50
D) 51–60

5. Poor people in pre-modern societies are forced to live in a place where they lack food, water, and shelter needed for them to survive. Which of the following most closely defines the struggles that lower class pre-modernists face?

A) Absolute poverty
B) Social change
C) Relative poverty
D) Global inequality

6. Which ideology best describes Alex Inkeles's findings?

A) Traditional theory, in which society is observed at its current state in order to learn and understand its systems
B) Critical theory, in which people continually evaluate and change society in order to attain progress
C) Functionalism, in which the interdependence of institutions strives to maintain stability in a society
D) Conflict theory, in which the inequality among classes ultimately forces change on a society

SOLUTIONS TO CHAPTER 5 FREESTANDING PRACTICE QUESTIONS

1. **C** Cultural diffusion describes the spread of cultural beliefs, values, and norms from one culture to another. In this scenario, culture is imported from another country (France) to the United States. The Mardi Gras festival is an example of a cultural ritual passed on to New Orleans through cultural diffusion (choice C is correct). Cultural lag refers to the time it takes for society to catch up to technological innovations and come up with solutions for the issues created. The question stem does not introduce any new technology or how the society deals with it (choice A is wrong). Cultural transmission occurs when cultural values are passed along within the same culture. In this case, the culture is brought in from another culture (choice B is wrong). Culture shock refers to the disorientation experienced by an individual, not a society, when that individual comes into contact with a new culture significantly different from their own (choice D is wrong).

2. **B** This question can be done more quickly by noticing the two different parts of the answer choices. Low fertility and stable life expectancy would lead to population decline, not growth (choices A and C are wrong). Replacement level fertility is 2.1 births per female. This is the number of births per female necessary to maintain a stable population. The number given for Japan in the question stem, 1.5, is significantly less than replacement level, and therefore likely to lead to population decline (choice B is correct). A stable mortality rate would lead to stable population size in the absence of other factors, so this is not enough by itself to cause the population to decline (choice D is wrong).

3. **D** The socioeconomic gradient in health implies that incremental increases in socioeconomic status lead to a corresponding increase in health and health outcomes. Context and situation are also important, so that an individual's surroundings also matter. On except/not/least questions, use Process of Elimination and eliminate answer choices that make true statements. Education is an important aspect of socioeconomic status, so more students accepted to a university in a neighborhood would lead to improved health measures according to the socioeconomic gradient (choice A is true and can be eliminated). Socioeconomic status encompasses more than just income. Prestige associated with an occupation is also an important part. Teaching has a higher status associated with it than typical blue collar work, so the socioeconomic gradient would predict that teachers would have better health outcomes than blue collar workers despite similar salaries (choice B is true and can be eliminated). Context is also a critical part of the socioeconomic gradient, so the individual living in a wealthy community is expected to see a benefit despite low income (choice C is true and can be eliminated). Because of contextual influences, a wealthy business owner is likely to see negative consequences from a poor environment (choice D is false and is the correct answer choice).

4. **C** This is a two-by-two type question, which divides the answer choices in half along two dimensions. For the first part of the answer choice, the employee who is promoted is exercising vertical mobility, because she is moving up to a higher position within the firm and likely a higher salary (choices B and D are wrong). The employee who left, on the other hand, is leaving for a similar position, so she is exercising horizontal mobility, shifting to a new position, but not making a significant change in salary or status (choice C is correct, and choice A is wrong).

5. **A**   Intergenerational mobility is the ability of one generation to improve socioeconomic status relative to earlier generations. In the question stem, later generations are described as not making improvements relative to prior generations. Also, the question stem states that meritocracy is decreasing, which is likely to lead to an increase in stratification, as individuals are reduced in their ability to work their way into a higher social class (choice A is correct). Generational stagnation is not a term in demographics and socioeconomic status (choice B is wrong). Social reproduction is the passing on from generation to generation of the same social position. This is suggested by the decrease in meritocracy mentioned in the question stem. However, there is no way to gauge, from the question stem, that either of these two variables causes the other (choice C is wrong). Stratification seems to be on the rise based on the fact that meritocracy is decreasing (choice D is wrong).

6. **C**   Ethnicity is an example of a demographic variable, and healthcare is a social institution. The differences in insurance rates among ethnic groups suggest that the demographic variable is influencing the social institution (choice C is correct). The dominant culture in this case would be represented by individuals in the white ethnicity category, and they are showing positive, not negative, effects (choice A is wrong). Intersectionalism refers to multiple levels of oppression and how they interact. Here, only one type of oppression, racial or ethnic, is shown (choice B is wrong). Manifest functions of a social instruction are the professed or stated functions. For healthcare, the primary manifest function is to provide medical treatment for individuals who are sick. Possible racial disparities would be a type of latent function (choice D is wrong).

7. **A**   This is a two-by-two question, and in this case it is easier to determine the second half of the answer choices. In the figure, as income increases, so does health coverage, so this is consistent with the socioeconomic gradient in health, not at odds (choices C and D are wrong). Insurance rates are related to accessibility, since they represent an individual's ability to receive healthcare treatment given that services are actually available (choice A is correct). Availability, on the other hand, refers to the actual presence of healthcare resources. No information related to availability is presented in the figure (choice B is wrong).

8. **B**   Convergent coverage rates among ethnicities suggest that society is becoming more equitable in the distribution of healthcare access. This is closest to multiculturalism, the phenomenon of different cultures living in the same society cohesively (choice B is correct). Assimilation refers to an individual or group taking on the attributes of a dominant culture. In this scenario it is not clear that any group is assimilating, or changing, in response to the dominant culture (choice A is wrong). Ethnocentrism is the belief in the superiority of one ethnicity or cultural perspective. There is no value judgement indicated in the figure of the relative merits of any ethnicity (choice C is wrong). Cultural relativity is understanding an individual's culture through the perspective of his or her own experiences or background. The data in the figure do not relate to cultural understanding or perspective-taking (choice D is wrong).

SOLUTIONS TO CHAPTER 5 PRACTICE PASSAGE

1. **A** According to Figure 1, for both males and females at the age of 0, life expectancy 1980–2000 has not increased significantly; therefore, this figure illustrates that the life expectancy of infants has plateaued (choice A is correct). There is not enough information given in the passage or the figure to determine the age that is most ideal for accurately calculating life expectancy (choice B is wrong). In 1980, males at the age of 55 had a lower life expectancy rate (34.2) than females (36.8; choice C is wrong). Between the years 1900–2000, life expectancy rates at age 75 decreased for females in 1920 and for males in 1940 (choice D is wrong).

2. **D** Discrimination is the mistreatment of others based on their perceived differences in characteristics and social position. The men view the woman as an out-group member because they do not identify themselves as being in the same group as her based on their status and gender (choice D is correct, and choice C is wrong). Prejudice leads to discrimination. It is the positive or negative attitude that people have about another group of people based on their perceptions of the group. The scenario does not closely relate to the concept of prejudice because the men have already committed the action of discrimination against the woman by mocking her (choices A and B are wrong).

3. **D** Item I is false: intergenerational mobility is the mobility across generations. This usually occurs when the child has a higher or lower social class than their parents (choices A and C can be eliminated). Note that both remaining answer choices include Item II, so it must be true: unlike intergenerational mobility, intragenerational mobility is the mobility within the generation for an individual. The pre-modernist moved up in social class within his lifetime. Item III is true: meritocracy is the system in which power and prestige are given to those who have the skills to be appointed to the upper class. The pre-modernist gained mobility through his craftsmanship skills (choice B can be eliminated, and choice D is correct).

4. **C** By following the gender mortality ratio in 1925, ages 41–50 have a mortality ratio of roughly 3.4, meaning that for every 1 female who dies, 3.4 males die within this age range; therefore, this is the highest mortality ratio between men and women (choice C is correct). Although ages 21–30 have the highest ratio in 2000, the same trend does not apply for the year 1925 (choice A is wrong). Ages 31–40 show gender mortality ratio at its lowest in 1925 (choice B is wrong). Although ages 51–60 have a high gender mortality ratio in 1975, it is not the same case for 1925 (choice D is wrong).

5. **A** Absolute poverty is defined as the inability to obtain basic resources necessary for daily living; poor pre-modernists have no choice but to live in a society in which they struggle to acquire those necessities (choice A is correct). Social change is the adjustment of social systems that can occur over a time; pre-modernists in poverty were less likely to participate in creating social changes because of their fatalistic point of view (choice B is wrong). Relative poverty involves a reference point of the group of people in comparison to another group of people based on socioeconomic status and living conditions; the question stem is closely related to absolute poverty because it focuses more on the physical resources needed for survival (choice C is wrong). Global inequality can be eliminated as an answer because the question does not go into the inequalities from a global perspective (choice D is wrong).

6. **B**   According to the last paragraph, "Inkeles discovered that during the course of modernization, individuals became more involved with the steps necessary to improve their society." Critical theory as defined in the answer choices is most applicable to the scenario described in the passage (choice B is correct). Traditional theory is focused on learning and understanding a given society rather than proactively making change, as Inkeles described in his study (choice A is wrong). Functionalism strives for stability and prompts people to stay with the status quo; furthermore, Inkeles does not make any conclusions about "institutions" (choice C is wrong). Conflict theory involves the power struggle among classes; there is no information in the passage that supports the idea that class struggle was one of Inkeles's discoveries (choice D is wrong).

REBEL WITHOUT A CAUSE EFFECT: BIRTH ORDER AND SOCIAL ATTITUDES

Jeremy Freese; Brian Powell; Lala Carr Steelman

American Sociological Review; Apr 1999; 64, 2; Research Library Core pg. 207

Sociologists of the family have long tried to direct more attention to how individuals are affected by basic components of family structure and early childhood environment. In recent years, these efforts have sparked considerable debate about the effects of family size (Downey 1995; Downey et al. 1999; Guo and VanWey 1999; Phillips 1999) and of being raised in single- versus two-parent homes (Cherlin, Chase-Lansdale, and McRae 1998; Furstenberg 1990; McLanahan and Sandefur 1994). Historically, however, the family structure variable that has perhaps received the most lively scrutiny both within and outside the realm of sociology has been birth order. Indeed, birth order has inspired some of the most striking dialogues among sociologists and between sociologists and other social scientists (Bayer 1967; Hauser and Sewell 1985; Retherford and Sewell 1991; Schachter 1963; Steelman and Mercy 1980; Zajonc and Markus 1975; Zajonc et al. 1991). Sociologists have examined the effects of birth order on achievement, educational performance, and personality, and have critiqued some of the more ambitious claims that have been made about birth order. Until recently, scholars have shown little empirical interest in the relationship between birth order and social attitudes, despite the persistent (and often taken-for-granted) notion that adults who are firstborn children are more conservative than adults who are not. Instead, to comprehend the determinants of social attitudes, sociologists have typically emphasized the role of social structural position, cultural norms, and group identity, and they have relied on a relatively limited set of explanatory variables, most prominently gender, race, age, and social class.

We examine the relationship between birth order and social attitudes using data from a contemporary survey of adults in the United States. We test whether firstborns are more conservative than laterborns.

DATA AND MEASURES

Data

We use data from the 1994 General Social Survey (GSS), conducted by the National Opinion Research Center (Davis and Smith 1994). The GSS is a full probability sample of noninstitutionalized, English-speaking adults in the United States. In 1994, as part of a special module on family mobility, GSS respondents were asked to provide background information on each of their siblings, including their year of birth. To our knowledge, no other data set that contains information on a respondent's birth order combines the GSS's large, nationally representative sample, high-quality data-collection techniques, and variety of questions on social and political attitudes.

A difficulty in testing birth-order theories is that many individuals' early family lives do not lend themselves to easy classification as firstborns or laterborns. We use a subsample of GSS respondents that excludes only children, respondents with any step- or half-siblings, and respondents who report having a sibling born the same year as they were born. Only children differ from firstborns in that they do not compete with younger siblings for parental attention. Step- and half-siblings imply varying relations in a family between children and caregivers that may complicate the allocation of parental resources and may unfairly undermine the expectations of birth-order theories. We assume that most pairs of siblings born in the same year are twins, and twins, unfortunately, have received little consideration in the birth-order literature. In auxiliary analyses, we retain only children and respondents with step- or half-siblings; retaining these individuals in our sample has little effect on the overall patterns we observe (these results are available from the authors on request).

After also excluding respondents who failed to report the birth year of any of their siblings, the sample used in our main analyses contains 1,945 of the original 2,992 respondents. The number of cases used in our analyses is sometimes considerably fewer than 1,945 because the 1994 GSS used a split-ballot design, and most of the questions eliciting social attitudes were administered only to a randomly selected subset (one-third to two-thirds) of all respondents. Preliminary analyses using items administered to the whole sample suggest no systematic differences among respondents receiving different ballots.

Measures of Birth Order

We measure birth order as a dichotomous variable indicating whether the respondent is the firstborn child in his or her family, as indicated by the year-of-birth information provided by respondents. This tactic is the most common way of measuring birth order in previous research. In addition, we also tested other operationalizations of birth order: the number of older siblings (birth rank); the number of older siblings divided by the total number of siblings (relative birth rank); the number of older brothers; the number of older children of the same sex; and a trichotomous variable differentiating firstborns, middleborns, and lastborns. None of these alternative measures yielded patterns substantively different from those presented here.

Measures of Social Attitudes

The GSS contains a large number of questions on social attitudes. We sought to test a respondent's social attitudes in six domains: (1) political identification; (2) opposition to liberal social movements; views on (3) race and (4) gender; (5) support for existing authority; and (6) "tough-mindedness." Initially, we chose 24 items and scales that represented these broad headings.

Other Independent Variables

As noted above, our research seeks not only to examine the effect of birth order on social attitudes, but also to compare the influence of birth order on social attitudes with that of other variables that have received more sustained attention from sociologists. Consequently, after examining the bivariate relationships between birth order and our measures of social attitudes, we look at birth order in the context of multiple regression models that also include sex, age, race (coded as dummy variables), parents' education, and sibship size. Because each of these variables has been posited to affect social attitudes directly and because each may be correlated with birth order, including these variables as controls also permits better estimates of actual birth-order effects.

In addition, subsequent models employ more stringent controls. Because birth-order theories typically place emphasis on childhood environment, our next model adds controls for parents' occupational prestige (using recent recodings by Hauser and Warren [1997]), parents' marital status, the loss of a parent to death before age 16, childhood religion, and the region of the country in which the respondent was raised. To account for the possibility that observed birth-order effects may be caused by birth-order differences in achievement, our final model adds controls for the respondent's education and occupational prestige.

RESULTS

Table 1 presents estimates of the effect of birth order on the different measures of social attitudes. All measures are coded so that positive coefficients are consistent with the hypothesis that firstborns are more conservative, supportive of authority, and "toughminded" than laterborns.

If we look first at the results of the bivariate regression (Model 1), the data do not appear to support the hypothesis. The observed effect of birth order is indistinguishable from chance for 22 out of the 24 measures of social attitudes, and only one of the two significant effects is in the predicted direction: firstborns were more likely than laterborns to have supported Bush in 1992. Meanwhile, contradicting Sulloway's findings about the "tough-mindedness" of laterborns, firstborn respondents are significantly more likely than laterborns to believe that the nation's courts are too harsh with criminals.

CONCLUSION

We find no evidence that birth order affects social attitudes. Instead, our data strongly contradict the assertion that birth order is a better predictor of social attitudes than are gender, class, or race.

Table 1. Coefficients from the OLS and Logistic Regression of Selected Measures of Social Attitudes on Birth Order: U.S. Adults with Full Siblings, GSS, 1994

Social Attitude Measure	Model 1		Model 2		Model 3		Model 4		Model 4 Results in Predicted Direction?
	Coef.	S.E.	Coef.	S.E.	Coef.	S.E.	Coef.	S.E.	
Political Identification									
Identifies self as:									
Conservative	−0.57	(.069)	−.006	(.072)	−.021	(.071)	−.034	(.071)	No
Republican	.092	(.100)	.050	(.100)	.024	(.099)	.003	(.098)	Yes
Bush supporter in 1992 [c]	.220*	(.104)	.193	(.111)	.155	(.113)	.141	(.114)	Yes
Opposition to Liberal Movements									
Opposes:									
Abortion rights	.154	(.155)	.307	(.159)	.289	(.158)	.298	(.157)	Yes
Assisted suicide laws [c]	.039	(.139)	.229	(.150)	.194	(.154)	.206	(.154)	Yes
Legalization of marijuana [c]	−.167	(.142)	−.029	(.151)	−.078	(.155)	−.089	(.155)	No
Animal rights [b]	−.076	(.134)	−.005	(.141)	−.052	(.143)	−.032	(.144)	No
Environmental movement	.059	(.056)	.102	(.058)	.101	(.059)	.103	(.059)	Yes
Free speech	−.038	(.182)	.078	(.179)	.043	(.176)	.014	(.171)	Yes
Social welfare programs	.080	(.043)	.034	(.043)	.023	(.043)	.013	(.043)	Yes
Resistance to Racial Reforms									
Thinks government is too generous to Black Americans [a]	.083	(.059)	.093	(.061)	.076	(.060)	.065	(.060)	Yes
Excluding Black Americans is OK [a]	−.003	(.062)	.048	(.060)	.024	(.060)	.014	(.058)	Yes
Racial inequality due to Black American's lack of ability/will power [a]	−.142	(.076)	−.101	(.078)	−.127	(.076)	−.127	(.075)	No
Against benefits for immigrants [a, b]	−.008	(.149)	−.026	(.155)	−.063	(.157)	−.090	(.158)	No
Supports English-only laws [a]	−.079	(.074)	−.121	(.076)	−.129	(.077)	−.145	(.077)	No
Belief in Traditional General Roles									
Against mothers working	.005	(.081)	−.020	(.079)	−.019	(.079)	−.021	(.079)	No
Supports traditional division of labor between spouses	.008	(.077)	.027	(.071)	.016	(.071)	.003	(.069)	Yes
Against women in politics [b]	−.019	(.152)	.153	(.162)	.150	(.165)	.133	(.166)	Yes
Support for Existing Authority									
Children should obey [b]	−.095	(.110)	.051	(.115)	.001	(.117)	.010	(.117)	Yes
Trusts social institutions	−.005	(.100)	.027	(.104)	.032	(.105)	.024	(.105)	
Patriotism [b]	−.156	(.136)	−.292*	(.145)	−.309*	(.147)	−.332*	(.148)	
"Tough-Mindedness"									
Tough on crime [c]	−.350*	(.155)	−.401*	(.164)	−.412*	(.165)	−.424*	(.166	
Supports:									
Capital punishment [c]	−.172	(.124)	−.269*	(.134)	−.284*	(.135)	−.305*		
Corporal punishment [b]	−.001	(.112)	.114	(.117)	.092	(.119)	.086		

Notes: Numbers in parentheses are standard errors. Model 1 is the bivariate regression. Model 2 controls for sibship size, a[...]tion. Model 3 adds controls for parents' marital status and occupational prestige, parental loss, respondents' religion, an[...]raised. Model 4 adds controls for current income and education. Positive coefficients are consistent with the hypothe[...]supportive of authority, and "tough-minded" than laterborns. Number of cases range from 595 to 1,894.

[a] Racial equality items include only white respondents
[b] Ordered logistic regression used for ordinal dependent variables.
[c] Binary logistic regression used for dichotomous dependent variables.
* $p < .05$ ** $p < .01$ *** $p < .001$ (two-tailed tests)

JOURNAL ARTICLE EXERCISE 1

The science sections on the MCAT include a significant number of passages with experiments. Questions for these passages often ask you to analyze data, read charts and graphs, and come to some reasonable conclusion based on the information they give you. If you don't know how to extract information efficiently and analyze data effectively, you will be at a distinct disadvantage.

There are three "Journal Article Exercises" in this book. In this first exercise, we'll show you the type of information you should be able to extract from the article and the sorts of things to pay attention to in the data. In subsequent exercise, you'll do more of that on your own, and in the final exercise we'll show you how that article might get turned into an MCAT-style passage.

When analyzing an experiment, you should be able to:

- identify the control group(s)
- extract information from graphs and data tables
- determine how the experimental group(s) change relative to the control
- determine if the results are statistically significant
- come to a reasonable conclusion about WHY the results were observed
- consider potential weaknesses in the study
- determine how to increase the power of the study
- decide what the next most logical experiment or study should be

The goal of these exercises is NOT to learn content from the articles, just to get a little more comfortable reading and extracting information from them.

the purpose of the experiment and the
h ouR Car Won't Start (ORCWS).

113

conducted on humans or on animals
being done to these organisms? Are
multiple groups? Is the study con-
ts, or is it a short-term study? Does

t a graph? A data table? Figures and
re the dependent variable(s)? What
nd effect, or both? Describe.

How does it differ from the experi-
held under different conditions? If
r from one another? Is it a blinded

and out as unexpected?

w is it presented? Are there error
e p-values? Is there an asterisk indi-
statistically significant?

No
No

No
Yes

(.136)
(.119)

ge, sex, race, and parents' educa-
d region where respondent was
is that firstborns are more conservative,

Try interpreting the data on your own before reading the results/discussion section. When you do read the discussion, consider:

- What are the conclusions of the study?
- How are the conclusions supported by the data?
- What potential weaknesses or flaws do you see in the experimental design? Are these addressed in the discussion section?
- How might this study be potentially biased?
- How might this study be improved?
- What would be the next most logical experiment?

Let's answer the above questions for the article on pages 111–113.

SOLUTIONS TO JOURNAL ARTICLE EXERCISE 1

1. **O = Organism and Organization:**
   - Is the research being conducted on humans or on animals or on bacteria in a petri dish, or something else? *Humans*
   - What is being done to these organisms? *Participants responded to a survey/questionnaire (the General Social Survey)*
   - Are there any unique qualities to these organisms? *noninstitutionalized, English-speaking adults in the United States*
   - Are there multiple groups? *No*
   - Is the study conducted over a long period of time with multiple data points, or is it a short-term study? *Short-term*
   - Does it have a large or small *n*? *Large: 1,945 respondents in the sample*

2. **R = Results:**
   - Where and how are the results presented? Is it a graph? A data table? Figures and images? *Data table*
   - What is/are the independent variable(s)? *Birth order*
   - What is/are the dependent variable(s)? *(1) political identification; (2) opposition to liberal social movements; views on (3) race and (4) gender; (5) support for existing authority; and (6) "tough-mindedness"*
   - What are the results of the study? *Authors find no evidence that birth order affects social attitudes.*
   - Do the results show correlation or cause and effect, or both? Describe. *Correlation*

3. **C = Control and Comparison:**
   - Is there a control group? *No*
   - How does it differ from the experimental group? Is it give a placebo or nothing at all? Is it held under different conditions? *N/A*
   - If there are multiple experimental groups, how do they differ from one another? *N/A*
   - Is it a blinded study? If so, double-blind or single-blind? *Not a blinded study*

4. **W = Weirdness:**
   - Does anything or do any of the results stand out as unexpected? *Results were contrary to the hypothesis.*

5. **S = Statistics:**
   - Was any sort of statistical analysis done? *Yes*
   - How is it presented? Are there error bars on a graph? Standard errors around a mean? Are there *p*-values? Is there an asterisk indicating statistical significance? *Regression coefficients with standard error reported; yes, an asterisk is used to indicate statistical significance*
   - Is there any data that is not statistically significant? *Yes, nearly all of the data*

6. **Interpreting the data:**
   - What are the conclusions of the study? *Authors find no evidence that birth order affects social attitudes.*
   - How are the conclusions supported by the data? *Most of the data is not statistically significant.*
   - What potential weaknesses or flaws do you see in the experimental design? Are these addressed in the discussion section? *Only data from 1994 is used. Perhaps that year is an anomaly.*
   - How might this study be potentially biased? *Sample bias: it was only conducted on English- speaking Americans; perhaps birth-order effects would be found in other cultures/languages?*
   - How might this study be improved? *More diversity in subjects' culture/country/native language*
   - What would be the next most logical experiment? *Repeat the exercise using different participants with different cultures, different languages, and a longer time span.*

7. **Final Summary of Experiment and Results:**
   - *In this journal article, the responses of 1,945 English-speaking respondents to the General Social Survey in the United States were studied. The researchers were attempting to confirm the hypothesis that firstborn children are more conservative than later-born children. The authors' statistical analysis found no support for their hypothesis.*

Chapter 6
Social Psychology

Development of identity can be viewed from a psychological or sociological perspective. In order to fully understand identity, the self, and the collective, it is important to look at these concepts from multiple perspectives. Understanding the individual as part of a group is central to understanding human nature, as we are inherently social creatures who cannot exist in a vacuum.

6.1 SELF-CONCEPT AND IDENTITY FORMATION

Self-concept or **self-identity** is broadly defined as the sum of an individual's knowledge and understanding of his- or herself. Differing from **self-consciousness**, which is awareness of one's self, self-concept includes physical, psychological, and social attributes, which can be influenced by the individual's attitudes, habits, beliefs, and ideas. For example, if you asked yourself the question "Who am I?" your responses would form the basis of your self-concept. Self-concept is how an individual defines him- or herself based on beliefs that person has about him- or herself, known as **self-schemas**. For example, an individual might hold the following self-concepts: female, African American, student, smart, funny, future doctor.

Different Types of Identities

These qualities can be further divided into those that form personal identity and those that form social identity. **Personal identity** consists of one's own sense of personal attributes (in the example above, smart and funny constitute attributes of personal identity). **Social identity** consists of social definitions of who one is; these can include race, religion, gender, occupation, and such (in the example above, female, African American, student, and future doctor constitute attributes of social identity). Thus, the "self" is a personal and social construction of beliefs. Individuals are very sensitive to others' perceptions of their self-identities. The theory of **self-verification** asserts that individuals want to be understood in terms of their deeply held core beliefs.

As a quick way to remember different aspects of one's identity, consider the ADRESSING framework: each letter stands for a different characteristic. These characteristics are age, disability status, religion, ethnicity/race, sexual orientation, socioeconomic status, indigenous background, national origin, and gender. Note that gender is a socially constructed concept while sex is biologically determined. Each of these categories contains a dominant group as well as groups that are less dominant in society. For example, here is the breakdown (generally) in American society:

Table 1 ADRESSING Framework

Cultural Characteristics	Power	Less Power
Age	Adults	Children, adolescents, elders
Disability status	Temporarily able-bodied	Persons with disabilities
Religion	Christians	Jews, Muslims, other no Christians
Ethnicity/race	Euro-American	People of color
Sexual orientation	Heterosexuals	LGBTQ+
Socioeconomic class	Owning and middle classes (those with access to higher education)	Poor and work
Indigenous background	Non-native	Native
National origin	U.S. born	Immig
Gender	Male	Fem

Old information that is consistent with one's self-concept is easy to remember, and new information coming in that is consistent with one's self-schemas is easily incorporated. This tendency to better remember information relevant to ourselves is known as the **self-reference effect**. Inconsistent information is more difficult. For example, if someone considers herself to be intelligent but receives an extremely low score on an exam, this would oppose her self-concept. Therefore, this person may choose to externalize the new information from her self-concept by attributing it to a lack of sleep or an unfair test. It is often easier to externalize information that opposes a self-concept by attributing it to an outside factor than it is to internalize the information and adjust one's self-concept.

When people have positive self-concepts (I am intelligent), they tend to act positively and have more optimistic perceptions of the world. When people have negative self-concepts (I am stupid), they tend to feel that they have somehow fallen short, and they are usually dissatisfied and unhappy.

Carl Rogers, founder of the **humanistic psychology** perspective, pioneered a unique approach to understanding personality and human relationships (see Chapter 7 for more on Carl Rogers). According to Rogers, personality is composed of the ideal self and the real self. The **ideal self** is constructed out of your life experiences, societal expectations, and the traits you admire about role models. The ideal self is the person *you ought to be*, while the real self is the person *you actually are*. When the ideal self and the real self are similar, the result is a positive self-concept. However, Rogers suggests that the ideal self is usually an impossible standard to meet, and that when the real self falls short of the ideal self, the result is **incongruity**.

Self-Esteem, Self-Efficacy, and Locus of Control in Self-Identity

In addition to how the "self" is defined, there are three powerful influences on an individual's development of self-concept. These are self-efficacy, locus of control, and self-esteem.

and effectiveness. It's how capable we believe

... factor; studies have shown that simply

Self-efficacy can vary from task to

low self-efficacy for juggling.

locus of control believe

...ions. Those with an

...de forces. Someone with

...elligence and hard work.

...me that the test was especially

...ich people are exposed to situ-

...ct because they believe it will

...sses and they find themselves once

...s lack of action may persist. This

...been shown that believing more in

...d to proactivity. An external locus of

...many depressed and oppressed people,

6. Social Psychology

3) **Self-esteem** is one's overall evaluation of one's self-worth. This may be based on different factors for different individuals, depending on which parts of a person's identity he or she has determined to be the most important. For some, self-esteem may rest on intelligence. How would you value yourself if you had low versus high intelligence? For others, it may rest on athletic ability, beauty, or moral character. Self-esteem is related to self-efficacy; self-efficacy can improve self-esteem if one has it for an activity that one values. However, if the activity is not one that is valued, it may not help self-esteem. For example, a person may have high self-efficacy as a soldier, but still struggle with low self-esteem if this is not her desired occupation. Low self-esteem increases the risk of anxiety, depression, drug use, and suicide. However, inflated self-esteem is also present in gang members, terrorists, and bullies, and may be used to conceal deep-seated insecurities. Unrealistic self-esteem to either extreme can be painful.

Stages of Identity Development

Identity formation or individuation is the development of a distinct individual personality. Identity changes throughout different life stages, but includes the characteristics an individual considers his or her own, which distinguish the individual from others. Erik Erikson's theory of psychosocial development (see Chapter 7) includes a series of crises and conflicts experienced throughout a person's lifetime that help to define and shape identity. According to Erikson, the particular stage relevant to identity formation takes place during adolescence (roughly ages 12–20): the "Identity versus Role Confusion" stage. In this stage, adolescents try to figure out who they are and form basic identities that they will build on throughout the rest of their lives. Other psychological theories concur with Erikson's that adolescence is an important time for establishing identity. Some theories posit that in order to establish identity, an individual has to explore various possibilities and then make commitments to an occupation, religion, sexual orientation, and political viewpoint. Gender, moral, psychosexual, and social development are all important elements of identity development. For a review of psychosexual development, see the discussion of Freud in Chapter 7. Interactions with individuals, as well as socialization into broader cultural groups, also affect the development of identity.

Influence of Social Factors on Identity Formation

Influence of Individuals

Charles Cooley, an American sociologist, posited the idea of the **looking-glass self**, which is the idea that a person's sense of self develops from interpersonal interactions with others in society and the perceptions of others. According to this idea, people shape their self-concepts based on their understanding of how others perceive them. The looking-glass self begins at an early age and continues throughout life; we never stop modifying it unless all social interactions cease. **George Herbert Mead**, another American sociologist, developed the idea of **social behaviorism**: the mind and self emerge through the process of communicating with others. The idea that the mind and self emerge through the social process of communication or use of symbols was the beginning of the **symbolic interactionism** school of sociology. Mead believed that there is a specific path to development of the self. During the preparatory stage, children merely imitate others, as they have no concept of how others see things. In the play stage, children take on the roles of others through playing (as when playing house and taking on the role of "mom"). During the game stage, children learn to consider multiple roles simultaneously, and can understand the responsibilities of multiple roles. Finally, the child develops an understanding of the **generalized other**, the common behavioral expectations of general society. Mead also characterized the "me" and the "I." The "me" is how the individual believes the generalized other perceives him or her. The "me" could also be defined as the social self. The "I" is the response to the "me;" in other words, the "I" is the response of the individual to the attitudes of others. The "I" is the self as subject; the "me" is the self as object.

Influence of Culture and Socialization on Identity Formation

Socialization is the process through which people learn to be proficient and functional members of society; it is a lifelong sociological process by which people learn the attitudes, values, and beliefs that are reinforced by a particular culture. For older adults, this process often involves teaching the younger generation their way of life; for young children, it predominantly involves incorporating information from their surrounding culture as they form their personalities (the patterns for how they think and feel). It is socialization that allows a culture to pass on its values from one generation to the next.

Clearly, this is a process that occurs through socializing (interacting with others in society). The necessity for social organisms to have early social contact has been demonstrated through deprivation studies. For example, Harlow's monkeys (Chapter 9) were extremely socially deprived from infancy, and were therefore unable to re-integrate successfully with other monkeys. Disturbingly, there are some examples of extreme deprivation in humans as well. Termed **feral children**, these children are individuals who were not raised with human contact or care, and a large part of our understanding about the importance of socialization is derived from what has been learned about their experiences and the terrible consequences of growing up without proper human care and contact.

Norms

Every society has spoken and unspoken rules and expectations for the behavior of its members, called **norms**; social behaviors that follow these expectations and meet the ideal social standard are described as **normative behavior**. Such behavior is strongly encouraged in everyday social interactions by **sanctions**—rewards and punishments for behaviors that are in accord with or against norms. For example, in some nations, it is considered the norm to offer your food to others when eating in a public place. To offer food to a stranger on a bus in the United States, though, would likely result in a sanction such as a disapproving or uncomfortable look.

Norms can be classified in multiple ways, and one way is by formality. **Formal norms** are generally written down; laws are examples of formal norms. They are precisely defined, publicly presented, and often accompanied by strict penalties for those who violate them. **Informal norms** are generally understood but are less precise and often carry no specific punishments. One example is not covering one's nose and mouth when sneezing in a public setting. Not to do so does not carry a fine, but it may affect how others perceive the sneezing individual.

Another way of classifying norms is based on their importance. **Mores** ("more-ays") are norms that are highly important for the benefit of society and so are often strictly enforced. For example, animal abuse and treason are actions that break mores in the United States and carry harsh penalties. **Folkways** are norms that are less important but shape everyday behavior (for example, styles of dress, ways of greeting). Although there is a strong relationship between mores and formal norms, and folkways and informal norms, this division is not absolute. Society may have a formal norm such as walking within a crosswalk when crossing the street; however, the lack of strong enforcement of this formal norm suggests that it is not that important and is more a folkway than a more.

In contrast, those behaviors that customs forbid are described as **taboo**. In the case of a taboo, the endorsement of the norm is so strong that its violation is forbidden and oftentimes punishable through formal or non-formal methods. Taboo behaviors, in general, result in disgust toward the violator. There is often a moral or religious component to the taboo, and violation of the norm poses the threat of divine penalties. For example, in accordance with religious laws, Muslims denounce the consumption of pork; thus, in Muslim countries, eating such products would be considered taboo. More widespread examples of taboo behaviors include cannibalism, incest, and murder. Furthermore, forms of prejudice and discrimination might be viewed as taboo, depending on the perspective. Modern research suggests that taboo behavior is a social construct that varies around the world; the idea of taboo changes in response to changes in social structure and there is no universal taboo.

Anomie

The normative effects of social values contribute to social cohesion and social norms are involved in maintaining order. In some cases, societies lack this cohesion and order. This is referred to as **anomie**, a concept that describes the social condition in which individuals are not provided with firm guidelines in relation to norms and values and there is minimal moral guidance or social ethics. For this reason, anomie is often thought of as a state of *normlessness*. The concept was developed through the work of the famous sociologist Émile Durkheim (section 4.1). In researching patterns of suicide in the context of nineteenth-century Europe, Durkheim used the term anomie as an explanation for the differences in suicide rates between Catholics and Protestants. His research suggested that suicide rates were lower in cultures that valued communal ties, as this provided a form of support during times of emotional distress. Anomie, then, is characteristic of societies in which social cohesion is less pronounced; for example, anomie may be more likely to occur in societies where individualism and autonomous decision-making predominate, even at the expense of the greater social order. Anomie suggests the disintegration of social bonds between individuals and their communities, which causes the fragmentation of social identities in exchange for an emphasis on personal success. Discrepancies between personal and social values are thought to contribute to moral deregulations.

Deviance

Complex social processes regulate social behaviors by positioning social norms as the correct method of action. However, there are cases where individuals do not conform to the expectations implicit in social structures. In contrast to normative behavior, **non-normative behavior** is viewed as incorrect because it challenges shared values and institutions, thus threatening social structure and cohesion. These behaviors are seen as abnormal and thus discouraged. Actions that violate the dominant social norms, whether formal or informal, are described as forms of **deviance**. In some cases, deviant behavior is seen as criminal, in which case it violates public policies; thus, studies of deviance are popular among criminologists.

The construction of deviance has important social functions. For example, the process of creating deviant labels affirms and reinforces social norms and values through the dichotomous presentation of the acceptable (normative) behavior and unacceptable (non-normative) behavior. The distinction between normal and deviant behavior is maintained through the punishment of transgressions through both formal and informal methods, such as means of criminal justice (for example, court hearings) and unofficial social processes (for example, public condemnation causing humiliation and shame).

However, the concept is problematic because deviance, similar to taboo, is a social construct. There are no behaviors in which deviance is inherent; instead, deviance is situational and contextual. For example, in most circumstances, murder is considered an illegal deviant behavior. However, this non-normative behavior is considered acceptable in certain contexts, such as warfare and self-defense when governments permit it. Furthermore, because social norms are subject to change, examples of deviance are also subject to change, both across time and cultures. For example, in the United States it is considered acceptable for interviewers and interviewees to shake hands, regardless of gender differences; in fact, it is considered a form of respect. However, in some Eastern cultures, this non-verbal form of communication would be offensive because of the different perspectives on relationships between men and women. Thus, it is important to consider differences in cross-cultural communication and the cultural meanings of behaviors in determining their appropriateness.

It is common that deviance is studied through the lens of crime; however, there are additional institutions in societies responsible for controlling deviance. In fact, deviance is an important concept in the context of health care. The purpose of the medical institution is to maintain health and control illness, which involves more than biological concerns. For example, according to the functionalist perspective, individuals experiencing illness are considered deviant because their condition violates conforming behavior and threatens social cohesion by limiting the individual's social contributions.

Functionalism, conflict theory, and symbolic interactionism all provide different descriptions of deviant behavior based on their respective premises (section 4.1). In addition to these three perspectives, the following are specific theories often used in the discussion of deviance.

1) Edwin Sutherland's **differential association**: This perspective asserts that deviance is a learned behavior resulting from interactions between individuals and their communities (for example, the communication of ideas). The process of learning deviance involves learning the techniques of deviant behaviors as well as the motives and values that rationalize these behaviors, and it is no different from other learning processes in its mechanism. The principal source of exposure is an individual's closest personal groups, whether formal groups, such as professional business associates, or informal groups, such as urban gangs. These groups determine the specific behaviors learned (for example, corporate, organized crime such as fraud, insider trading, or tax evasion versus gang-related offenses such as vandalism or violence). In either case, when an individual participates in communities that condone deviant behaviors, it becomes easier for the individual to learn these behaviors and thus become deviant themselves. The extent of learning is dependent on certain features, such as the frequency and intensity of the interactions. In social situations, it is inevitable that individuals will encounter others with both favorable and unfavorable views of deviance. Sutherland posits that individuals become deviant when their contacts with favorable attitudes toward deviance outweigh their contacts with unfavorable attitudes.

A criticism of differential association is the idea that individuals are reduced to their environments; instead of considering people as independent, rational actors with personal motivations, this perspective suggests that deviant behavior is learned from one's environment without choice. It fails to consider individual characteristics and experiences and how these considerations affect a person's reaction to deviant influences in their current surroundings.

2) Howard Becker's **labeling theory**: This perspective suggests that deviance is the result of society's response to a person rather than something inherent in the person's actions; behaviors become deviant through social processes (it assumes the act itself is not deviant for intrinsic moral reasons). This approach is one of the most important theories in understanding

deviance from a social perspective. The use of negative labels can have serious consequences, both on our perception of the deviant person and the person's self-perception. For example, individuals might internalize labels and redefine their concept of the self, which can lead to **self-fulfilling prophecies** (section 6.2). Because of the societal preoccupation with labels, the individual might begin to exhibit more deviant behaviors to fulfill the expectations associated with specific ascribed labels (a form of conforming behavior). Furthermore, because deviance is a social construct, there is no absolute set of characteristics that are viewed as deviant; instead, deviance is contextual. In fact, across the same social context, there are often double standards: the same behavior might be viewed as acceptable in one group and unacceptable in another (for example, the virgin woman versus the virgin man).

Because this perspective views deviance as a social construct, it is often used in interactionist arguments. However, the use of social labels also concerns conflict theorists. Those with the most power in societies, such as politicians, are able to impose the most severe labels, while those with the least power in societies, such as criminals, are those whom labels are most often directed toward. In general, it is often the dominant groups (majorities) labeling the subordinate groups (minorities); for example, men labeling women as "less capable" in professional contexts or the upper class labeling the lower class as "less motivated" to achieve economic success. In fact, social structures often contribute to this by allowing the dominant groups the power to enforce the boundaries of normal behavior and thus define the difference between non-deviant and deviant behaviors, perhaps institutionalizing these differences through legal policies. These groups are often referred to as **agents of social control** because of their ability to attach stigmas to certain behaviors (for example, a doctor can define obsessive-compulsive behavior as a mental illness, a form of deviance). The creation of stigmatic roles, in turn, reinforces the power structures and hierarchies inherent in most societies and serves to limit deviant behavior. Furthermore, there is also a functional component to labels, as labeling satisfies the social need to control behaviors and maintain order.

A criticism of the labeling theory is the idea that deviance is assumed to be an automatic process: individuals are seen to be influenced through the use of labels, which ignores their abilities to resist social expectations.

3) Robert Merton's **structural strain theory:** This perspective posits that deviance is the result of experienced strain, either individual or structural. Modern societies have shared perceptions of the ideal life (social goals). These societies also have accepted means of achieving these established goals. In expanding upon Durkheim's research, Merton specified that anomie is the state in which there is a mismatch between the common social goals and the structural or institutionalized means of obtaining these goals. In this state, individuals experience social strain; because existing social structures are inadequate, there is pressure to use deviant methods to prevent failure. When the social goals and means are balanced, deviance is not expected.

For example, economic success is a common goal for most individuals and societies and the legitimate means for obtaining this goal include continued education and professional positions that compensate well. However, in the United States, it is known that there is not equal access to resources among social groups (see section 4.2 for more details on social inequalities). For example, individuals born into lower class families have less financial resources available to obtain an education. Because the means are not serving these individuals in accomplishing the goal of economic success, the result is structural strain, which in turn leads to deviance. Merton's perspective, then, suggests that lower class individuals are more expected to use deviant methods of reaching economic success (for example, stealing, selling drugs).

A criticism of the structural strain theory is the fact that some deviant behaviors, and in particular criminal behaviors, are seemingly excessive and serve no useful purpose. Merton's perspective is applicable to fraud and theft, for example, in the cases where the economic structure is not serving individuals as best as possible (such as the means of earning is not the best option for the goal of obtaining financial assets). However, it is less applicable to deviant behaviors that are malicious and violent in nature, such as forms of sexual assault. Furthermore, this perspective is more applicable to material, rather than social, goals.

Collective Behavior

In addition to normative or conforming behaviors and non-normative or deviant behaviors, there is a third form of social behavior that is described through the separate and distinct concept of **collective behavior**, in which social norms for the situation are absent or unclear. This concept describes the actions of people operating as a collective group; however, it is important to distinguish collective behavior from group behavior. In general, collective behavior is more short-lived and less conventional values influence the group's behavior and guidelines for membership. Examples of collective behavior, as opposed to those of group behavior, do not reflect the existing social structure but are instead spontaneous situations in which individuals engage in actions that are otherwise unacceptable and violate social norms. Research on collective behavior has suggested that there are characteristics of the behavior that cannot be compared to the independent effect of numerous individual actions. Instead, with collective behavior, there is a loss of the individual and independent moral judgment in exchange for a sense of belonging to the group. This can be destructive (for example, mobs and riots) or harmless (for example, fads and popular catchphrases), depending on the diverse episode. It is important to understand collective behavior to limit its negative consequences—in particular, those negative consequences which are the result of human response rather than unpreventable circumstances. For example, an understanding of collective behavior could help establish effective and safe crowd management and design planning to accommodate for potential issues.

The classification of collective behavior is a point of contention. However, **Herbert Blumer**, a sociologist whose ideas were foundational in the understanding of collective behavior, identified four main forms of collective behavior:

1) **Crowds:** The **crowd** is defined as a group that shares a purpose. The crowd is the most agreed-upon example of collective behavior and is the most common in modern life (for example, orchestras, theaters, and other performances). In general, crowds are thought to be emotional; often, in the context of the crowds, there is a non-permanent loss of rational thought and the crowd influences individual behaviors, sometimes referred to as **herd behavior**. However, not all crowd behavior is irrational. For example, although the thought of stampedes suggests chaos, in the face of threats, such as during bombings or fires, it is not irrational for individuals to run, rather than walk, to the nearest exit as a response to fear. Crowds can be classified based on their specific intention: acting crowds gather for a specific cause or goal (for example, protesters or revolutionaries), casual crowds emerge spontaneously and include people who are not really interacting (for example, people waiting in line for something), conventional crowds gather for a planned event (for example, football fans or religious congregants), and expressive crowds aggregate to express an emotion (for example, funeral attenders or rock-concert goers). Crowds can be further classified based on the closeness of the individuals (for example, compact or diffuse crowds) and the emotions caused (for example, fear in the panic, happiness in the craze, and anger in the hostile outburst). The idea of panic is a common theme in examples of collective behavior; **panic** is a situation in which fear escalates to the point that it dominates thinking and thus affects entire groups (for example, during disaster situations). A **mob** is a specific example of a crowd in which emotion is heightened and behavior is directed toward a specific and violent cause. Historical examples of mobs include lynching.

2) **Publics:** A **public** is defined as a group of individuals discussing a single issue, which conflicts with the common usage of the term. This form of collective behavior begins as the discussion begins and ceases as the discussion ceases and there can exist various publics to reflect various discussions. People in publics share ideas.

3) **Masses:** A **mass** is defined as a group whose formation is prompted through the efforts of mass media; masses consist of a relatively large number of people who may not be in close proximity but nevertheless share common interests.

4) **Social movements:** A **social movement** is defined as collective behavior with the intention of promoting change. There are two main categories of social movements: **active movements**, which attempt to foster social change (for example, revolutions), and **expressive movements**, which attempt to foster individual change (for example, support groups). There are numerous forms of social movements identified in sociological tradition: global or local (range), old or new (origin), peaceful or violent (method), etc. In contrast to other forms of collective behavior, social movements can become established and permanent social institutions.

There are additional aspects of collective behavior with which you should be familiar. A **fad**, also known as a **craze**, is an example of a collective behavior in which something (1) experiences a rapid and dramatic boost in reputation, (2) remains popular among a large population for a brief period, and (3) experiences a rapid and dramatic decline in reputation. The enthusiasm for the particular thing is driven through methods such as peer pressure and social media and through actors such as peers and famous celebrities. Examples of fads include clothing, food, language, and other novel ideas that often fade not long after catching on. Internet phenomena are an excellent example of fads; viral videos that have lost momentum include dances such as Gangnam Style and the Harlem Shake. It is important to note that fads are separate from **trends**, which are longer-lived and often lead to permanent social changes; for example, the hippie movement created visible trends, such as peace signs, but also prompted widespread social change.

Another aspect of collective behavior is the concept of **mass hysteria**, which is a diagnostic label that refers to the collective delusion of some threat that spreads through emotion (for example, fear) and escalates until it spirals out of control (for example, panic). Mass hysteria is the result of public reactions to stressful situations; common examples include medical problems and supernatural occurrences, such as periodic interest in crop circles. In these situations, the collective behavior is often irrational as a result of emotional excesses and thus mass hysteria has been described as a form of groupthink (section 6.2). For example, in the context of medical problems, there might be a spontaneous spread of related diseases. Those affected might manifest similar medical symptoms, such as fatigue, headaches, or nausea. It is curious that these popular signs are also connected to high levels of stress. In most cases, the illness cannot be linked to an external source, such as an infectious agent.

It is thus important to distinguish this form of collective behavior from the concepts of **outbreaks**, **epidemics**, and **pandemics**. These cases involve an unexpected increase in the incidence of an infectious disease in a given region, with outbreaks being the most limited and pandemics being the most widespread. For example, the Bubonic plague is a well-known historical epidemic; in modern times, the extent of the dangerous COVID-19 virus reached pandemic proportions, spreading across the world. In contrast, famous examples of mass hysteria include larger movements without clear medical explanation, such as the Salem witch trials. This series of trials and prosecutions began as the result of a group of adolescent girls experiencing "fits" that were thought to exceed the power of the more common epileptic fits. This caused a **moral panic**—a specific form of panic as a result of a perceived threat to social order—which lead to numerous executions.

Riots are a third example of collective behavior. Riots are a form of crowd behavior (see page 128). Most riots occur as the result of general dissatisfaction with social conditions, with examples including food and bread, police, prison, race, religion, sports, student, and urban riots. In general, collective behavior is often thought to be irrational. However, some research suggests that riots are not irrational as there are examples where the source of dissatisfaction is less political and more fundamental; for example, some riots begin as a response to a lack of basic needs (for example, hunger riots). The most famous historical examples include reactions to government oppression, poor living conditions, racial or religious conflicts, and other serious social issues. In these cases, riots can have serious measurable consequences for economics and politics; these effects are often complex. For example, the Arab Spring was a revolution that included riots. It first began in Tunisia but spread across the Arab world, causing civil uprisings that contributed to the eventual fall of governments. The power of riots has led to increased public attention and participation, due in part to mass media coverage, and certain representations, which were once intended to conceal identities and offer protection (such as facemasks and scarves), have become iconic.

In general, riots are chaotic and disorganized due to a sudden onset, often described as states of civil disorder, civil distress, or civil unrest. There is an increase in criminal behaviors, such as vandalism and violence. The target of this destruction can include both private and public properties, depending on the source of the grievance, but often include institutions such as government or religious buildings. Because of the state of distress common in riots, crowd control is an important consideration. Police measures tend to be non-lethal in nature (for example, arrest or tear gas), but police intervention does lead to occasional injuries and deaths.

Agents of Socialization

There are many different social forces that influence our lives and the development of culture over time. Six of these "agents of socialization" are family, school, peers, the workplace, religion/government, and mass media/technology.

1) *Family*
   The lifelong process of socialization begins shortly after birth and is generally driven first by family members. Family members attend to a baby's physical needs but also to social development. First relationships heavily influence how an individual will interact in future relationships. Family members teach children the customs, beliefs, and traditions of their cultures through both instruction and modeling. They also influence the situations to which children are exposed, especially in the early years of life.

2) *School*
   Like family, schools explicitly teach children the norms and values of their culture. Schools can also affect children's self-identities by accentuating those intellectual, physical, and social strengths that society endorses. For example, schools may differ in how they value logic and linear thinking versus creativity, and can influence children toward one or the other. Finally, schools can reinforce divisive aspects of society, because the quality and availability of schooling is influenced by socioeconomic status.

3) *Peer Groups*
   As children grow older, the family typically becomes less important in social development and peer groups become more significant. Fashion, style of speech, gender-role identity, sexual activity, drug/alcohol use, and other behaviors are affected by peers and by the influence of hierarchies such as popularity.

4) *Workplace*

People typically spend a good portion of their time at work. The workplace influences behavior through written codes and rules as well as through informal norms. There is pressure to fit in at the workplace that often alters behavior; occupation can also be a large part of one's identity.

5) *Religion/Government*

Both government and organized religion influence the course of cultural change by creating "rites of passage." In religion, this might include traditional milestones and celebrations such as coming of age and marriage. Government sets legal ages for drinking, voting, joining the military, and so on. Laws both influence and are influenced by the societies to which they apply. For example, in the United States, stricter laws apply to crack than to cocaine, and this affects society's perceptions of these drugs and of drug addicts.

6) *Mass Media/Technology*

Mass media and technology have extended themselves to influence almost everyone on the planet, through television, movies, the Internet, cell phones, and other communications. The impact of television on culture through displays of sex, violence, and impossible-to-achieve ideals has been much debated. It has also affected culture in ways that most people agree are positive, such as educational programming and introductions to other cultures and lifestyles. The Internet can similarly help shrink the world and increase social influences through tools such as online social networking and blogs.

Cultural Assimilation

Assimilation and amalgamation are two possible outcomes of interactions among multiple cultures in the same space. **Assimilation** is the process by which an individual forsakes aspects of his or her own cultural tradition to adopt those of a different culture. Generally, this individual is a member of a minority group who is attempting to conform to the culture of the dominant group.

$$A + B + C \rightarrow A$$

In the diagram above, A is the dominant group that minority groups B and C work to imitate and become absorbed by. In order to assimilate, members of the minority group may make great personal sacrifices, such as changing their spoken languages, their religions, how they dress, and their personal values. In the United States, minority groups attempting to assimilate not only must learn English if it is not their native language, but must adopt the values of a capitalist society with a heavy emphasis on the individual and independence—a tough transition for those from collectivist cultures. In addition, assimilation does not guarantee that one will not be the victim of discrimination.

Amalgamation occurs when majority and minority groups combine to form a new group.

$$A + B + C \rightarrow D$$

In this case, a unique cultural group is formed that is distinct from any of the initial groups.

Multiculturalism

Multiculturalism or **pluralism** is a perspective that endorses equal standing for all cultural traditions. It promotes the idea of cultures coming together in a true melting pot, rather than in a hierarchy. The United States, despite the common description as a melting pot, includes elements of hierarchy. For example, English is the dominant language, and national holidays tend to reflect Eurocentricism.

$$A + B + C \rightarrow A + B + C$$

In true multiculturalism, each culture is able to maintain its practices. It is especially apparent in cities such as New York where there exist pockets of separate cultures (Chinatown, Little Italy, Koreatown). As a practice, multiculturalism is under debate. Supporters say it increases diversity and helps empower minority groups. Opponents say it encourages segregation over unity by maintaining physical and social isolation and hinders cohesiveness within a society.

Subcultures

Bike enthusiasts, bartenders, and medical personnel are examples of groups that can be called subcultures. A **subculture** is a segment of society that shares a distinct pattern of traditions and values that differs from that of the larger society. As the name suggests, a subculture can be thought of as a culture existing within a larger, dominant culture. Members of a subculture do participate in many activities of the larger culture, but also have unique behaviors and activities that are specific to their subculture. This often includes having unique slang, such as that used by medical personnel (for example, *cabbage* for "coronary artery bypass graft"). Sometimes, subcultures are the result of countercultural backlash, an opposition to views widely accepted within a society. Hippies in the late 1960s and early 1970s would be considered a counterculture, because they opposed certain aspects of the dominant culture, such as middle class values and the Vietnam War.

Moral Development

Moral development is an important aspect of socialization and identity formation. Lawrence Kohlberg, an American psychologist, expanded upon Jean Piaget's theory (Chapter 11) of moral development in children. **Kohlberg's stages of moral development** include six identifiable developmental stages of moral reasoning, which form the basis of ethical behavior. Kohlberg's stages are grouped into three levels with two stages each (see Table 2). According to Kohlberg, stages cannot be skipped. Each stage provides a new and necessary moral perspective, and the understanding from each stage is retained and integrated at later stages. Interestingly, most adults attain but do not surpass the fourth stage, in which morality is dictated by outside forces (laws, rules, social obligations). Few people attain a post-conventional level of moral reasoning. In fact, though Kohlberg insisted that stage 6 exists, he found it difficult to identify people who operated at that level.

Table 2   Kohlberg's Stages of Moral Development

| Level 1 | Pre-conventional level of moral reasoning: morality judged by direct consequences to the self (no internalization of "right" and "wrong")

Typical of children | Stage 1: Obedience and punishment orientation | Individuals focus on the direct consequences to themselves of their actions ("How can I avoid punishment?") |
|---|---|---|---|
| | | Stage 2: Self-interest orientation | Individuals focus on the behavior that will be in their best interests, with limited interest in the needs of others ("What's in it for me?") |
| Level 2 | Conventional level of moral reasoning: morality judged by comparing actions to society's views and expectations (acceptance of conventional definitions of "right" and "wrong")

Typical of adolescents and adults | Stage 3: Interpersonal accord and conformity | Individuals focus on the approval and disapproval of others, and try to be "good" by living up to expectations ("What will make others like me?") |
| | | Stage 4: Authority and social-order maintaining orientation | Beyond a need for individual approval, individuals feel a duty to uphold laws, rules, and social conventions ("What am I supposed to do?") |
| Level 3 | Post-conventional level of moral reasoning: morality judged by internal ethical guidelines; rules viewed as useful but malleable guidelines

Many people never reach this abstract level of moral reasoning | Stage 5: Social contract orientation | Individuals see laws as social contracts to be changed when they do not promote general welfare ("The greatest good for the greatest number of people") |
| | | Stage 6: Universal ethical principles | Morality is based on abstract reasoning using universal ethical principles; laws are only valid if they are grounded in justice |

6.2   POSITIVE AND NEGATIVE ELEMENTS OF SOCIAL INTERACTION

Attribution

Attribution theory is rooted in social psychology and attempts to explain how individuals view behavior, both our own behavior and the behavior of others. Given a set of circumstances, individuals attribute behavior to internal causes (**dispositional attribution**) or external causes (**situational attribution**). Driving tends to be a situation that generates plenty of salient examples. Imagine you are driving and someone cuts you off. You might think, "Wow, that driver is a real jerk." This would be a dispositional attribution, because the driver's behavior is attributed to an internal cause (he is a jerk). On the other hand, you could alternatively think, "Wow, that driver must be in a hurry because of an emergency; maybe he just found out his mom is in the hospital." This would be a situational attribution (there is an emergency).

How often do you think that someone who cut you off might have had a good reason to do so? People tend to assign dispositional attributions to others (they are just jerks), but give themselves the benefit of situational attributions. For example, the last time you cut someone off while driving, did you feel like you had a good reason to do so? Did you then think to yourself, "Wow, I am a real jerk"?

What determines whether we attribute behavior to internal or external causes? There are three factors that influence this decision: consistency, distinctiveness, and consensus. To consider these, imagine a simple situation: you are walking past your friend, who looks angry and walks past you without saying hello.

1) **Consistency:** is anger consistent with how your friend typically acts? If it is, then you might explain it with internal causes (dispositional). If not, you might think there are external factors that explain it (situational).

2) **Distinctiveness:** is your friend angry toward everyone or just toward you? If your friend is angry toward everyone, the cause likely has to do with your friend (dispositional). If your friend is just angry toward you, it may be situational; perhaps you did something irritating.

3) **Consensus:** is your friend the only one angry or is everyone angry? If your friend is the only one angry, then it is more likely that the anger has something to do with your friend (dispositional). If everyone is angry, then it might be situational (the team lost the playoffs).

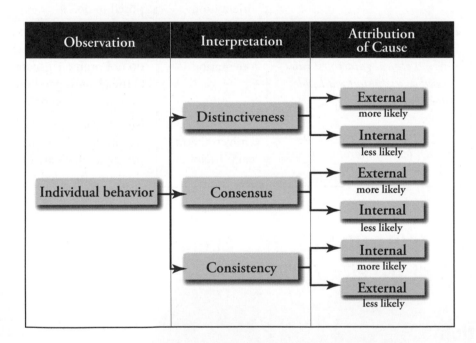

Figure 1 Attributing behavior to external or internal causes

Attributional Biases

Despite the apparent logic in our methods of identifying whether someone's behavior is due to internal or external causes, we are frequently wrong in our analysis of others. We often make the **fundamental attribution error**, which is that we tend to underestimate the impact of the situation and overestimate the impact of a person's character or personality. Another way of saying this is that we tend to assume that people *are* how they act. Thus, we are more likely to think that the driver who cuts us off is a jerk in general, rather than assuming the driver acted that way because he has to rush to the hospital to be with his ailing mother. Remember, when we attribute our own actions to something, we tend to attribute to external rather than internal causes. So if I cut someone off, it is because I had a good reason to. This tendency to blame our actions on the situation and blame the actions of others on their personalities is also called the **actor-observer bias**.

People tend to give themselves much more credit than they give others. We are wired to perceive ourselves favorably. The **self-serving bias** is the tendency to attribute successes to ourselves and our failures to others or the external environment. If we perform well academically, it is because we are smart and worked hard. If we perform poorly academically, it was because the test was unfair or the teacher graded too hard.

Similarly, we have a tendency to be optimistic and want to believe that the world is a good place. We want to believe that life is predictable and that actions influence outcomes. The **optimism bias** is the belief that bad things happen to other people, but not to us. This goes hand-in-hand with the fact that we want to believe that life is fair, which also impacts how we think about others. The **just world phenomenon** is a tendency to believe that the world is fair and people get what they deserve. When bad things happen to others, it is the result of their actions or their failure to act, not because sometimes bad things happen to good people. Similarly, when good things happen to us, it is because we deserved it. **Hindsight bias,** or the knew-it-all-along effect, is the tendency to believe that an event that has already occurred was predictable.

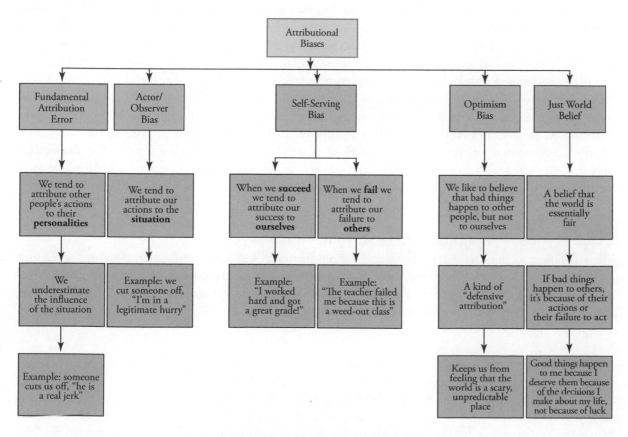

Figure 2   Attributional biases

Another type of error that occurs when we make assumptions about others is the halo effect (or halo error). The **halo effect** is a tendency to believe that people have inherently good or bad natures, rather than looking at individual characteristics. Our overall impression of a person is influenced by how we feel or think about his or her character. For example, your overall impression of your neighbor might be "he is nice," therefore, you make other assumptions about him ("he must be a good dad"). The **physical attractiveness stereotype** is a specific type of halo effect; people tend to rate attractive individuals more favorably on personality traits and characteristics than they do those who are less attractive.

Culture Affects Attributions

There are cultural differences that influence how attributions are made. Western cultures tend to endorse an individualistic attitude: "You can do anything you put your mind to!" This influences people toward more internal attributions for success and failure. Unemployment is sometimes explained as laziness or stupidity. In Eastern Asian cultures, external attribution is more predominant. Thus, the system as a whole is scrutinized more than the individual. If an insider trading scandal occurs, this attitude would emphasize controlling the financial organization, rather than finding and prosecuting the guilty individuals.

Self-Perceptions Shape Our Perceptions of Others

Social perception involves the understanding of others in our social world; it is the initial information we process about other people in order to try to understand their mindsets and intentions. **Social cognition** is the ability of the brain to store and process information regarding social perception. Social perception is the process responsible for our judgments and impressions about other people, and it allows us to recognize how others impact us, and predict how they might behave in given situations. We rely upon our social perception and cognition in order to interpret a range of socially relevant information, such as verbal and non-verbal communication, tone, facial expressions, and an understanding of the social relationships and social goals present in situations. Using social perception, we try to figure out what others are thinking. Sometimes our tendencies lead us to mistakes in social perception. A **false consensus** occurs when we assume that everyone else agrees with what we do (even though they may not). A **projection bias** happens when we assume others have the same beliefs we do. Since people have a tendency to look for similarities between themselves and others, they often assume them even when this is unfounded.

Stereotypes, Prejudice, and Discrimination

Many people may not know the differences between the terms stereotype, prejudice, discrimination, and racism, but from a sociological perspective, it is important to know their meanings. **Stereotypes** are oversimplified ideas about groups of people, based on characteristics (race, gender, sexual orientation, religion, disability). Stereotypes can be positive ("X group is successful because they are hard workers") or negative ("Y group is poor because they are lazy").

Prejudice refers to the thoughts, attitudes, and feelings someone holds about a group that are not based on actual experience. As the name implies, prejudice is a prejudgment or biased thinking about a group and its members. The group that one is biased against can be one defined by race, age, gender, religion, or any other characteristic. Some forms of prejudice are blatant or overt, such as the prejudice used to justify the actions taken by Hitler and his regime against the Jews and other groups during World War II. Other forms are more subtle, such as the finding that employers in a study considered more resumes for employment from candidates with "white-sounding names" than "Black-sounding names." In this situation, an employer may not even be aware of his or her prejudice. In fact, prejudice has been found at a subconscious level when studying individuals' reactions to pleasant and unpleasant words. For example, when primed with a Black face rather than a white face, people are more likely to predict the subject is carrying a gun rather than another object, such as a tool or wallet.

While prejudice involves thinking a certain way, **discrimination** involves acting a certain way toward a group or group member. People can discriminate against any number of characteristics and, unfortunately, American history is rife with examples of discrimination. Moreover, traditions, policies, ideas, practices, and laws that are discriminatory still exist in many institutions. Attempts to limit discrimination, such as **affirmative action** (policies that take factors like race or sex into consideration to benefit underrepresented groups in admissions or job hiring decisions) have been used to benefit those believed to be current or past victims of discrimination. However, these attempts have been controversial, and some have deemed these practices "discrimination against the majority," or **reverse discrimination**.

Prejudices and actions that discriminate based on race, or hold that one race is inferior to another, are called **racism**. While the exact definitions of "race," "ethnicity," and "racism" have been subject to much debate over the years, racism tends to be seen when the dominant or majority group (usually white) holds a prejudice or engages in discrimination, whether intentional or not, against non-dominant or minority groups (usually non-white). Sometimes racism is used to describe discrimination on an ethnic or cultural basis, independent of whether these differences are described as racial. The confusion largely stems from confusion about the definitions of the terms "race" and "ethnicity."

Institutional discrimination refers to unjust and discriminatory practices employed by large organizations that have been codified into operating procedures, processes, or institutional objectives. An example of institutional discrimination was the "don't ask, don't tell" policy of the U.S. military, which frowned upon openly gay men and women serving in the armed forces. In general, members of minority groups are much more likely to encounter institutional discrimination than members of majorities.

A society's prescriptions for which groups attain more power, prestige, and social standing can account for prejudice toward those on the lower rungs of that society. In general, any unequal status sets the stage for prejudice. These symbols of status are all relative, so in order to be of a higher status, one needs other people to be of a lower status. Thus, some people at the "top" are motivated to try to justify and maintain these differences, sometimes using prejudice as a tool. For example, very wealthy individuals may justify their wealth by insinuating that poorer members of society are lazy, and they seek to maintain this gap by voting against welfare programs for this group. Social institutions can also be designed to maintain these differences. For example, in the United States, good, well-funded schools are in wealthier neighborhoods and below-average, poorly-funded schools are in poorer neighborhoods.

In the United States, wealth is an important source of power and class, with the wealthiest shaping the laws and agenda of the society. Prestige is often based on occupation. Doctors get more respect than janitors, not just in their occupations but also as people. Higher prestige positions are usually taken by members of the dominant groups in societies, as can be seen by the disparate number of men compared to women in many of these prestigious roles.

Emotion and Cognition in Prejudice

Prejudice is an attitude. Remember that attitudes have three components (the ABCs): affect (feelings), behavioral inclinations/tendencies, and cognition (beliefs). Therefore, emotion and cognition both play roles in contributing to prejudice. In addition, there are several social sources of prejudice. Let's consider each of these contributing factors.

Emotion can play a role in feeding prejudices. At the core of prejudice is often fear or frustration. When someone is faced with something intimidating or unknown, especially if it is presumed to be blocking that person from some goal (frustration), hostility can be a natural reaction. There is a tendency to want to direct that hostility at someone, and history shows that displaced aggression often falls on marginalized people. **Scapegoats** are the unfortunate people at whom displaced aggression is directed. Many Germans blamed the Jews for the economic struggles that preceded the genocide of World War II. In the United States, fear and hostility were redirected onto women who were accused as "witches" in the 1600s. In subtler forms, scapegoats for an economic collapse can be those who are impoverished and on welfare.

This is not to say that one has to be some kind of "monster" to experience feelings of prejudice. Although in some of the above examples, drastic actions were taken, the underlying emotions can also influence those who do not take action. For example, when seated next to someone who is clearly very different from them on a bus, even people who do not see themselves as prejudiced may be uncomfortable. When a person sees an unfamiliar person of another race, emotion processing centers in the brain become more active automatically. It is only through active self-monitoring and reflection that people are able to inhibit prejudiced responses despite the presence of prejudiced feelings. Some may feel guilty for having the feelings at all, though they are not unusual. These self-inhibition abilities weaken with age, so many older adults find it hard to inhibit the prejudiced thoughts that they may have suppressed during their younger years.

There are also some aspects of normal thinking and information processing that contribute to prejudice. Our brains seek to categorize and organize data based on similarities, as a shortcut. We create conceptual categories such as "white" just as we do categories like "furniture" and "toys." These conceptualizations can lead to stereotypes. Stereotypes, both positive and negative, stem from our mental shortcuts that simplify our conceptualizations of the world.

Our brains also hone in on differences. Even babies are more interested in new objects presented in their field of vision than they are in things they've seen before. Thus, people who are seen as distinctive draw more attention and are often likely to be seen as representative of groups. For example, all Black people may be incorrectly considered good athletes based on examples of distinctive Black athletes like Michael Jordan. There is an **illusory correlation** created between a group of people and a characteristic based on unique cases.

Attributional biases (described above), particularly the optimism bias and just-world belief, also suggest that we are more likely to believe that the world is fair and predictable, things happen for a reason, and people get what they deserve. Thus, the sick or disadvantaged often face prejudice because others believe that they have done something wrong that led them to be in their position. Thus, someone with HIV may face prejudice, including the assumption that he or she contracted the disease through irresponsible behavior, despite how the disease was actually transmitted.

Self-Fulfilling Prophecy and Stereotype Threat

These stereotypes can lead to behaviors that affirm the original stereotypes in what is known as a **self-fulfilling prophecy**. For example, if a college guy believes that the girls in a certain sorority are snobby and prudish, he may avoid engaging in conversations with the girls from that sorority at parties. Because he does not engage them in conversation, his opinion of them as snobby and prudish will probably be reinforced. People may also be affected by stereotypes they know others have of a group to which they belong. **Stereotype threat** refers to a self-fulfilling fear that one will be evaluated based on a negative stereotype. For example, the idea that males are better at math than females is a negative stereotype. In studies where females are asked to complete a math test, if the female is first told that males do better than females on the math test, the female's performance on the test is lower than if she was not first presented with this information. Similarly, if the female is being tested on math concepts with males present, she will perform more poorly than if there are no males present. This phenomenon helps to explain the dearth of women in math and engineering fields.

Ethnocentrism Versus Cultural Relativism

On a broader level, when different cultures interact, there is often a tendency to judge people from another culture by the standards of one's own culture, a phenomenon known as **ethnocentrism**. It is an example of favoritism for one's in-group over out-groups (see Groups below). For example, the tension that exists between those who live in the city and those who live in rural areas is often due to judgments about each other's ways of life. City dwellers may look down on those in rural areas based on their standards of occupation and wealth. Those in the country may look down on city dwellers based on standards of morality, practicality, and quality of life. An alternative to ethnocentrism is **cultural relativism**: judging another culture based on its own standards. This can be very difficult to do, especially when the values of another culture clash with the values of one's own. For example, in India, child labor is common and is often seen as a way in which children can help their families. This may be a difficult viewpoint to accept for someone from a culture in which childhood is equated with a carefree time of play, and child labor is seen as abusive. However, practicing cultural relativism would involve judging this practice in the context of that culture's values.

Groups

A **group** is a collection of any number of people (as few as two) who regularly interact and identify with each other, sharing similar norms, values, and expectations. A team of neurologists may be considered a group, while the entire hospital staff may not be considered a group if there is little interaction between departments. The concept of social groups is complex, and groups come in numerous varieties. There are sociologists who might view societies as large groups in the context of cohesive social identities. Within a social structure, groups are often the setting for social interaction and influence. Groups help clearly define social roles and statuses.

Groups can be further divided into primary groups and secondary groups. **Primary groups** play a more important role in an individual's life; these groups are usually smaller and include those with whom the individual engages with emotionally, in-person on a long-term basis. A **secondary group** is larger and more impersonal, and may interact for specific reasons for shorter periods. Primary groups serve **expressive functions** (meeting emotional needs) and secondary groups serve **instrumental functions** (meeting pragmatic needs). A family would be an example of a primary group (regardless of how family is defined), whereas the MCAT study group would be an example of a secondary group.

In-groups and out-groups are subcategories of primary and secondary groups. An **in-group** is a group that an individual belongs to and believes to be an integral part of who she is. A group that an individual does not belong to is her **out-group**. Social identity theory asserts that when we categorize other people, we identify with some of them, whom we consider our in-groups, and see differences with others, whom we consider our out-groups. We tend to have favorable impressions of our in-groups because they bolster our social identities and self-esteem. People tend to have positive stereotypes about their own in-groups ("we are hard-working"). It feels good to have a sense of belonging, and feel positive about the groups to which you belong. On the other hand, we may have more negative impressions of members of out-groups. Different can be seen as worse (for example, "I feel sorry for those who don't believe the same things I do"). People also tend to have more negative stereotypes about out-groups ("they are lazy"). In-groups and out-groups help to explain some negative human behaviors like exclusion and bullying. When certain groups of people are defined as different, they may also be seen as inferior (when people assume that their in-group is the best, everyone in the out-group is somehow less); therefore, in-groups may engage in sexism, racism, ethnocentrism, heterosexism, and other such behaviors. (These ideas are discussed in more detail below.)

A **reference group** is a standard measure to which people compare themselves. For example, peers who are also studying for the MCAT might be a reference group for you. This is a group to which you might compare yourself. What are the people in this group studying? What classes are they taking? When are they taking the exam? To which medical schools are they applying? An individual can have multiple reference groups, and these different groups may convey different messages. For example, you might view your friends in class who are all taking the MCAT as one reference group, and your older sibling, who is in medical school, and his or her medical school friends as another reference group.

Furthermore, there are descriptions of **group size**. The number of people present within the group has consequences for group relations. The smallest social group, known as the **dyad**, contains two members. Dyadic interaction is often more intimate and intense than that in larger groups because there is no outside competition. However, the small size also requires active cooperation and participation from both members to be stable. In some cases of dyads, such as within marriages, there are laws that enforce the strength of the pair. Dyads can involve equal relationships, such as with monogamous romantic partners, or unequal relationships, such as with master-servant relationships. The next largest group, known as the **triad**, contains three members. In the dyad, there is a single relationship, but in the triad, there are three relationships, one between each pair of members. For this reason, triads can be more or less stable. It is possible for the group to become more stable because there is an additional person to mediate tension; it is possible for the group to become less stable because it is an observed rule that two people will tend to unite, causing conflict with the final group member. Triads can also be equal or unequal, and a common example of hierarchical triads involves groups in which there is a single dominant member, such as in an MCAT tutoring group (one tutor and two students).

People who exist in the same space but do not interact or share a common sense of identity make up an **aggregate**. For example, an MCAT study group that meets after class regularly at a coffee shop to prepare for the exam is a group. All of the people that frequent that coffee shop on a regular basis (but do not interact or share a common identity) are an aggregate. Similarly, people who share similar characteristics but are not otherwise tied together would be considered a **category**. All of the people studying for the MCAT this year make up a category of people.

Bureaucracy is a term used to describe an administrative body and the processes by which this body accomplishes tasks. Bureaucracies arise from an advanced division of labor in which each worker does his or her small task. These tasks are presided over and coordinated by managers. Bureaucracies can be a very efficient way to complete complicated tasks because each member of the organization has a specific role. A major theory of bureaucracy was developed by sociologist Max Weber, who considered bureaucracy to be a necessary aspect of modern society. Weber outlined the following characteristics of an ideal bureaucracy:

1. It covers a fixed area of activity.
2. It is hierarchically organized.
3. Workers have expert training in an area of specialty.
4. Organizational rank is impersonal, and advancement depends on technical qualification, rather than favoritism.
5. Workers follow set procedures to increase predictability and efficiency.

One major concept related to bureaucracy is rationalization. Rationalization describes the process by which tasks are broken down into component parts to be efficiently accomplished by workers within the organization. Because the workers follow set procedures in completing tasks, it is easy to predict the outcome of the process. Manufacturers have taken advantage of these aspects of bureaucracy when designing production processes. One of the first manufacturers to popularize this process was Henry Ford, who implemented assembly lines in his automobile plants. Ford rationalized the process of building a car by breaking it down into component parts and assigning the assembly of each part to a worker. In this way, he was able to have cars efficiently assembled and each car was exactly the same as the ones coming before and after it. Sociologist George Ritzer studied a similar process—the design of McDonald's restaurants to produce food quickly, and to produce uniform products across all franchises. He describes the rationalization of fast food production as **McDonaldization**. This process has four components that reflect the principles of bureaucracy: efficiency, calculability (assessing performance through quantity and/or speed of output), predictability, and control (automating work wherever possible in order to make results more predictable).

While a bureaucracy, in its ideal form, may be the most efficient way to accomplish complicated tasks, this organizational form can have several drawbacks. First, because workers follow set procedures, this can cause the organization to struggle when adapting to challenges that require it to change its way of coordinating tasks. Second, workers may become overly attached to their individual task and lose sight of the organizational mission as a whole. Third, workers may become overly attached to the set procedures and not respond flexibly to new challenges on an interpersonal level.

One paradoxical feature of organizations is that, although they may be founded to tackle new challenges in revolutionary ways, as their organizational structure becomes more complex, it also becomes more conservative and less able to adapt. Thus, revolutionary organizations inevitably become less revolutionary as their organizational structures develop and become entrenched. This pattern is known as the **Iron Law of Oligarchy**. Oligarchy means rule by an elite few, and it comes about through the very organization of the bureaucracy itself. Bureaucracies depend on increased centralization of tasks as one moves up the hierarchy. That is, there are many layers of managers in a bureaucracy, each one responsible for coordinating (centralizing) a set of tasks. The individuals who are responsible for coordinating the coordinators have the most power, and those individuals become an oligarchy at the top of the organizational structure. Furthermore, these oligarchs become specialized at their task (management), just as other members of the organization become specialists in their tasks. As discussed above, one downside to bureaucracy is that workers will fight to maintain control over their task and their established way of carrying it out. Thus, managers defend their position at the top of the organizational structure, thereby entrenching the oligarchy.

Social Facilitation

Social psychology seeks to understand how people influence one another through their interactions. The most basic level of experience between members of society is "mere presence." **Mere presence** means that people are simply in one another's presence, either completing similar activities or apparently minding their own business. For example, the task of grocery shopping usually involves the mere presence of other shoppers, without direct engagement. What's fascinating is that it turns out that the mere presence of others has a measurable effect on an individual's performance.

People tend to perform simple, well-learned tasks better when other people are present. For example, people can do simple math problems more quickly and run slightly faster when in the presence of others. People's color preferences are even stronger when they make judgments in the presence of others (a task that has no competitive influence). This finding has been called the **social facilitation effect**, and it may help explain why some of us study in the library (in the presence of others) or walk faster when in the presence of other pedestrians. However, the social facilitation effect only holds true for simple or practiced tasks. The presence of others can impair performance when completing complex or novel tasks. Thus, people do not complete complex math problems as quickly and may have a harder time navigating in novel environments when others are present.

The prevailing explanation for these phenomena involves arousal. The presence of others stimulates arousal, which serves to activate our dominant responses (the practiced responses that come most easily to us). When completing tasks that are easy and well-practiced, these dominant responses are exactly what is called for; thus, performance improves with arousal stimulated by the presence of others. When completing tasks that are more complex or novel, the dominant responses are likely to be incorrect for the situation; thus, performance declines with arousal, and in the presence of others. A basketball player who is a good, well-practiced shooter will experience an improvement in performance when there is an audience, because making baskets is his or her dominant response. A player who does not often shoot the ball will suffer with an audience, because shooting is not his or her dominant response.

There are other factors that also impact one's performance in the presence of others. Overwhelming fear of evaluation reduces performance even on behaviors that were previously automatic, because self-consciousness and doubt can lead to overanalysis. Athletes struggle if they tend to overthink their body movements at critical times. Distraction is also a factor, with the presence of others sometimes serving to divert our attention from tasks. This can be due to external events, such as others' behavior, or internal events, such as our thoughts of what others might be thinking or doing.

Deindividuation

When situations provide a high degree of arousal and a very low sense of responsibility, people may act in startling ways, surprising both to themselves at a later time and to others who know them closely. In these situations, people may lose their sense of restraint and their individual identity by identifying with a group or mob mentality, a situation called **deindividuation**. Its effects can be seen in examples ranging from atrocious acts during wartime to mosh pits at concerts. Deindividuation involves a lack of self-awareness and is the result of a disconnection of behavior from attitudes.

The confluence of several factors creates the ideal conditions for deindividuation to occur. These factors include:

- Group size: larger groups create a diminished sense of identity and responsibility, and may allow people to achieve anonymity by getting "lost in the crowd"
- Physical anonymity: using face paint, masks, or costumes (or communicating anonymously online) makes one less identifiable
- Arousing activities: rather than beginning with a frenzy, deindividuating circumstances usually start with arousing activities that escalate

The bottom line is that factors that reduce self-awareness increase a sense of deindividuation. This can further include social roles (as evidenced by Zimbardo's prison study) and the use of drugs or alcohol, which serve to disinhibit and reduce self-consciousness.

Bystander Effect

The **Kitty Genovese** case involved the stabbing of a woman in New York City late at night. Research spawned by this event revealed what is known as the **bystander effect**: the finding that a person is less likely to provide help when there are other bystanders. This occurs because the presence of bystanders creates a diffusion of responsibility—the responsibility to help does not clearly reside with one person in the group. When faced with circumstances in which one is the only individual available to assist, one may be more likely to act. Interestingly, the likelihood that someone will stop to help is inversely correlated with the number of people around; therefore, if you ever find yourself in a life-threatening emergency, you would be better off in a small town with a few folks around than in the middle of Times Square with thousands of people around.

Social Loafing

The bystander effect involves a diffusion of responsibility when in the presence of others. Taken further, this effect extends to circumstances in which people are working together toward common goals. In these situations, there is a tendency for people to exert less effort if they are being evaluated as a group than if they are individually accountable, a phenomenon called **social loafing**. It is something that you may have experienced in your everyday life, and it does not necessarily mean that the "loafer" is someone who is lazy or irresponsible. For example, as an audience member in a small group of five, you are likely to clap louder for a presenter than if you were in an audience of 500 people. This is thought to occur because there can be less pressure on individuals as parts of a group on some tasks, leading to a tendency to take a little bit of a free ride, getting the benefit from the group while putting less effort in than one might on one's own.

Social facilitation and social loafing are both responses to the group situation and the task at hand. Which one tends to occur is based in part on evaluation. When being part of a group increases concerns over evaluation, social facilitation occurs. When being part of a group decreases concerns over evaluation, social loafing occurs. In order to fight against the threat of social loafing, companies in which people work in groups often use measures of group performance (for example, a store's total revenue) as well as of individual performance (for example, individual sales).

Group Polarization

We've seen how groups can influence one's performance, either by facilitating or hindering it based on circumstances. But how does group influence affect beliefs and opinions? It turns out that groups tend to intensify the preexisting views of their members—that is, the average view of a member of the group is accentuated. This tendency is called **group polarization**. It does NOT indicate that the group becomes more divided on an issue, but rather, suggests that the entire group tends toward more extreme versions of the average views they initially shared before discussion.

Group polarization occurs at every level in society—in families, schools, political parties, communities, and such. Consider a political debate on whether a wetland area should be converted into a shopping center. Although they likely each initially held a belief in the importance of conserving the wetlands, members of an environmental political party who interact with each other end up adopting a more extreme stance toward conservation than previously held by the average member. Similarly, members of another political party that focuses on the importance of jobs would emphasize this focus even more after discussions within the group. Thus, each group adopts a more extreme stance than its initial position. This creates more divisiveness between the two groups. When you consider the group polarization phenomenon together with the fact that people tend to preferentially interact with like-minded people, you can see why group negotiations are so difficult.

There are two reasons why group polarization occurs. The first is **informational influence**; in group discussion, the most common ideas to emerge are the ones that favor the dominant viewpoint. This serves to persuade others to take a stronger stance toward this viewpoint and provides an opportunity to rehearse and validate these similar opinions, further strengthening them. In fact, just thinking about an opinion for a couple of minutes can strengthen your support of it, because we tend to mostly think of facts that support it. The second reason is **normative influence**, which is based on social desirability, that is, wanting to be accepted or admired by others. If you want to identify with a particular group, then you may take a stronger stance than you initially would have in order to better relate to and internalize the group's belief system. The influence of **social comparison** (evaluating our opinions by comparing them to those of others) extends far beyond high school.

Groupthink

Pressure not to "rock the boat" in a group by providing a dissenting opinion can lead to what is known as groupthink. Although **groupthink** is a state of harmony within a group (because everyone is seemingly in a state of agreement), it can lead to some pretty terrible decisions. Groupthink manifests in a group when certain factors come together. Groups that are at risk tend to be overly friendly and cohesive, isolated from dissenting opinions, and inclined to favor the decisions of a directive leader.

There are certain symptoms that are often clues to the presence of groupthink:

- the group is optimistic about its capabilities and has unquestioned belief in its stances—an overestimation of "might and right"
- the group becomes increasingly extreme by justifying its own decisions while demonizing those of opponents
- some members of the group prevent dissenting opinions from permeating the group by filtering out information and facts that go against the beliefs of the group (a process called **mindguarding**)
- there is pressure to conform, and so individuals censor their own opinions in favor of consensus, which creates an illusion of unanimity

Stigma and Deviance

As discussed earlier in this chapter, **deviance** involves a violation of society's standards of conduct or expectations. Deviant behavior can range from being late to an interview to smuggling drugs. In the United States, there are many groups who are classified as deviants, including drug pushers and gang members. However, more harmless groups can also be labeled deviants, including the obese and the mentally ill. Deviance can even involve positive acts, for example, Rosa Parks and other African Americans who refused to sit in the back of the bus were acting deviantly in an attempt to change norms they saw as unfair.

Society often devalues deviant members by assigning demeaning labels, called **stigma**. Entire groups may be labeled based on physical or behavioral qualities. For example, the term "fob" (for "fresh off the boat") has been used to refer to recent immigrants. Once these identities have been assigned, they can follow individuals and affect their lives based on the reactions other people have when they discover the labels. How might your behavior toward an individual change (for example, how likely would you be to hire the person) if you learned that he or she carried the label "felon"?

Conformity and Obedience

Behavior can often be contagious; for example, have you ever walked past someone on the street who is staring up at something on a tall building or in the sky? If you have never had this experience, try it and see what happens—more than likely other people around you will also start looking up. People, as social creatures, tend to do what others are doing. This can have an interesting impact on behavior. There are two well-known experiments that sought to investigate the influence of conformity and obedience.

Solomon Asch wanted to test the effects of **group pressure** (or **peer pressure**) on individuals' behavior, so he designed a series of simple experiments where subjects would be asked to participate in a study on visual perception. In the experiment, subjects were asked to determine which of three lines was most similar to a comparison line (there was one line that was clearly identical to the comparison line and the other two were clearly longer). When subjects completed this task alone, they erred less than 1% of the time. When subjects were placed in a room with several other people who they thought were also participating in the study, but who were actually **confederates** (meaning that they were part of the experiment), the results were quite different. On the first few tests, all of the confederates responded correctly. However, after a little while, the confederates began all choosing one of the incorrect lines. What's interesting is that Asch found that more than one-third of subjects conformed to the group by answering incorrectly. They chose to avoid the discomfort of being different, rather than trust their own judgment in answering. The phenomenon of adjusting behavior or thinking based on the behavior or thinking of others is called **conformity**.

Another commonly referenced experiment is **Stanley Milgram**'s study of obedience involving fake shocks. The participants in this study believed that they were in control of equipment that delivered shocks to another subject (the "learner") who was attempting to pass a memory test. No shocks were actually used. A researcher was in the room and directed the participant to administer increasing levels of shock to this purported subject, a confederate, by turning a dial whenever he or she answered incorrectly. The only contact the participant had with the learner was to hear the student's voice from the other room. When shocks were given at particular levels, the participants would hear moans, shouts of pain, pounding on the walls, and after that, dead silence. Milgram found that participants in the study were surprisingly obedient to the researcher's demands that they continue to administer the shocks. Out of 40 subjects, few questioned the procedure before reaching 300 volts and 26 of the subjects continued all the way to the maximum 450 volts. Milgram conducted many variations on his original experiment, to see how various independent variables affected obedience. He found that decreased distance of the "learner," increased distance of the authority figure, more casual wardrobe of the authority figure, and a shabbier office location all decreased obedience among subjects. While this series of experiments has long been considered a seminal study in the area of obedience research, many have sharply questioned not only Milgram's ethics (this experiment would never be permitted today) but also his methodology and the importance of his findings. Many note that only one variation of the original experiment yielded the oft-cited high rates of obedience. Moreover, there is evidence that many subjects did not believe they were actually administering shocks to the learner.

6.3

There are three ways that behavior may be motivated by social influences:

1) *Compliance*: compliant behavior is motivated by the desire to seek reward or to avoid punishment. There is likely to be a punishment for disobeying authority. Compliance is easily extinguished if rewards or punishments are removed.

2) *Identification*: identification behavior is motivated by the desire to be like another person or group. A participant who conformed in Asch's experiment likely did not want to be disapproved of for choosing a different answer than the rest of the group. Identification endures as long as there is still a good relationship with the person or group being identified with and there are not convincing alternative viewpoints presented.

3) *Internalization*: internalized behavior is motivated by values and beliefs that have been integrated into one's own value system. Someone who has internalized a value not to harm others may have objected to the shocks administered in Milgram's study. This is the most enduring motivation of the three.

When the motivation for compliance is desire for the approval of others and to avoid rejection, this is called **normative social influence**. With normative social influence, people conform because they want to be liked and accepted by others. This often leads to public compliance, but not necessarily private acceptance of social norms. **Informational social influence** is the process of complying because we want to do the right thing and we feel like others "know something I don't know." Informational social influence is more likely to apply to new situations, ambiguous situations, or situations in which an obvious authority figure is present.

There are several factors that influence conformity:

1) *Group Size:* a group doesn't have to be very large, but a group of 3–5 people will elicit more conformity than one with only 1–2 people.

2) *Unanimity:* there is a strong pressure not to dissent when everyone else agrees. However, if just one person disagrees, others are more likely to voice their real opinions.

3) *Cohesion:* an individual will more likely be swayed to agree with opinions that come from someone within a group with which the individual identifies.

4) *Status:* higher-status people have stronger influence on opinions.

5) *Accountability:* People tend to conform more when they must respond in front of others rather than in closed formats in which they cannot be held accountable for their opinions.

6) *No Prior Commitment:* once people have made public commitments, they tend to stick to them. For example, once someone has taken a pledge to become a fraternity brother, he is more likely to follow the norms of that group.

6.3 SOCIAL INTERACTION AND BEHAVIOR

All social interactions take place within social structures, which are composed of five elements: statuses, social roles, groups (previously discussed), social networks, and organizations. These five elements are developed through the process of socialization, discussed earlier. Social interactions include behaviors such as expressing emotion, managing others' impressions, and communicating.

Social Structures

Statuses and Roles

Status is a broad term in sociology that refers to all the socially defined positions within a society. These can include positions such as "president," "parent," "resident of Wisconsin," and "Republican." Needless to say, one person can hold multiple statuses at the same time. Some of these statuses may place someone in a higher social position while others may imply a lower position. One's **master status** is the one that dominates the others and determines that individual's general position in society. For example, an A-list movie star's life is typically completely dominated by the master status of "famous celebrity;" few people ever consider her other statuses, such as "wife," "mother," "American," etc. Sometimes the master status is not one the individual prefers; someone with a disability may be strongly identified by others as holding that status, with less attention paid to her other statuses, which she may find more important and fulfilling.

Statuses may be ascribed or achieved. **Ascribed statuses** are those that are assigned to a person by society regardless of the person's own efforts. For example, gender and race are ascribed statuses. **Achieved statuses** are considered to be due largely to the individual's efforts. These can include statuses such as "doctor," "parent," or "Democrat."

Roles

Social roles are expectations for people of a given social status. It is expected that doctors will possess strong medical knowledge and be intelligent. Role expectations can also come with ascribed statuses. There may be an expectation that a female is more likely to be a babysitter than a male. Roles help contribute to society's stability by making things more predictable.

However, roles can also be sources of tension in multiple ways. **Role conflict** happens when there is a conflict in society's expectations for *multiple statuses* held by the same person (for example, a male nurse or a gay priest). **Role strain** occurs when a *single status* results in conflicting expectations. For example, a homosexual man may feel pressure to avoid being "too gay" and also "not gay enough." **Role exit** is the process of disengaging from a role that has become closely tied to one's self-identity to take on another. Some examples include the transition from high school student to more independent college student living on campus with peers. Another would be transitioning from the workforce to retirement. These transitions are difficult because they involve the process of detaching from something significant, as well as embarking on something new and unknown.

Networks and Organizations

Networks

Think about the people you know. Now think about the people that those people know. As you keep extrapolating to more distant connections, you can get a sense of your **social network**. A social network is a web of social relationships, including those in which a person is directly linked to others as well as those in which people are indirectly connected through others. Facebook is a popular online social network. Social networks are often based on groups to which individuals belong. Network ties may be weak, but they can be powerful resources for meeting people (for example, using a network like LinkedIn to find a job).

Organizations

Large, more impersonal groups that come together to pursue particular activities and meet goals efficiently are called **organizations**. They tend to be complex and hierarchically structured. Formal organizations can include businesses, governments, and religious groups. Organizations serve the purpose of increasing efficiency, predictability, control, and uniformity in society. They also allow knowledge to be passed down more easily, so that individual people become more replaceable. As an example, consider going to a McDonald's. Because this corporation is an organization, one may expect a particular experience and menu options regardless of who is actually working at that particular restaurant.

There are three types of organizations. **Utilitarian organizations** are those in which members get paid for their efforts, such as businesses. **Normative organizations** motivate membership based on morally relevant goals, for example, Mothers Against Drunk Driving (MADD). **Coercive organizations** are those for which members do not have a choice in joining (for example, prisons). Like groups, organizations are influenced by statuses and roles and also help define statuses and roles.

Social Interactions

Expressing and Detecting Emotion

The physiological basis of emotion will be discussed in Chapter 7. Emotion is also vital in explaining how we react to situations and others. Emotions arise based on our (typically unconscious) appraisals of situations. The ability to quickly appraise situations using emotion has evolutionary significance: if we hear something and feel fearful, we might have the opportunity to escape a threatening situation faster than if we were to wait to see what was causing the noise, and then make a decision about whether it would be a good idea to escape. Some emotional responses, such as likes, dislikes, and fears, involve no conscious thought. More complex emotions, like hatred, love, guilt, and happiness, can have important influences on our memories, expectations, and interpretations. Take a simple example: if you are having an awful day and are in a really crummy mood when your mother calls you, you might have an expectation that she is calling to nag you about something, even when she is actually calling for some other reason.

We detect emotion in others using clues: their body language, tone and pitch in their voices, and expression on their faces, which can display an impressive array of emotions that humans are precisely wired to detect (Chapter 7). For example, through experiments it was determined that if we glimpse a face for a mere tenth of a second, we can accurately judge the emotion it portrays. The eyes and mouth are the two areas of the face that convey the most emotion: we can detect fear and anger in the eyes and happiness in the mouth. Some of our facial muscles can actually betray our emotions if we are trying to conceal our feelings. For example, lifting the inner part of the eyebrow conveys distress or concern. Raising the eyebrows and pulling them together conveys fear. Muscles in the eyes and cheeks convey happiness through smiling. Some people are more sensitive to emotional cues than others, and introverts are better at reading others' emotions, while extroverts are generally easier to read.

Gender Shapes Expression

Some studies suggest that women surpass men at reading emotional cues. Women's greater sensitivity to nonverbal cues perhaps explains their greater emotional literacy, or ability to describe their emotions. Men tend to describe emotions in simpler ways, while women are generally capable of describing more complex emotions. Women also demonstrate greater emotional responsiveness in positive and negative situations, with the one exception being anger. Anger is the one emotion that seems to be considered by most a "masculine" emotion. For example, when shown pictures of a gender-neutral face that was either smiling or angry, people were more likely to assume the face was male if it was angry, and female if it was smiling. **Empathy**, the ability to identify with others' emotions, is relatively equal between the sexes. Both men and women can "put themselves in someone else's shoes" and feel that person's pain or elation. But women are more likely than men to *express* empathy by crying or reporting genuine distress at another's misfortune. In studies, women tend to experience emotional events more deeply, with greater brain activation in the areas that process emotion, and are better able to remember emotional events later.

Culture Shapes Expression

Culture provides an additional filter for interpreting emotion. In other cultures, common emotions like fear and happiness are expressed in ways that Americans may find difficult to interpret. Gestures (movements of the hands and body that are used to express emotion) vary widely among cultures. For example, the use of a thumbs-up sign indicates to an American that things are "okay," but is used as an insult in some other cultures, whereas the extension of just the middle finger expresses anger or discourtesy in America, but is a neutral symbol in several other cultures. Certain facial expressions, however, seem to be universal; babies and blind people make the same universal emotional expressions with their faces. While cultures do share universal facial expressions, the degree to which emotion is expressed is influenced by culture. Cultures that promote individuality (such as Western cultures) also encourage emotional expressiveness. Like many other facets of human interaction, emotion is best understood by considering its biological, psychological, and sociological aspects.

Impression Management

In sociology and psychology, **impression management** or **self-presentation** is the conscious or unconscious process whereby people attempt to manage their own images by influencing the perceptions of others. This is achieved by controlling either the amount or type of information, or the social interaction. People construct images of themselves and want others to see them in certain lights. There are multiple impression management strategies that people employ. Assertive strategies for impression management include the use of active behaviors to shape our self-presentations, such as talking oneself up and showing off flashy status symbols to demonstrate a desired image. Defensive strategies for impression management include avoidance or self-handicapping. **Self-handicapping** is a strategy in which people create obstacles and excuses to avoid self-blame when they do poorly. It is easier to erect external hindrances to explain our poor performances than to risk considering, or having others consider, an internal characteristic to be the cause of a poor performance. A classic example is the student who loudly lets everyone know before an exam that she did not study. Her strategy is such that if she receives a poor grade on the exam, it can't be blamed on her intelligence (an internal characteristic that is likely an important element of her self-esteem), but must rather be blamed on an external factor, the fact that she didn't study.

Front Stage Versus Back Stage Self

The **dramaturgical perspective** in sociology stems from symbolic interactionism and posits that we imagine ourselves as playing certain roles when interacting with others. This perspective uses the theater as a metaphor for the way we present ourselves; we base our presentations on cultural values, norms, and expectations, with the ultimate goal of presenting an acceptable self to others. Dramaturgical theory suggests that our identities are not necessarily stable, but dependent on our interactions with others; in this way, we constantly remake who we are, depending on the situations we are in. Social interaction can be broken into two types: front stage and back stage. On the **front stage**, we play a role and use impression management to craft the way we come across to other people. On the **back stage**, we can "let down our guard" and be ourselves. For example, the way you dress and behave at work (front stage) is potentially very different from your dress and behavior at home (back stage).

Verbal and Nonverbal Communication

Nonverbal communication involves all of the methods for communication that we use that do not include words. Because humans are inherently visual creatures, a majority of these cues are visual, but we employ other cues as well. Nonverbal communication includes gestures, touch, body language, eye contact, facial expressions, and a host of finer subtleties. The act of communicating verbally also employs a lot of nonverbal cues, such as pitch, volume, rate, intonation, and rhythm. In a society in which written communication is exploding in popularity (for example, emails and text messaging), we also employ nonverbal cues in our writing, such as emoticons and emojis, use of capitalization and punctuation, and spacing. Consider the following three text messages. Each uses the same three words, yet they each express slightly different ideas:

OH MY GOSH!!!!!

Oh. My. Gosh.

Oh my... Gosh?

Social Behavior

Social behavior occurs between members of the same species within a given society. Communication occurs between members of the same species, and not usually between different species. Specific social behaviors include attraction, aggression, attachment, and social support.

Attraction

Attraction between members of the same species is a primary component of love, and explains much about friendship, romantic relationships, and other close social relationships. Researchers in social psychology are particularly interested in studying human attraction because it helps to explain how much we like, dislike, or hate others. Research into human attraction has found that the following three characteristics foster attraction: proximity, physical attractiveness, and similarity.

Proximity

Proximity (geographic nearness) is the most powerful predictor of friendship. Think of the people you consider your closest friends. How many of them shared a grade school classroom or a neighborhood with you growing up? How many people from your freshman dorm or living situation do you still consider to be close friends? People are more inclined to like, befriend, and even marry others from the same class, neighborhood, or office. People prefer repeated exposure to the same stimuli; this is known as the **mere exposure effect**. With certain exceptions, familiarity breeds fondness. This partially explains the common affinity for celebrities, and the fact that many people vote based on name recognition alone, regardless of whether or not they know much about a candidate. The tendency to like those in close proximity probably has an evolutionally foundation; for our ancestors, the familiar faces were likely the ones that could be trusted.

Appearance

Appearance also has a powerful impact on attraction. Physical attractiveness is an important predictor of attraction; in fact, studies show that people rate physically attractive people higher on a number of characteristics and traits, indicating that physically attractive people are somehow more likeable. While many aspects of attractiveness vary across cultures, some appear to be culturally universal, such as youthful appearance in women (perhaps reflecting a biological constraint of fertility), and maturity, dominance, and affluence in men. Humans also tend to prefer average, symmetrical faces. Attractiveness is also influenced by personality traits; people believed to have positive personality traits are judged more attractive.

Similarity

Similarity between people also impacts attraction. Friends and partners are likely to share common values, beliefs, interests, and attitudes. The more alike people are, the more their liking for each other endures over time.

Aggression

While attraction is an important unifying force in society, aggression is the opposite: a potentially destructive force to social relations. **Aggression** is broadly defined as behavior that is forceful, hostile, or attacking. In sociology, aggression is considered something that is intended to cause harm or promote social dominance within a group. Aggression can be communicated verbally or by actions or gestures. While aggression is employed for a variety of reasons by humans today (competitive sports, war, getting ahead at work), in non-human animals it is generally employed as a means for protecting resources, such as food, territory, and mates. Indeed, aggression was likely employed for similar reasons by prehistoric humans, and as our society evolved, we began using aggression in additional ways.

Aggression is considered an instinct, but biology and society can influence aggression. There are three types of predictors for aggressive behavior: genetic, neural, and biochemical. Identical twin studies suggest that there is some genetic predisposition toward aggressiveness; if one twin has a temper, the other tends to as well. Humans and other animals are naturally wired both to inhibit and to exhibit aggressive behavior. While no particular locus in the brain controls aggression, certain areas are thought to facilitate aggression, while other areas (in the frontal lobe) inhibit aggression. Many biochemical factors can alter the neural control of aggression. Alcohol, for example, can lower aggression inhibition, making someone more aggressive while drunk. Animals also tend to exhibit less aggression when they are castrated.[1]

Many psychological and social factors are thought to trigger aggression in humans. The **frustration-aggression principle** suggests that when someone is blocked from achieving a goal, this frustration can trigger anger, which can lead to aggression. Other frustrating stimuli, such as physical pain, unpleasant odors, and hot temperatures can also lead to aggression. Aggression is more likely to occur in situations in which prior experience has somehow promoted aggression. For example, if a child acts aggressively toward another child and ends up getting what she wants (lunch money, for example), she is more likely to behave in an aggressive manner in the future. People who are ostracized are also more likely to behave aggressively, which may partially explain some of the mass shootings that have occurred in schools and public spaces. While it would be a mistake to oversimplify the roots of aggression, it seems clear that biology, experience, and society combine to provide the fodder for aggression.

---

[1] Though castration does not *completely* remove aggression, as territorial battles between "fixed" housecats illustrate.

6.3

Social Support

Social support is a major determinant of health and wellbeing for humans and other animals. Family relationships provide comfort, and close relationships are predictive of health outcomes. Happily married people live longer, healthier lives, regardless of age, sex, and race. People who have social support have been shown to engage in healthier behaviors; they are less likely to smoke, more likely to exercise, and report a better capacity to cope with adversity and stress. Interestingly, social support is not confined to human-human interactions. People with dogs or other pets also reap some of the benefits of social support.

Biological Explanations of Social Behavior in Animals

Many animals also exhibit a wide range of social behavior. Some species (such as ants, bees, and wasps) engage in highly organized and hierarchical social behaviors, with each individual playing a specific role within the group. Most mammals also engage in social behavior, and many interesting phenomena have been elucidated by studying how mammals interact with members of their own species.

Foraging Behavior

Foraging behavior describes the search for and exploitation of food resources by animals. Securing food can come at a high energetic cost, which is an important consideration for organisms; the amount of energy it requires a lion to track, chase, and kill an antelope, or the amount of energy it takes an antelope to search for and graze upon enough foliage to sustain itself matters greatly to that organism's patterns of behavior. Ethologists believe that organisms employ learning behavior in the search for food. Since an organism's environment is constantly changing, it is important that foraging behavior be adaptable. Many organisms employ observational learning of older members in the group to learn behaviors such as knowing what is safe to eat.

Mating Behavior and Mate Choice

Mating behavior involves the pairing of opposite-sex organisms for the purposes of reproduction and the propagation of genes. Mating behaviors include courtship rituals, copulation, the building of nests, and the rearing of offspring for specific periods. For animals, mating strategies include random mating, disassortative mating, and assortative mating. In random mating, all members of a species are equally likely to mate with each other, meaning that there are no spatial, genetic, or behavioral limitations on mating. This ensures the largest amount of genetic diversity, and protects against genetic drift and bottlenecking. Assortative mating is a nonrandom mating pattern in which individuals with similar genotypes or phenotypes mate with each other more frequently than would be expected with random mating. In negative assortative mating, also known as disassortative mating, individuals with more disparate traits mate more frequently than would be expected with random mating.

Inclusive Fitness and Altruism

The **inclusive fitness** of an organism is defined by the number of offspring the organism has, how it supports its offspring, and how its offspring support others in a group. The inclusive fitness theory proposes that an organism can improve its overall genetic success through altruistic social behaviors. An **altruistic behavior** is one that helps ensure the success or survival of the rest of a social group, possibly at the expense of the success or survival of the individual. For example, the ground squirrel, a social mammal that lives in dens underground, will sound an alarm call if it sees a predator near the group. The alarm call does two things: first, it alerts the rest of the group to danger, and second, it calls the predator's attention to the particular squirrel that makes the noise. Therefore, in many instances, alerting the group results in the demise of the individual that sounded the alarm. Even though the alerter has not survived to reproduce, it has helped promote the survival of the rest of the clan, many of whom are probably close genetic relatives. In this way, the altruistic behavior of the ground squirrel has increased its own inclusive fitness by ensuring the survival of its siblings and other genetic relatives.

Applying Game Theory

Evolutionary **game theory** is used to try and predict large, complex systems, such as the overall behavior of a population. Evolutionary game theory has been used to explain many complex and challenging aspects of biology, such as how altruistic behaviors work in the context of Darwinian natural selection. While it may seem that large groups of animals and large crowds of people are too complex to accurately predict behavior, game theory suggests that it might be possible to do so. This type of analysis might be useful, for instance, in predicting the behavior of a large crowd of people in an enclosed space during a disaster. While this field is still emerging, it may be quite possible to accurately predict behavior in complex living systems in the future.

6.4 SOCIAL COGNITION AND INTELLIGENCE

Attitudes are an important part of what makes us human and what makes us unique. Our attitudes about people, places, and things are shaped by experience, but can be highly mutable. Attitude and behavior are intimately related, and it is important to understand how both develop and change over time.

Elaboration Likelihood Model

Persuasion is one method of attitude and behavior change. When you change your beliefs about something, there are a few factors that likely come into play. For example, say you are listening to two speeches about the importance of expanding the ban on smoking in public spaces. The first orator is attractive, but his argument is not well-formulated. The second orator's speech has better, more logical arguments, but he is not as attractive. Whose argument will persuade you more? The **elaboration likelihood model** explains when people will be influenced by the content of the speech (or the logic of the arguments), and when people will be influenced by other, more superficial characteristics like the appearance of the orator or the length of the speech.

Since persuasion can be such a powerful means for influencing what people think and do, much research has gone into studying the various elements of a message that is likely to be highly persuasive. The three key elements are message characteristics, source characteristics, and target characteristics.

1) The **message characteristics** are the features of the message itself, such as the logic and number of key points in the argument. Message characteristics also include more superficial factors, such as the length of the speech or article and its grammatical complexity.
2) The **source characteristics** of the person or entity delivering the message, such as expertise, knowledge, and trustworthiness, are also of importance. People are much more likely to be persuaded by a major study described in the *New England Journal of Medicine* than in the pages of the local supermarket tabloid.

6.4

3) Finally, the **target characteristics** of the person receiving the message, such as self-esteem, intelligence, mood, and other such personal characteristics, have an important influence on whether a message will be perceived as persuasive. For instance, some studies have suggested that those with higher intelligence are less easily persuaded by one-sided messages.

The two **cognitive routes** that persuasion follows under this model are the central route and the peripheral route. Under the **central route,** people are persuaded by the *content* of the argument. They ruminate over the key features of the argument and allow those features to influence their decisions to change their points of view. The **peripheral route** functions when people focus on superficial or secondary characteristics of the speech or the orator. Under these circumstances, people are persuaded by the attractiveness of the orator, the length of the speech, whether the orator is considered an expert in his field, or other features. The elaboration likelihood model asserts that people will choose the central route only when they are both motivated to listen to the logic of the argument (they are interested in the topic), and they are not distracted, thus focusing their attention on the argument. If those conditions are not met, individuals will choose the peripheral route, and, if persuaded at all, will be persuaded by more superficial factors. Messages processed via the central route are more likely to have longer-lasting persuasive outcomes than messages processed via the peripheral route.

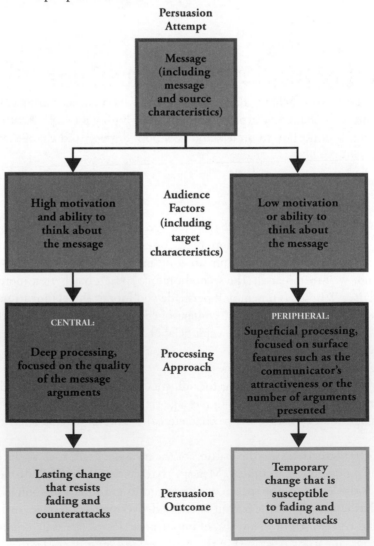

Figure 3 Elaboration likelihood model: central vs. peripheral processing routes

Social Cognitive Theory

The social cognitive perspective incorporates elements of cognition, learning, and social influence. **Social Cognitive Theory** is a theory of behavior change that emphasizes the interactions between people and their environment. However, unlike behaviorism (where the environment controls us), cognition (how we process our environment) is also important in determining our behavior. Social cognitive theory focuses on how we interpret and respond to external events and how our past experiences, memories, and expectations influence our behavior. According to social cognitive theory, **social factors**, observational learning, and environmental factors can also influence a person's attitude change. The opinions and attitudes of your friends, family members, and other peer groups often have a major influence on your beliefs.

Reciprocal determinism is the interaction between a person's behaviors (conscious actions), personal factors (individual motivational forces or cognitions; personality differences that drive a person to act), and environment (situational factors). There are three different ways that individuals and environments interact.

1) People choose their environments which in turn shape them. For example, the college that you chose to attend had some sort of unique impact on you.
2) Personality shapes how people interpret and respond to their environment. For example, people prone to depression are more likely to view their jobs as pointless.
3) A person's personality influences the situation to which she then reacts. Experiments have demonstrated that how you treat someone else influences how they will treat you. For example, if you call customer service because you are furious about something, you are more likely to receive a defensive or aggressive response on the phone.

In these three ways people both shape, and are shaped by, their environments.

Behavioral Genetics

Genetics plays an important role in the behavior of humans and other animals. **Behavioral genetics** attempts to determine the role of inheritance in behavioral traits; the interaction between heredity and experience determines an individual's personality and social behavior.

Almost every cell in the body contains DNA [which cells in humans do not contain DNA?[2]], and this DNA contains genes, some 20,000 or so in humans. Genes encode the information for creating proteins, the building blocks of physical development. To help determine what makes us different (for example, why one person suffers from schizophrenia while his brother does not), it is vital to understand the variations in both our genes and our environments. The **genotype** is the genetic makeup of an organism, while the **phenotype** is the observable characteristics and traits. Behavioral genetics seeks to understand how the genotype and environment affect the phenotype.

Most phenotypes are influenced by several genes and by the environment; for example, tallness in humans is the result of the interaction between several genes, and is also the result of proper nutrition at key developmental stages. If someone is born with genes for tallness, but is malnourished as a child, they will not grow nearly as tall as their genotype might indicate. Therefore, in order to determine the influence of genes versus the environment (the old "nature versus nurture" argument!), behavioral genetics uses two types of studies in humans: twin studies and adoption studies.

---

[2] Mature red blood cells do not contain DNA.

Twin studies compare traits in monozygotic (identical) and dizygotic (fraternal) twins. Monozygotic (MZ) twins have essentially identical genotypes[3] and an almost identical environment (assuming they are reared together), starting from the womb[4]. Dizygotic (DZ) twins share roughly 50% of their DNA (they are genetically no more similar than ordinary siblings), and an arguably similar environment, starting in the womb. The classic twin study attempts to assess the variance of a phenotype (behavior, psychological disorder) in a large group in order to estimate genetic effects (heritability) and environmental effects (both from shared environment or experiences and unshared/unique environment or experiences). If identical twins share the phenotype more than fraternal twins (which is the case for most traits), genes likely play an important role. For example, if one MZ twin develops Alzheimer's disease, the other MZ twin has a 60% chance of developing it as well. Alternatively, if one DZ twin develops the disease, the other only has a 30% chance of developing it. By comparing hundreds of twin pairs, researchers can understand more about the roles of genetic effects, shared environment, and unique environment in shaping behavior.

Adoption studies present another unique way to study the effects of genetics and environment on phenotype. Adoption creates two groups: genetic relatives and environmental relatives. Adopted individuals can be compared with both groups to determine if they are more similar to their genetic relatives or their environmental relatives. The advantage of adoption studies over twin studies is that they can help to elucidate the impact of both heredity and environment on phenotype. Twin studies can only examine the impact of genetics because the environment is so similar for each twin. Interestingly, hundreds of studies have shown that people who grow up together do not much resemble one another's personalities. Adopted children have personalities more similar to their biological parents than their adopted parents; traits such as agreeableness, extraversion, introversion, etc. tend to pass from parents to biological offspring. However, adopted children are more similar to their adoptive families in terms of attitudes, values, manners, faith, and politics.

There have been some cases of identical twins separated at birth and raised independently by different adopted families. Psychologists have noted that these individuals, despite being raised in completely different environments with no contact with each other while growing up, are remarkably similar in terms of their tastes, physical abilities, personality, interests, attitudes, and fears.

Using twin and adoption studies, behavioral geneticists can mathematically estimate heritability for many phenotypes. Heritability does not pertain to an individual, but rather to how two individuals differ. For example, the estimated heritability of intelligence (the variation of intelligence scores attributable to genetic factors) is roughly 50%. This does not mean that your genes are responsible for 50% of your intelligence, rather, it means that heredity is responsible for 50% of the variation in intelligence between you and someone else. In fact, it means that genetic differences account for 50% of the variation in intelligence *among all people*.

---

[3] Though MZ twins have the same genes, they don't always have the same number of copies of a gene; this may help to explain why one develops a disease, while the other does not. Furthermore, X inactivation in female somatic cells is not identical between MZ female twins; therefore, female MZ twins are actually not *quite* as identical as male MZ twins!

[4] About 70% of MZ twins share a placenta in the womb, and in some instances, one twin will receive more blood flow, resulting in differential nutrition and growth between the two. Additionally, approximately 30% of MZ twins develop separate placentas and therefore may have slightly different prenatal conditions, as well.

Figure 4 The heritability of intelligence, estimated using twin studies and adoption studies

In animals, the interaction between genotype and phenotype is easier to study because genes and environment can be more tightly controlled. Researchers can use **transgenesis** (the introduction of an exogenous[5] or outside gene) or knockout genes to alter genotype while controlling for environment. Transgenic animal models are useful for helping researchers understand what happens when a certain gene is present. For example, transgenic mice that have had human cancer genes introduced can help researchers study how and when cancer develops, and how cancer responds to various treatments in the mouse model (before trying the treatments on humans). Knockout animal models are useful for helping researchers understand what happens when a gene is absent. For example, knockout mice that are missing a specific gene known to protect against cancer can also help researchers understand how and why cancer develops, and how it responds to treatment.

One of the most important aspects of all life—from single-celled organisms to human beings—is the capacity for adaptation. Genes and environment work together; not only do genes code for proteins, but they also respond to the environment. Genes might be turned on in one environment and turned off in another. For example, in response to an ongoing stressor, one gene might begin producing more of a neurotransmitter involved in overeating, which then leads to obesity. The gene itself was not hard-wired to produce obesity, but an interaction between the gene and the environment resulted in obesity.

Genes and environment interact. Consider the example of **temperament** (emotional excitability): infants who are considered "difficult" have a temperament that is more irritable and unpredictable, while infants who are considered "easy" have a more placid, quiet, and easygoing temperament. While heredity might predispose infants toward these temperament differences, an easy baby will be treated differently than a difficult baby, and studies have shown that temperament persists through childhood and beyond. Do difficult babies grow up to be aggressive, pugnacious teenagers because their temperament is genetically wired, or because their parents reacted to their irritability and unpredictability in infancy with frustration and unsupportive caregiving? It is difficult to say, but it is important to understand that both heredity and environment play an important role in many complex human traits, such as personality (of which temperament is one aspect), intelligence, and motivation.

---

[5] In Greek, "exo" means "outside" and "gignomi" means "to come to be."

Intellectual Functioning

Multiple Definitions of Intelligence

What is intelligence? We often think of it as something objective that can be measured like height and weight, but the concept of intelligence is a human creation. A common definition is the ability to learn from experience, problem-solve, and use knowledge to adapt to new situations. But there is no neurological trait that defines intelligence. Consider the concept of athleticism. Athleticism can be broadly defined as physical prowess. However, it becomes difficult to define details since athleticism could be defined by one's speed, agility, ability to lift weights, or visual motor skills. Based on the criteria, a golfer or a football player may or may not be considered an athlete.

Theories of Intelligence

Francis Galton first proposed a theory of general intelligence in the mid 1800s. Galton believed intelligence had a strong biological basis and could be quantified by testing certain cognitive tasks. Galton's book, *Hereditary Genius*, argues that intelligence is genetically determined. In the early 1900s, **Alfred Binet** administered intelligence tests to schoolchildren in France, with the goal of developing a measure to determine which children were in need of special education. The intelligence test, better known as an IQ (intelligence quotient) test, created by Binet (and his collaborator, Theodore Simon) was later revised by a psychologist at Stanford University and renamed the Stanford-Binet Intelligence Scale. Also in the early 1900s, **Charles Spearman** first coined the term **general intelligence** (also referred to as "Spearman's g"); Spearman, like Binet, believed that intelligence could be strictly quantified through cognitive tests, and those who possessed high general intelligence would do well on lots of different measures of cognitive ability.

In the mid-twentieth century, psychologist **Raymond Cattell** proposed two types of intelligence: fluid intelligence (Gf), which is the ability to "think on your feet" and solve novel problems, and crystallized intelligence (Gc), which is the ability to recall and apply already-learned information (which is the majority of what you are expected to do in school—learn and memorize information, then apply it on test day). In the 1980s, **Howard Gardner** put forth a theory on multiple intelligences, which breaks intelligence down into eight different modalities: logical, linguistic, spatial, musical, kinesthetic, naturalist, intrapersonal, and interpersonal intelligences. This theory is a nice counter to the idea that intelligence is a single general ability that can be conveniently measured and quantified by an IQ test. While Gardner was not the first to consider the importance of social intelligence (**Edward Thorndike** first proposed the idea of social intelligence in the 1920s, defined as the ability to manage and understand people), the theory of multiple intelligences did renew interest in the concept of social intelligence. This renewed interest led to the idea of emotional intelligence in the 1990s. Emotional intelligence involves being well attuned to one's own emotions, being able to accurately intuit the emotions of others, and using this information as a guide for thinking and acting. Studies suggest that both emotional intelligence and social intelligence are correlated with good leadership skills, good interpersonal skills, positive outcomes in classroom situations, and better functioning in the world.

Influence of Heredity and Environment on Intelligence

Is it natural ability, or is it the environment and experiences that determine one's intellectual abilities? As you might expect, it's a little bit of both. Studies of twins, family members, and adopted children indicate that there is significant heritability of intelligence. Scores on intelligence tests taken by identical twins correlate highly, while those of adopted children more closely resemble scores of their birth parents than of their adoptive parents. However, although genes are a predisposing factor, life experiences affect one's performance on intelligence tests. Malnutrition, sensory deprivation, social isolation, and trauma can affect normal brain development in childhood. On the other hand, early intervention and schooling can increase intelligence scores.

Also remember that intelligence is a social construct. The way it is measured is determined by cultural context. In many Western cultures, intelligence is often thought of as superior performance on academic and cognitive tasks. Some of these tasks emphasize speed, because it is valued in those societies. However, other cultures may emphasize emotional and spiritual knowledge, or social skills.

Variations in Intellectual Ability

Some differences have been found in how various groups perform on intelligence tests. These differences have often been attributed to biases within the tests themselves or related to outside confounding factors. For example, controversial but well-established findings are that racial groups differ in their average scores on intelligence tests, and that high-scoring people are more likely to attain high levels of education and income. However, these differences are potentially due to environmental factors, such as the availability of quality schooling.

Intellectual abilities at the upper and lower extremes have profound social and functional implications. At the lower extreme are individuals whose intelligence scores fall below 70. On intelligence tests, a score of 70 is two standard deviations below the average score of 100. Individuals who not only have a score below 70, but also have difficulty adapting to everyday demands of life are classified as having an **intellectual disability**. Sometimes, intellectual disability is the product of a physical cause, such as Down's syndrome or an acquired brain injury. Students with mild intellectual disabilities are educated in the least restrictive environments in which they can learn, and they are integrated into regular classrooms with accommodations if possible. At the upper extreme, high intelligence scores (130+) often serve as selection criteria for gifted education.

Experience and Behavior

While it is true that our genes play an important role in our behavior, our individual experiences and our social experiences also shape our behavior in important ways. The **life course perspective**, or **life course approach** looks at how key events in a person's life such as marriage, professional milestones, and the birth of children unfold over time and lead to a person's development. As social animals, we learn ways of thinking and behavior from our families and peer groups. An individual's development, then, is determined by a complex interplay of biology, psychology, society, and culture. Biological influences include the inherited genome, prenatal development, sex-related genes, hormones, and physiology. Psychological influences include gene-environment interactions, significant experiences, responses evoked in others by our own traits (such as our temperament or gender), and beliefs, feelings, and expectations. Social and cultural influences include families, peers, friends, cultural ideals, cultural mores, and cultural norms.

Chapter 6 Summary

- Culture refers to the beliefs and practices that a social group shares.

- Socialization is the process by which people learn the norms, values, attitudes, and beliefs necessary to become proficient members of society.

- Norms are spoken or unspoken rules and expectations for the behavior in society.

- Cultural assimilation occurs when an individual forsakes their own culture to completely adopt another culture; amalgamation occurs when majority and minority groups combine to form a new group.

- Multiculturalism or pluralism endorses equal standing for all cultural traditions within a society.

- A subculture is a segment of society that shares a distinct pattern of traditions and values that differs from that of the larger society.

- Self-concept or self-identity is the sum of an individual's understanding of him- or herself, including physical, psychological, and social attributes.

- Personal identity includes personal attributes (such as age, disability status, ethnicity/race), while social identity consists of social definitions (such as religion, gender, occupation).

- Self-efficacy is a belief in one's own competence and effectiveness, while self-esteem is an individual's evaluation of his or her overall worth.

- Those with an internal locus of control believe they are able to influence outcomes through their own effort; those with an external locus of control believe outcomes are controlled by outside forces.

- Multiculturalism or pluralism endorses equal standing for all cultural traditions within a society.

- Kohlberg described six stages of moral development; most adults reach stage 4, but few reach stage 6.

- In order to determine whether behavior should be attributed to internal or external causes, consistency, distinctiveness, and consensus must be considered.

- The fundamental attribution error occurs when people tend to underestimate the impact of the situation and overestimate the impact of a person's character or personality on observed behavior.

- The self-serving bias is the tendency to attribute our successes to ourselves and our failures to others or to the external environment.

- The optimism bias is the belief that bad things happen to other people, but not to us; the just world phenomenon is a tendency to believe that the world is fair and people get what they deserve.

- Stereotypes are oversimplified ideas about groups of people, based on characteristics (race, gender, sexual orientation, religion, disability, etc.).

- A self-fulfilling prophecy occurs when stereotypes lead to behaviors that affirm the original stereotypes; stereotype threat refers to a self-fulfilling fear that one will be evaluated based on a negative stereotype.

- The social facilitation effect occurs when people perform simple, well-learned tasks better when other people are present.

- Deindividuation occurs in situations that provide a high degree of arousal and a very low sense of responsibility, when people lose their sense of restraint and their individual identity by identifying with a group or mob mentality.

- The bystander effect predicts the finding that a person is less likely to provide help when there are other bystanders.

- Social loafing is the tendency for people to exert less effort when they are being evaluated as a group than when they are individually accountable.

- Group polarization occurs when group members adopt more extreme versions of their original viewpoints as the result of group membership.

- Groupthink is a phenomenon that occurs within a group when the desire for harmony or conformity in the group results in a consensual perspective without much thought of alternative viewpoints.

- Deviance is a violation of society's expectations or standards of conduct.

- Behavior is motivated by social influences when there is compliance, identification, and internalization.

- Several factors influence conformity: group size, unanimity, cohesion, status, accountability, and lack of prior commitment.

- The elaboration likelihood model of persuasion is the theory that attitudes are formed by dual processes: the central processing route (which includes high motivation and deep processing of the message) or by the peripheral processing route (which includes low motivation and superficial processing of the messenger).

- Behavioral genetics attempts to determine the role of inheritance in behavioral traits; the interaction between heredity and experience determines an individual's personality and social behavior.

CHAPTER 6 FREESTANDING PRACTICE QUESTIONS

1. Agent(s) of socialization include:

   I. parents.
   II. teachers.
   III. friends.

   A) I only
   B) I and II
   C) II and III
   D) I, II, and III

2. Eli studies really hard for his chemistry class but keeps getting poor scores on quizzes and lab assignments. Eventually, he begins to feel like nothing he does will improve his performance in chemistry. When faced with future chemistry assignments, Eli doesn't even bother trying because he feels destined to fail at chemistry. This can best be described as:

   A) learned helplessness.
   B) an internal locus of control.
   C) incongruity.
   D) the fundamental attribution error.

3. Marcia wears clothing that she thinks are appropriate but that are also sharply criticized by her community. Upon learning of the criticism, Marcia is overcome with guilt and feelings of shame. As a result, she vows never to wear that type of clothing again. According to Kohlberg, Marcia is most likely at which level/stage of moral development?

   A) Preconventional morality
   B) Stage 1: Punishment and obedience orientation
   C) Conventional morality
   D) Stage 6: Universal ethical principles

4. When new members of a society eventually become indistinguishable from the rest of society, adopting the language, norms, and customs, which process has occurred?

   A) Multiculturalism
   B) Amalgamation
   C) Assimilation
   D) Groupthink

5. A researcher randomly surveys people, asking them how they found out about their most recent job: either through an acquaintance or through a close friend. The researcher concluded that the results proved the social network theory, which suggests:

   A) more respondents found their jobs from an acquaintance rather than a close friend.
   B) more respondents found their jobs from a close friend rather than an acquaintance.
   C) half of the respondents found their jobs from an acquaintance, while the other half of the respondents found their jobs from a close friend.
   D) a majority of respondents found their jobs on their own.

6. A doctor does a checkup on a 40-year-old patient and talks to him in a serious and professional manner. A few moments later, the same doctor goes to a different room to do a routine checkup on a 5-year-old patient. The doctor makes funny faces throughout the checkup in order to make the patient laugh. This scenario is most closely related to which concept?

A) Deviance
B) Impression management
C) Conflict theory
D) Symbolic interactionism

7. College students have started an environmental awareness club on their campus. At the first meeting, they gave out a questionnaire, which indicated that the students in attendance strongly favored policies protecting the environment. At the end of the school year, the questionnaire was re-administered to the same students. The results indicated that the membership had become even more strongly in favor of environmental protection policies. This scenario most likely illustrates which of the following phenomenon?

A) Groupthink
B) Group polarization
C) Deindividuation
D) Peer pressure

8. Despite having a stake in an upcoming election, a citizen eligible to vote declines to go to the polls, declaring that her vote is too insignificant to make a difference and she knows her candidate will win anyway. Her behavior is most demonstrative of which of the following?

A) Social loafing theory
B) Opponent-process theory
C) Regression to the mean
D) Group polarization

CHAPTER 6 PRACTICE PASSAGE

When people want to establish a new form of identity, they undergo an exiting process to transition from their ex-role to their new role. The exiting process from their ex-role will be satisfied once society gives acknowledgment to the individual's change in identity. This is a difficult transition because society has already set expectations for the individual based on their ex-role. Through a series of interviews with people who have undergone role exiting, ranging from ex-nuns to ex-convicts, researchers found several issues that individuals encounter in the process of creating new roles.

The first issue that individuals face is the presentation of self. Individuals use external and internal indicators to publicly show others that they would like to be treated differently from their past selves. For example, transgender individuals, who identify with a gender that is the opposite of their biological sex, alter their clothes and mannerisms based on what they believe society considers acceptable for the sex they want to convey in their new role. It is the responsibility of others in society to recognize the individual's new identity through the newly acquired props and mannerisms the individual employs.

Social reaction is another issue for those exiting an old role and assuming a new one. During the exiting process, individuals are affected by reactions they receive from society based on their ex-role. Role exits are either socially desirable (such as being a drug user turning into an ex-drug user) or socially undesirable (such as being a doctor and turning into an ex-doctor). People continue to hold positive or negative expectations about the old role that an individual is trying to break away from as they continue through the exiting process. However, the more society expects certain behaviors from an individual, the more likely the individual will act in a way they are expected to act. For instance, if parents and teachers continue to treat a student like a delinquent, it is likely that the student will continue to misbehave because he is fulfilling the role assigned. The presentation of self and social reaction to the ex-role together determine the difficulty of adapting to the new role for the individual.

Another challenge is the change of friendship networks for the individual. People who shift identities are inclined to distance themselves from their old peers in order to be surrounded with a network that would encourage and facilitate their new role. For example, individuals who are married surround themselves with other married couples. However, if they become "ex-spouses," they are likely to begin associating with single people and fellow divorcées because their interactions with other married couples are different and uncomfortable. Additionally, while in their old role, individuals formed bonds with other people. After role-exiting, individuals have to manage their relationships with people who continue to be a part of their ex-role as well as those who are part of their new role.

Finally, individuals face role residuals, which can also be known as "hangover identity." This concept describes the number of aspects that persist for an individual from an ex-role even after completing the exiting process to their newly formed identity. Overall, the more involved an individual was in his former role, the more likely he is to have a higher role residual compared to someone who was not as committed to his previous role.

Source: Adapted from H.R.F. Ebaugh, *Becoming an Ex: The Process of Role Exit*. ©1988 by The University of Chicago Press

1. Which of the following theories best describes the process of presentation of self in creating an ex-role?

A) Social facilitation
B) Dramaturgy
C) Social support
D) Peer pressure

2. Which of the following scenarios describes the self-serving bias?

A) An employee who receives a bonus believes this reward was well-deserved because of how hard she worked and all of the extra hours she put into her job.
B) A man who is ignored by a salesperson at a high-end suit store believes the salesperson is just a rude jerk.
C) A survey finds that most people think that attractive celebrities are good people.
D) An employee receives a promotion and feels lucky to have been "in the right place at the right time."

3. Based on the passage, which of the following types of social identities do transgender individuals try to express through their self-presentation?

   I. Sexual orientation
   II. Gender
   III. Biological sex

A) I only
B) II only
C) III only
D) II and III

4. A felon fails to find a job because potential employers are aware of his role as a convict. Which of the following concepts best describes this social reaction?

A) Social stigma
B) Social support
C) False consensus
D) Socialization

5. All of the following are ways that an individual's behavior may be motivated by social influences, EXCEPT:

A) compliance.
B) identification.
C) aggregation.
D) internalization.

6. Which of the following individuals would most likely experience "hangover identity?"

A) A biological male who identifies as a female, but has not yet begun the transition to the female gender
B) An alcoholic who was sober for six months and then relapsed
C) Someone who was married for six weeks and then gets a divorce
D) A recent retiree who worked at the same company for 45 years, had a tight group of friends at work, participated in the company Thursday night bowling league, and volunteered with her colleagues every holiday season in a neighborhood soup kitchen

SOLUTIONS TO CHAPTER 6 FREESTANDING PRACTICE QUESTIONS

1. **D** Item I is true: family, including parents, are considered agents of socialization (choice C can be eliminated). Item II is true: educators, like teachers, are agents of socialization (choice A can be eliminated). Item III is true: peers and friends are also agents of socialization (choice B can be eliminated; choice D is correct).

2. **A** Learned helplessness occurs when someone tries hard but fails repeatedly at a task. Eventually, the individual believes that they have no control over the outcome, develops an external locus of control (choice B is wrong), and stops trying (choice A is correct). Incongruity refers to the idea that the real self has fallen short of the ideal self; while this might pertain to the situation described in the question stem, there is not enough evidence to assume that succeeding in chemistry is part of Eli's idealized self (choice C is wrong). The fundamental attribution error occurs when an individual attributes the actions of others (but not their own actions) to dispositional factors (choice D is wrong).

3. **C** The question asks how far Marcia appears to have progressed in terms of Kohlberg's stages of moral development. Marcia views her behavior as bad if other people view it as bad, feeling shame and guilt when others criticize her. Thus, she is in the "conventional" level of morality. More specifically, she is most likely in stage 3 (the "good boy/girl" stage) in which morality is determined by others' approval (choice C is correct). If you didn't remember Kohlberg, you can use POE to eliminate some of the choices. Marcia seems to be past the stage 1: preconventional level of moral development in which good = avoidance of punishment (this is common among very young children). Marcia genuinely feels guilty and ashamed because she believes she did something wrong; she's not simply conforming to escape some punishment (choices A and B can be eliminated). Stage 6: universal ethical principles wouldn't seem to fit here either. Marcia sees an action as "wrong" because others see it that way, not because it violates some higher universal moral code that she's developed (choice D can be eliminated).

4. **C** Assimilation occurs when a new member forgoes her own culture in order to adapt to the dominant culture. When new members of society eventually become indistinguishable from the rest of society, assimilation has occurred (choice C is correct). Multiculturalism asserts that different cultures can live harmoniously without newcomers feeling the need to adjust or adapt to the dominant culture (choice A is wrong). Amalgamation occurs when two cultures combine to form a new culture, different from both of the original cultures (choice B is wrong). Groupthink is the phenomenon whereby a cohesive group establishes a consensual perspective without much thought to alternative viewpoints (choice D is wrong).

5. **A** The social network theory posits that people's networks are important and necessary for the spread of ideas and resources; there is much strength in weak ties because weak ties allow the sharing of new resources to a vast network. It is more likely for participants to find jobs through an acquaintance (weak tie) than a close friend (strong tie; choice A is correct). Although having strong ties has an advantage with respect to people's networks, there is a sense of redundancy with the information and resources provided; generally people's strong ties have information that the person is already aware of since they are a part of the same

cluster (choice B is wrong). Since the researcher concluded that the results "proved the social network theory," it wouldn't make sense for the results to be half and half (choice C is wrong), nor would it make sense that most respondents found their jobs on their own (choice D is wrong).

6. **B** Impression management involves expressing different aspects of oneself, depending on the person on the receiving end of the interaction. The doctor acts differently toward the 40-year-old patient and the 5-year-old patient (choice B is correct). Deviance occurs when an individual is violating social norms. It is socially acceptable for the doctor to act professionally with the adult and silly with the child (choice A is wrong). Conflict theory is the belief that inequality exists due to an uneven distribution of power and resources in society; this theory is unrelated to the scenario described in the question (choice C is wrong). Symbolic interactionism asserts that the way individuals interpret interactions affects how they choose to interact. In comparison with impression management, symbolic interactionism is not more closely related to the scenario and does not fully explain the doctor's different behavior toward the two patients (choice D is wrong).

7. **B** The key words are "strongly favored policies protecting the environment" and "even more strongly in favor of environmental protection policies." The correct answer choice will be a concept in social psychology that explains how like-minded people, when they have been meeting over time, tend to become even more intensely aligned with their original points of view. That is choice B, group polarization (choices A, C, and D do not match the scenario and are incorrect).

8. **A** According to social loafing theory, people working in groups will exert less effort when they are not held individually accountable, downplaying the importance of their own contribution while assuming that someone else will take up the slack. Because the citizen described does have a stake in the election, but decides not to vote because she believes her vote won't make a difference (she assumes that the candidate will win because everyone else will vote for that candidate), her behavior can best be explained by social loafing (choice A is correct). The opponent-process theory has to do with color perception, not group behavior (choice B is wrong) and regression to the mean is a statistical phenomenon, not a social one (choice C is wrong). Group polarization describes the phenomenon whereby a group's views become more extreme; it does not explain the scenario presented in the question stem (choice D is wrong).

SOLUTIONS TO CHAPTER 6 PRACTICE PASSAGE

1. **B**   In the second paragraph, the mention of "props" is a strong indicator that dramaturgy is implicated, which is the concept that individuals' lives are a stage and they use the appropriate props to portray their respective roles (choice B is correct). Social facilitation is the idea that an individual will perform better on simple or familiar tasks because of the presence of other people; this concept does not apply to the process of presentation of self (choice A is incorrect). Social support involves having a strong network to assist the individual in times of need; this does not best explain the process of presentation of self (choice C is incorrect). Peer pressure involves peers influencing one another to conform; the passage implies that the individuals choose to change themselves as opposed to being pressured into doing so (choice D is incorrect).

2. **A**   Self-serving bias occurs when we attribute our successes to ourselves and our failures to external factors; the employee who attributes her promotion to her own hard work is the best example of the self-serving bias (choice A is correct). Self-serving bias does not attribute success to external factors like luck (choice D is wrong). The man who believes a salesperson is a rude jerk after he is ignored by the salesperson is committing a fundamental attribution error, by attributing the salesperson's actions to some internal element of personality (choice B is wrong). The physical attractiveness stereotype explains why people tend to believe that attractive people are also "good" people (choice C is wrong).

3. **B**   Item I is false: sexual orientation describes an individual's sexual attraction and preference; while this is a social identity, transgender individuals are not attempting to convey information about their sexual preferences through presentation of self (choice A can be eliminated). Item II is true: gender is a social identity; transgender individuals express their self-perceived gender through the use of ~~outward indicat~~ors. The passage specifies that transgender indi-
    ~~viduals use clothing and~~ ~~or~~ to adjust to gender norms of society (choice C
    ~~can be eliminated). Item I~~ ~~cal sex is not a social identity; rather, it is based~~
    ~~on biolog~~ ~~cuses on the act of presenting the individual's~~
    ~~~~ ~~r than body parts (choice D can be eliminated,~~

    des toward an individual or group due to some
    ~~~~ons have high social stigma since their former
    ~~~~ society (choice A is correct). Social support
    ~~~~th each other, typically within a family; the
    ~~~~s not demonstrate social support (choice B is
    ~~~~ individual believes that everyone else agrees
    ~~~~ consensus has no relevance to the scenario
    ~~~~ocess of creating an individual identity based
    ~~~~s, and customs; socialization does not explain
    ~~~~incorrect).

5. **C** There are three ways that an individual's behavior may be motivated by social influences. Compliance is a desire to seek rewards or avoid punishment (choice A is a motivating factor and can be eliminated). Identification is the desire to be like another person or group (choice B is a motivating factor and can be eliminated). Internalization happens when values and beliefs are integrated into a person's own value system and then drives their behavior (choice D is a motivating factor and can be eliminated). However, aggregation is not a term in sociology; an *aggregate* describes people who exist in the same space but do not share a common sense of identity (choice C is not a motivating behavior and is the correct answer choice).

6. **D** A "hangover identity" (also known as a role residual) can occur when several aspects persist for an individual from an ex-role even after completing the exiting process to a newly formed identity. According to the final paragraph, "the more involved an individual was in his former role, the more likely he is to have a higher role residual compared to someone who was not as committed to his previous role." Therefore, a newly retired individual who worked at the same company for a long time and was very involved with her coworkers would be most likely to experience "hangover identity" upon transitioning into her new role as retiree (choice D is correct). A biological male who has not begun the process of transitioning to female has not yet abandoned his former role (choice A is wrong), and neither the alcoholic nor the married person was committed to the role at issue for a significant amount of time (choices B and C are wrong).

Chapter 7
Personality, Motivation, and Emotion

Many different qualities make up an individual; our personalities are a big part of who we are (some might say *all* of who we are!). Each of us has a personality shaped over time by both internal and external factors. We all develop our own unique sets of attitudes and opinions and are driven by different motivating forces: these are also important aspects of who we are as individuals.

7.1 PERSONALITY

Theories of Personality

Personality, while very hard to precisely define, is essentially the individual pattern of thinking, feeling, and behavior associated with each person. Personalities are nuanced and complex. Various theories and perspectives on personality have evolved to help explain this fundamental aspect of individuality, including the psychoanalytic perspective, the humanistic perspective, the behaviorist perspective, the social-cognitive perspective, the trait perspective, and the biological perspective. Therapies to treat personality disorders are based on the first four perspectives (psychoanalytic therapy, humanistic or person-based therapy, behavioral therapy, and cognitive behavioral therapy).

Psychoanalytic Perspective

According to **psychoanalytic theory**, personality (made up of patterns of thoughts, feelings, and behaviors) is shaped by a person's unconscious thoughts, feelings, and memories. These unconscious elements are derived from past experiences, particularly interactions with primary early caregivers. What a person is conscious of is quite limited, like the tip of an iceberg compared with his or her vast unconscious stores of experiences, memories, needs, and motivations below the surface. According to psychoanalytic theory, the existence of the unconscious is inferred from behaviors such as dreams, slips of the tongue, posthypnotic suggestions, and free associations.

Within classical psychoanalytic theory as developed by **Sigmund Freud**, two instinctual drives motivate human behavior. The **libido**, or life drive, generates behaviors focused on survival, growth, creativity, pain avoidance, and pleasure. Note that libido is commonly defined as "sex drive," but libido includes more than just sexual energy. The **death drive** generates aggressive behaviors fueled by an unconscious wish to die or to hurt oneself or others.

Sigmund Freud

Psychic energy is distributed among three personality components that function together: id, ego, and superego.

1) The largely unconscious **id** is the source of energy and instincts. Ruled by the **pleasure principle**, the id seeks to reduce tension, avoid pain, and gain pleasure. It does not use logical or moral reasoning, and it does not distinguish mental images from external objects. According to Freud, young children function almost entirely from the id.

2) The **ego**, ruled by the **reality principle**, uses logical thinking and planning to control consciousness and the id. The ego tries to find realistic ways to satisfy the id's desire for pleasure.

3) The **superego** inhibits the id and influences the ego to follow moralistic and idealistic goals rather than just realistic goals; the superego strives for a "higher purpose." Based on societal values as learned from one's parents, the superego makes judgments of right and wrong and strives for perfection. The superego seeks to gain psychological rewards such as feelings of pride and self-love, and to avoid psychological punishment such as feelings of guilt and inferiority.

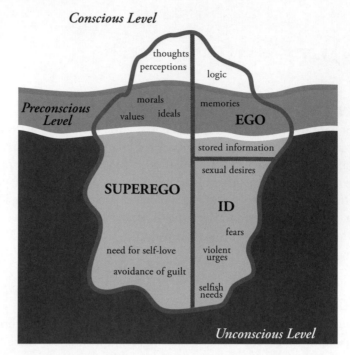

Figure 1   Freud's iceberg analogy to the human mind and personality

According to Freud, anxiety is a feeling of dread or tension, a warning of potential danger, that occurs when a person begins to become aware of repressed feelings, memories, desires, or experiences. To cope with this anxiety and protect the ego, all people develop **ego defense mechanisms** that unconsciously deny or distort reality. Ego defense mechanisms are therefore normal, and become unhealthy only when taken to extremes. The psychoanalyst Anna Freud published a book-length discussion of the ego and its defenses. Several (but not all) common ego defense mechanisms are described in Table 1.

Table 1   Some Common Ego Defense Mechanisms

Defense Mechanism	Description
Repression	Lack of recall of an emotionally painful memory
Denial	Forceful refusal to acknowledge an emotionally painful memory
Reaction Formation	Expressing the opposite of what one really feels, when it would feel too dangerous to express the real feeling (such as acting hateful toward someone to whom one is inappropriately sexually attracted)
Projection	Attributing one's own unacceptable thoughts or feelings to another person ("I'm not angry; you are!")
Displacement	Redirecting aggressive or sexual impulses from a forbidden action or object onto a less dangerous one (as when a person goes home and kicks the dog instead of expressing anger at a boss)
Rationalization	Denying the true motivations for one's behavior while believing false ones that are reassuring or otherwise self-serving (such as believing that embezzling from one's company was an act of politically-motivated "wealth distribution" as opposed to base greed)
Regression	Reverting to an earlier, less sophisticated behavior (as when a child reverts to bedwetting after a trauma)
Sublimation	Channeling aggressive or sexual energy into positive, constructive activities, such as producing art

According to psychoanalytic theory, at each developmental stage throughout the lifespan, certain needs and tasks must be satisfied. When these needs and tasks are not met, a person harbors unresolved unconscious conflicts that lead to psychological dysfunction. There are two different theories of developmental stages that you should be familiar with: Sigmund Freud's psychosexual stages and Erik Erikson's psychosocial stages.

Freud suggested that sexual energy is present from infancy, and that each person matures through **five psychosexual stages** (the oral, anal, phallic, latent, and genital stages), each corresponding to whichever part of the body is the focus of sensual pleasure. In the **oral stage**, the child seeks sensual pleasure through oral activities such as sucking and chewing. In the **anal stage**, the child seeks sensual pleasure through control of elimination. In the **phallic stage**, the child seeks sensual pleasure through the genitals. At this stage, the child is both sexually attracted to the opposite-sex parent and hostile toward the same-sex parent, who is seen as a rival. This is known as the **Oedipus complex** in a boy, and the **Electra complex** in a girl. Girls are also said to experience **penis envy** during the phallic stage (as they discover that they do not have penises). During the **latency stage**, sexual interests subside and are replaced by interests in other areas such as school, friends, and sports. The **genital stage** begins in adolescence, when sexual themes resurface and a person's life/sexual energy is not only directed toward various rewarding activities, but also toward members of the opposite sex outside the family unit.

According to Freud, adult personality is largely determined during the first three psychosexual stages. If parents either frustrate or overindulge the child's expression of sensual pleasure at a certain stage so that the child does not resolve that stage's developmental conflicts, the child becomes **psychologically fixated** at that stage, and will, as an adult, continue to seek sensual pleasure through behaviors related to that stage. For example, if an infant is not fed adequately he or she might become an orally-fixated adult, continually overeating, smoking cigarettes, and abusing alcohol.

Several prominent theorists emerged from the community around Sigmund and Anna Freud and developed their own versions of psychodynamic theory. These include Carl Gustav Jung, Alfred Adler, Karen Horney, and Melanie Klein, among others.

In particular, **Erik Erikson** extended Freud's theory of developmental stages in two ways. Erikson added social and interpersonal factors to supplement Freud's focus on unconscious conflicts within a person. And Erikson delineated eight developmental stages and conflicts in adolescence and adulthood to supplement Freud's focus on early childhood. Also, note that Erikson's stages are much less rigid than Freud's with respect to age range, and he accounted for considerable variability from person to person. The ages given (table, next page) are approximations.

Erik Erikson

1) In Erikson's first stage, the infant's task is to resolve the crisis of **trust versus mistrust**. If an infant's physical and emotional needs are not met, as an adult he or she may mistrust the world and interpersonal relationships.
2) In the second stage, the toddler must resolve the crisis of **autonomy versus shame and doubt**. If a toddler's need to explore, make mistakes, and test limits is not met, as an adult he or she may be dependent rather than autonomous.
3) In the third stage, the preschool-age child must resolve the crisis of **initiative versus guilt**. If a young child's need to make decisions is not met at this stage, as an adult he or she may feel guilty taking initiative and instead allow others to choose.
4) In Erikson's fourth stage, the school-age child must resolve the crisis of **industry versus inferiority**. If a child's need to understand the world, develop a gender-role identity, succeed in school, and set and attain personal goals is not met at this stage, as an adult he or she may feel inadequate.

5) The fifth stage occurs in adolescence and involves resolving the crisis of **identity versus role confusion**. If an adolescent does not test limits and clarify his or her identity, goals, and life meaning, he or she may develop role confusion.

6) The young adult faces the sixth stage: resolving the crisis of **intimacy versus isolation**. If a person does not form intimate relationships at this stage, he or she may become alienated and isolated.

7) In the seventh stage, which occurs in middle age, a person must resolve the crisis of **generativity versus stagnation**. If a person does not feel productive by helping the next generation and resolving differences between actual accomplishments and earlier dreams, he or she may become psychologically stagnant.

8) Finally, in later life, a person must resolve the crisis of **integrity versus despair**, Erikson's eighth and final stage. If a person looks back with regrets and a lack of personal worth at this stage, he or she may feel hopeless, guilty, resentful, and self-rejecting.

Table 2   Freud's and Erikson's Developmental Stages

Age	Psychosexual Stages (Freud)	Age	Psychosocial Stages (Erikson)
Birth to 1 year	Oral • Sensual pleasure in mouth area	Birth to 1.5 years	Infancy • Trust vs. mistrust • Physical and emotional needs met
1–3 years	Anal • Sensual pleasure in controlling elimination	1.5–3 years	Early childhood • Autonomy vs. shame and doubt • Explore, make mistakes, test limits
3–6 years	Phallic • Sensual pleasure in genital area • Incestuous desire for the opposite-sex parent	3–5 years	Preschool age • Initiative vs. guilt • Make decisions
6–12 years	Latency • Localized sensual pleasures disappear • Pursue school, friends, sports	6–12 years	School age • Industry vs. inferiority • Gender-role identity, school success, attain personal goals, understand the world
12 +	Genital • Sensual pleasure returns to genital area • Life/sexual energy fuels friendships, art, sports, careers, and relationships with the opposite sex	12–18 years	Adolescence • Identity vs. role confusion • Identity, goals, life meaning, limit-testing
		18–40 years	Young adulthood • Intimacy vs. isolation • Form intimate relationships
		40–65 years	Middle age • Generativity vs. stagnation • Help next generation and resolve the difference between dreams and accomplishments
		65+ years	Later life • Integrity vs. despair • Look back with no regrets and feel personal worth

Psychoanalytic therapy uses various methods to help a patient become aware of his or her unconscious motives and to gain insight into the emotional issues and conflicts that are presenting difficulties. Therefore, one of the goals of therapy is to help the patient become more able to choose behaviors consciously. Another goal of therapy is to strengthen the ego, so that choices can be based on reality rather than on instincts (id) or guilt (superego). Psychoanalytic therapy is sometimes referred to as "talk therapy" because therapy sessions usually focus on patients talking about their lives. The therapist will listen for patterns or significant events that may play a role in the client's current difficulties. Psychoanalysts believe that childhood events and unconscious feelings, thoughts, and motivations play a role in mental illness and maladaptive behaviors. Psychoanalytic therapy may also use other techniques such as free association, role-play, and dream interpretation.

Humanistic Perspective

In contrast to classical psychoanalytic theory, which tends to focus on conflicts and psychopathology, the **humanistic theory** focuses on healthy personality development. According to this theory, humans are seen as inherently good and as having free will, rather than having their behavior determined by their early relationships. In humanistic theory, the most basic motive for all people is the **actualizing tendency**, which is an innate drive to maintain and enhance the organism. Like a child learning to walk, a person will grow toward **self-actualization**, or realizing his or her human potential, as long as no obstacle intervenes.

According to humanistic theory, as developed by **Carl Rogers**, when a child receives disapproval from a caregiver for certain behavior, he or she senses that the caregiver's positive regard is conditional. In order to win the caregiver's approval and still see both self and caregiver as good, the child introjects the caregiver's values, taking them on as part of his or her own self-concept. The **self-concept** is made up of the child's conscious, subjective perceptions and beliefs about his or her self. The child's true values remain but are unconscious, as the child pursues experiences consistent with the introjected values rather than the true values. The discrepancy between conscious introjected values and unconscious true values is the root of psychopathology. This discrepancy between the conscious and unconscious leads to tension, not knowing oneself, and a feeling that something is wrong.

Carl Rogers

People choose behavior consistent with their self-concepts. If they encounter experiences in life that contradict their self-concepts, they feel uncomfortable **incongruence**. By paying attention to his or her emotional reactions to experiences, a person in an incongruent state can learn what his or her true values are, and then become healthy again by modifying the introjected values and self-concept and growing toward fulfillment and completeness of self. However, people usually find it easier to deny or distort such experiences than to modify their self-concepts.

The goal of **humanistic therapy** (also called **person-centered therapy**) is to provide an environment that will help clients trust and accept themselves and their emotional reactions, so they can learn and grow from their experiences. According to Rogers, the essential elements of such an environment are the therapist's trust in the client, and the therapist communicating genuineness (congruence), unconditional positive regard, and empathic understanding to the client. Using the term "client" rather than "patient" is meant to suggest the inherent health of the person and place the person on an equal level with the therapist.

Behaviorist Perspective

According to the **behaviorist perspective**, personality is a result of learned behavior patterns based on a person's environment. Behaviorism is **deterministic**, proposing that people begin as blank slates, and that environmental reinforcement and punishment completely determine an individual's subsequent behavior and personalities. This process begins in childhood and continues throughout the lifespan.

According to behaviorism, learning (and thus the development of personality) occurs through two forms of conditioning: classical conditioning and operant conditioning. In classical conditioning, a person acquires a certain response to a stimulus after that stimulus is repeatedly paired with a second, different stimulus that already produces the desired response. Classical conditioning is also called associational learning (see Chapter 9). In operant conditioning, behaviors are influenced by the consequences that follow them. An operant is a person's action or behavior that operates on the environment and produces consequences. Consequences are either reinforcements (which make it more likely that the operant will be repeated) or punishments (which make it less likely that the operant will be repeated). Both reinforcements and punishments can be positive or negative. In this context, the terms "positive" and "negative" are used to describe whether the consequence involves the presence or the absence of a particular stimulus. A positive reinforcement is the presence of a rewarding stimulus (e.g., money), and a negative reinforcement is the absence of an aversive stimulus (e.g., a respite from daily chores). A positive punishment is the presence of an aversive stimulus (e.g., an electric shock), and a negative punishment is the absence of a rewarding stimulus (e.g., taking away a teenager's car) (see Chapter 9 for more details on conditioning).

Table 3   Positive and Negative Reinforcement and Punishment

	Reinforcement	Punishment
Positive	Presence of rewarding stimulus	Presence of aversive stimulus
Negative	Absence of aversive stimulus	Absence of rewarding stimulus

Behavioral therapy uses conditioning to shape a client's behavior in the desired direction. Using the ABC model, the therapist first performs a functional assessment to determine the antecedents (A) and consequences (C) of the behavior (B). Therapy then proceeds by changing antecedents and consequences, using the least aversive means possible. Common applications of behavioral therapy include relaxation training and systematic desensitization to help clients manage fear and anxiety. In systematic desensitization, the client is helped to relax while repeatedly being exposed to real or imagined anxiety-producing stimuli, the intensity of which increase incrementally. This technique involves creating a hierarchy of fear-inducing versions of the disturbing object or situation (e.g., seeing a picture of a snake, seeing a snake across the room, holding a snake in one's hands, etc.).

Social Cognitive Perspective

According to the **social cognitive perspective**, personality is formed by a reciprocal interaction among behavioral, cognitive, and environmental factors. The behavioral component includes patterns of behavior learned through classical and operant conditioning, as well as **observational learning**. Observational, or **vicarious**, learning occurs when a person watches another person's behavior and its consequences, thereby learning rules, strategies, and expected outcomes in different situations. For example, studies found that children who watched aggressive and violent behavior in a video subsequently behaved with more aggression and violence toward a doll[1]. People are more likely to imitate models whom they like or admire, or who seem similar to themselves.

---

[1]   The infamous "Bobo doll" experiments conducted by Albert Bandura in the early 1960s will be covered in more detail in Chapter 9.

The cognitive component of personality includes the mental processes involved in observational or vicarious learning, as well as conscious cognitive processes such as self-efficacy beliefs (beliefs about one's own abilities). The environmental component includes situational influences, such as opportunities, rewards, and punishments.

Behavioral therapy is usually combined with a cognitive approach and called **cognitive behavioral therapy** (CBT). From the cognitive perspective, a person's feelings and behaviors are seen as reactions not to actual events, but to the person's thoughts about those events. Each person thus lives by self-created, subjective beliefs about him- or herself, other people, and the world, and these beliefs color the person's interpretations of events. Many of these beliefs are formed during childhood, and they are often unconscious. From the cognitive perspective, the roots of psychopathology are irrational or dysfunctional thoughts and beliefs. The goal of cognitive psychotherapy is to help the client become aware of these and substitute rational or accurate beliefs and thoughts, which will lead to more functional feelings and behaviors.

Table 4 Comparison of the Major Therapy Types

Therapy	Assumed Problem	Therapy Goals	General Method
Psychoanalytic (also known as psychodynamic or talk therapy)	Unconscious forces and deleterious childhood experiences	Reduction of anxiety through self-insight	Analysis and interpretation
Humanistic (also known as client-centered or person-centered)	Barriers to self-understanding and self-acceptance	Personal growth through self-insight	Active listening and unconditional positive regard
Cognitive Behavioral (CBT)	Maladaptive behavior and/or negative, self-defeating thoughts	Extinction and relearning of undesired thoughts/behaviors and healthier thinking and self-talk	Reconditioning, desensitization, reversal of self-blame

Trait Perspective

A **personality trait** is a generally stable predisposition toward a certain behavior. Trait theories of personality focus on identifying, describing, measuring, and comparing individual differences and similarities with respect to such traits.

Trait theorists distinguish between surface and source traits. **Surface traits** are evident from a person's behavior. For example, a person might be described as talkative or exuberant. There are as many surface traits as there are adjectives for describing human behavior. Conversely, **source traits** are the factors underlying human personality and behavior; source traits are fewer and more abstract (see Table 5). Each trait is not binary but rather a continuum ranging between two or more extremes, such as extroversion and introversion.

The **Five-Factor Model** described by McCrae and Costa is widely accepted. The five factors in their model are extroversion, neuroticism, openness to experience, agreeableness, and conscientiousness.

Table 5 McCrae & Costa Personality Traits

Big Five Personality Traits (McCrae & Costa)	
Source Traits	**Surface Trait Examples**
Extroversion	Reserved / Affectionate Loner / Joiner Quiet / Talkative Internal stimuli / External stimuli
Neuroticism	Calm / Worrying Even-tempered / Emotional Secure / Sensitive Confident / Nervous Emotionally stable / Unstable
Openness to experience	Down-to-earth / Imaginative Uncreative / Original Prefer routine / Prefer variety Cautious / Curious Consistent / Inventive
Agreeableness	Antagonistic / Acquiescent Ruthless / Softhearted Suspicious / Trusting Cold / Friendly Unkind / Compassionate Obstinate / Cooperative Not pleasing / Pleasing others
Conscientiousness	Lazy / Hardworking Aimless / Ambitious Quitting / Persevering Ineffectual / Efficient Careless / Organized

Personality traits are thought to help predict a person's performance and enjoyment in certain careers. Assessments of personality traits are often used for career counseling, and by human resources departments as an aid to hiring and promotion decisions. Trait-based personality assessments are also used to help people understand and accept themselves and others. Each personality type is seen as having its own strengths and weaknesses. No type is identified as pathological, and weaknesses are viewed as characteristics to be aware of and manage, rather than to change. Trait theories are generally not concerned with explaining why a person has particular traits, although some have proposed that certain traits are biologically based.

Biological Perspective

From the biological perspective, much of what we call personality is at least partly due to innate biological differences among people. Support for this view is found in the heritability of basic personality traits, as well as in correlations between personality traits and certain aspects of brain structure and function.

Hans Eysenck proposed that a person's level of extroversion is based on individual differences in the reticular formation (which mediates arousal and consciousness). In this view, introverts are more easily aroused and therefore require and tolerate less external stimulation, whereas extroverts are less easily aroused and are therefore comfortable in more stimulating environments. Eysenck also proposed that a person's level of neuroticism is based on individual differences in the limbic system (which helps mediate emotion and memory). Correlations have been found between extroversion and the volume of brain structures involved with processing rewards, and between neuroticism and the volume of brain regions involved with processing negative emotions and punishment. In addition, twin studies and adoption studies (discussed in Chapter 6) have found strong evidence for the heritability of extroversion and neuroticism.

Jeffrey Alan Gray proposed that personality is governed by interactions among three brain systems that respond to rewarding and punishing stimuli. In this view, fearfulness and avoidance are linked to the "fight-or-flight" sympathetic nervous system, worry and anxiety are linked to the behavioral inhibition system, and optimism and impulsivity are linked to the behavioral approach system. **C. Robert Cloninger** also linked personality to brain systems involved with reward, motivation, and punishment. Cloninger proposed that personality is linked to the level of activity of certain neurotransmitters in three interacting systems. In this view, low dopamine activity correlates with higher impulsivity and novelty-seeking, low norepinephrine activity correlates with higher approval-seeking and reward dependence, and low serotonin activity correlates with risk avoidance. Correlations have been found between novelty-seeking and grey matter volume in the cingulate cortex, between reward dependence and grey matter volume in the caudate nucleus, and between harm avoidance and grey matter volume in the orbitofrontal, occipital, and parietal cortices.

Situational Approach to Explaining Behavior

The **person-situation controversy** (also known as the **trait versus state controversy**) considers the degree to which a person's reaction in a given situation is due to their personality (trait) or is due to the situation itself (state). **Traits** are considered to be internal, stable, and enduring aspects of personality that should be consistent across most situations. **States** are situational; they are unstable, temporary, and variable aspects of personality that are influenced by the external environment. For example, extroversion is a trait, stress is a state. The primary question is whether personality is consistent over time and across situations and contexts. A fair amount of research suggests that while people's personality *traits* are fairly stable, their *behavior* in specific situations can be variable. In other words, people do not act with predictable consistency, even if their personality traits are predictably consistent. In unfamiliar situations, people tend to modify their behavior based on **social cues** (verbal or nonverbal hints that guide social interactions); therefore, specific traits may remain hidden. For example, a person who is normally quite extroverted may seem quiet and reserved in an unfamiliar formal situation. In familiar situations, people may "act more like themselves" (the same extroverted person may be considerably more talkative in a familiar situation with friends). Averaging behavior over many situations is the best way to reveal distinct personality traits.

7.2 MOTIVATION

Out of all the behaviors that are possible, what motivates us (and all animals) to act in particular ways in particular moments? This process can be as simple as being motivated to take a drink of water due to a feeling of thirst or as complex as being motivated to undertake a difficult studying regimen and training program in order to become a physician due to a desire to help others.

Factors that Influence Motivation

Instincts

There are several factors that are understood to influence motivation. The first is **instinct**: behaviors that are unlearned and present in fixed patterns throughout a species. An example is imprinting in chicks, who learn to follow objects or organisms that are present when they hatch. In humans, instincts in babies include sucking behaviors, naturally holding the breath under water, and demonstrating fear when approaching drops in elevation. Instincts represent the contribution of genes, which predispose species to particular behaviors.

Drives / Negative Feedback Systems

Physiological drives can also push organisms to act in certain ways, as is the case when we are thirsty. A **drive** is an urge originating from a physiological discomfort such as hunger, thirst, or sleepiness. Drives can be useful for alerting an organism that it is no longer in a state of homeostasis, an internal state of equilibrium. They suggest that something is lacking: food, water, or sleep, for example. Drives often work through negative feedback systems, which are abundant in human physiology. The process of **negative feedback** works by maintaining stability or homeostasis; a system produces a product or end result, which feeds back to stop the system and maintains the product or end result within tightly controlled boundaries. Biological examples of negative feedback include regulation of blood pressure, blood glucose levels, and body temperature. These biological systems can have an important impact on behavior. For example, if blood glucose drops because you haven't eaten in hours, you will feel hungry and have a strong drive to eat. If your temperature begins to drop, you will feel cold and have a strong drive to seek warmth.

Arousal

However, instincts and drives cannot explain some of the artistic accomplishments of humans or the exploratory behavior of infants and animals. Even a toddler whose needs have all seemingly been met will wander around the room, putting objects in his or her mouth. This suggests that some behaviors are motivated by a desire to achieve an optimum level of arousal. A toddler who is not stimulated enough may seek stimulation by exploring the surroundings. An adult who is feeling bored will do the same. On the other hand, feeling overstimulated can lead to feelings of stress, which may lead one to seek ways to relax or sleep. Different people may have different optimal levels of arousal.

Needs

While including basic biological needs (physiological drives), this category also includes higher-level needs than those previously discussed. Instincts, drives, and arousal do not explain why a student may aspire to become a physician. In addition to drives, one may experience various needs, including a need for safety, a need for belonging and love, and a need for achievement.

Theories that Explain How Motivation Affects Human Behavior

Drive Reduction Theory

Since drives are physiological states of discomfort, it follows that we are motivated to reduce these drives through behaviors such as eating and drinking. Drive-reduction theory suggests that a physiological need creates an aroused state that drives the organism to reduce that need by engaging in some behavior. If your blood glucose drops, you feel hungry (or light-headed), and have a drive to eat. The greater the physiological need, the greater the physiological drive (an aroused and motivated state).

Figure 2 Drive-reduction theory

Incentive Theory

While drives are internal physiological needs, **incentives** are external stimuli in the environment that either encourage or discourage certain behaviors. Incentives can be positive and drive us to do something, or they can be negative and repel us from doing something. For example, if you were offered a new job accompanied by a large increase in salary, the salary might serve as a positive incentive. If the job also involved an increase in work hours, the increased workload might serve as a negative incentive. In general, behaviors are most strongly motivated when there are physiological needs, strong positive incentives, and a lack of negative incentives. For example, if you were walking down the street and were very hungry, smelled delicious pizza, and found out it was being given away for free, you'd have a strong motivation to eat it.

Expectancy-Value Theory

Expectancy-value theory posits that the extent to which human beings are motivated to act in a certain way is a function of 1) **expectancy**: the likelihood that the action under consideration will bring about a desired result; and 2) **value**: the degree to which the individual desires the anticipated result. When either of these two factors is very low, there will be little or no motivation to act. For example, a woman who learns of an essay contest, with the first prize being a free trip to France, might want desperately to win that contest. If she knows she has little or no chance of doing so, however, she is unlikely to put in much effort and may not even submit an entry. Conversely, a professional writer who has an excellent chance of winning, but who has no desire to visit France, would be similarly unmotivated. A gifted writer with a passion for everything French, however, may very well make an arduous effort to win that contest.

Self-Determination Theory

The basic tenet of **self-determination theory** is that human beings are inherently motivated to achieve personal growth and well-being. This ideal state of psychological health is thought to come essentially from **intrinsic** sources (i.e., from inside the person) as opposed to **extrinsic** sources (i.e., from the external world). For example, a social worker who strives to perform well at her job in order to receive a raise in salary will not consequently grow as a person. However, if she does her best simply for the satisfaction of knowing that she is a noble human being who is helping society, she will truly benefit from her hard work. Self-determination theorists believe that three core factors facilitate personal growth: 1) **autonomy**: one must feel in control of one's actions and free to make his or her own choices; 2) **competence**: one must believe that he or she possesses skills and abilities capable of producing results; and 3) **connection**: one must feel a sense of relatedness to the world and to other people such that his or her actions matter. When these three critical needs are met, the process of self-determination can occur.

Maslow's Hierarchy of Needs

Abraham Maslow sought to explain human behavior by creating a hierarchy of needs (Figure 3). At the base of this pyramid are physiological needs, or the basic elements necessary to sustain human life. If these needs are met, we will seek safety; if the need for safety is met, we will seek love, and so on. His pyramid suggests that not all needs are equal; some needs take priority over others. For example, an individual who is struggling every day to work and put food on the table will place a higher value on meeting physiological needs than on fulfilling a cognitive need for belongingness by joining a community organization that hopes to increase awareness of global warming. Maslow's hierarchy is somewhat arbitrary—it comes from a Western emphasis on individuality, and some individuals have shown the ability to reorganize these motives (for example, hunger strikes or eating disorders). Nevertheless, it has been generally accepted that we are only motivated to satisfy higher-level needs once certain lower-level needs have been met. The inclusion of higher-level needs, such as self-actualization and the need for recognition and respect from others, also explains behaviors that the previous theories do not.

Figure 3   Maslow's hierarchy of needs

Application of Theories of Motivation to Understand Behaviors

Biological Factors that Regulate Motivation

As drive-reduction theory suggests, biological factors can play a large part in motivation. For many physiological processes, it is theorized that our bodies have a "set point" or a "sweet spot" at which things are in homeostasis. Our bodies also have mechanisms for detecting deviations from the set point and stimulating us to react either internally or behaviorally to regain the set point. Responses to body temperature variations, fluid intake, weight variations, and sexual stimulation are regulated to a large extent by biological processes.

Regulating body temperature is important for survival because it affects protein function, cellular membranes, and the like. Even small elevations in blood temperature can result in heat stroke. The hypothalamus is the primary control center for detecting changes in temperature and receives input from skin receptors. When the hypothalamus determines that the body is cold, it causes vasoconstriction and shivering. When the hypothalamus determines that the body is hot, it causes vasodilation and sweating. Behaviorally, we respond to heat by stretching out to maximize surface area and shedding layers of clothing, as on a hot summer day; we respond to cold by curling inward, snuggling up, and adding layers of clothing, as on a cold winter day.

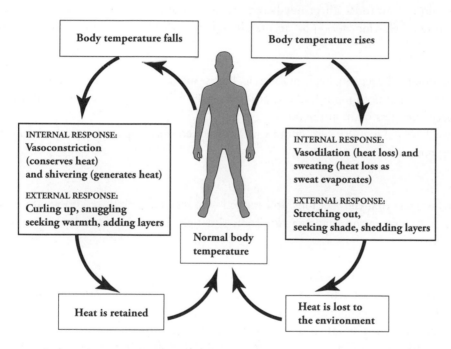

Figure 4 Physiological and behavioral processes regulating body temperature

Monitoring fluid levels includes the intake of fluids as well as excretion. The intake of fluids is stimulated by specialized osmoreceptors in the brain that detect dehydration. These receptors communicate with the pituitary gland to stimulate the release of antidiuretic hormone (ADH), which in turn communicates with the kidneys to reduce urine production by reclaiming water. When blood volume is low, including when one has sustained an injury and is losing a significant amount of blood, the desire for sodium is stimulated to increase the concentration of salt in the blood. Thirst is also stimulated to replace the lost fluid.

7.3 ATTITUDE AND BEHAVIOR

When psychologists refer to a person's **attitude**, they are referring to a person's feelings and beliefs about other people or events around them as well as their tendency to react behaviorally based on those underlying evaluations. Attitudes are useful in that they provide a quick way to size things up and make decisions. However, they can also lead us astray when they lead to inaccurate snap judgments or when they remain fixed beliefs in the face of disconfirming evidence.

Components of Attitudes

Attitudes are considered to have three main components (the ABCs): affect (emotion), behavioral tendencies, and cognition (thought).

The Link Between Attitudes and Behavior

Processes by Which Attitudes Influence Behavior

To what extent do our attitudes affect our behaviors? As is the case with most answers in psychology, it depends. At times, behavior does not accurately reflect attitudes. Consider the following common experiences:

- an individual believes in a healthy lifestyle, but is unable to sustain a healthy diet
- a man believes in not judging others, but finds himself avoiding eye contact and the seat next to a dirty homeless man on the bus
- a juror believes in a guilty verdict but finds himself conforming to the opinions of other jurors to vote "not guilty"

These scenarios suggest that the relationship between who we believe we are and what we do is complex. Social psychologists have found that there are some situations in which attitudes better predict behavior. Those are as follows:

1) *When social influences are reduced*
   Compared to attitudes, which are more internal, external behavior is much more susceptible to social influences. People are much more likely to be honest in a secret ballot process than if they must overtly express their opinions. This is in large part due to fear of criticism and the powerful influence of factors such as conformity and groupthink (discussed in Chapter 6).
2) *When general patterns of behavior, rather than specific behaviors, are observed*
   Our attitudes are better at predicting overall decision-making rather than specific behaviors. For example, one who believes in a healthy lifestyle will tend to make healthier decisions than someone who does not, yet this attitude does not necessarily prevent someone from occasionally reaching for a slice of cheesecake. This is known as the **principle of aggregation**; an attitude affects a person's aggregate or average behavior, but not necessarily each isolated act.
3) *When specific, rather than general, attitudes are considered*
   Belief in a healthy lifestyle can be a poor predictor of a specific behavior, such as eating properly. It would be wiser to compare the specific attitude that the individual has toward eating properly, because it will be a better predictor of this particular behavior. Thus, it is most accurate to consider specific attitudes closely related to the specific behavior of interest.

4) *When attitudes are made more powerful through self-reflection*

People are more likely to behave in accordance with their attitudes if they are given some time to prepare themselves to do so. When people act automatically, they may be impulsive and act in ways that do not match their beliefs. However, when given more time to deliberate over actions, they are more likely to act in ways that match. In addition, when people are made more self-conscious, often through the use of mirrors in experiments, they are more likely to behave morally. Self-awareness reminds us of the beliefs that we have attached to our identities.

Processes by Which Behavior Influences Attitudes

What is perhaps more interesting is the notion that behavior sometimes precedes and affects our attitudes. This comports with the James-Lange theory of emotion (section 7.4), which proposes that behaviors may precede and influence emotions. It has been found that just the act of smiling can somewhat boost mood, and that the act of running away may contribute to a sensation of fear.

There are several situations in which behaviors are likely to influence attitudes.

1) *Role-playing*

The most notable influence of behavior on attitudes is **role-playing**. Like a role in a play, a social role is a script for how to act. The most powerful demonstration of the power of roles is Zimbardo's **prison study** at Stanford. In this experiment, **Philip Zimbardo** randomly divided Stanford students into prisoners and guards in a mock prison. What happened over the course of the study was astonishing. After an initial lighthearted period, the guards and prisoners began really acting out their characters to the point that the guards were actively humiliating and degrading the prisoners. Some prisoners rebelled while others broke down or became apathetic. Participants in the study reported feeling a sense of confusion about reality and fantasy as they became caught up in their roles. The study, which was intended to be two weeks long, had to be discontinued after six days. While some have called Zimbardo's findings and methodology into question in recent years (e.g., only a few "guards" behaved abusively and some of them admit to posturing), the study demonstrates a powerful lesson about the influence that social roles can have.[2] Consider how social roles such as "soldier" and "slave" may have affected how people have acted over the course of history. In wartime, soldiers' beliefs about the enemy become dramatically altered over time, with feelings of ambivalence giving way to perceiving the enemy as "evil." Actions, such as singing the national anthem and saluting the flag, tend to increase patriotic beliefs. How does your own role of "student" affect your behavior? The same influences can stem from positive roles. Zimbardo has also researched positive roles, like that of "hero." Someone who identifies with the role of citizen, parent, or spiritual teacher may be influenced toward wholesome actions in order to better play out that role.

2) *Public Declarations*

In order to please others, people may feel pressure to adapt what they say. What's interesting is that saying something publicly—a **public declaration**—can cause the declarant to believe it in the absence of bribery, coercion, or some other blatant external motive. Since the individual may not be aware of the social pressure that might have influenced the statement, he

---

[2] Note that the Stanford Prison experiment, if conducted today, would violate modern ethical rules governing experimentation on human subjects.

or she may justify it by concluding that the statement is a personal belief. As we continue to express ourselves, we become more and more entrenched in believing what we say, a habit that is even stronger for statements made publicly. Consider a politician who voices an opinion on the issue of abortion that mirrors the belief of the majority of her supporters, although she is somewhat ambivalent about the issue herself. As she continues to express their opinion, she will find herself becoming more polarized toward that opinion and her feelings of ambivalence will start to subside. Because her statements were made publicly, think how hard it would be for the politician to shift positions if she had a change of heart through her own development. Thus, she will be more likely to maintain a belief that is consistent with the actions she has taken. An emphasis on "political correctness" has developed from the idea that saying can become believing. The use of a term such as "gay" in a derogatory manner can lead to the development of beliefs that justify use of the term; therefore, many people feel terms of that sort should not be used.

3) *Justification of Effort*

Just as people may modify their attitudes to match their language, they may also modify them to match other behavior. A prominent example of this phenomenon is **justification of effort**. For example, consider a student who works hard to study for the MCAT and earns a fantastic score, only to feel a calling toward becoming an actor rather than going to medical school at the end of the process. In order to justify the effort already put into the process, the student will feel pressure to go to medical school. Another interesting example of justification of effort is the finding that doing favors for someone increases feelings of liking for that person. The internal dialogue is something like: "I must really like this person; otherwise, why would I be doing so many favors for him?"

4) *Foot-in-the-Door*

Salespeople, political activists, and others trying to influence behavior often take advantage of what is known as the **foot-in-the-door** phenomenon. The strategy involves enticing people to take small actions, such as signing a free petition or joining a mailing list, at first. Upon obtaining this level of involvement, the stakes are raised to accepting bumper stickers or lawn signs. Then, further involvement is encouraged when donations or volunteer time is requested. While people may have agreed to the earlier steps because they required minimal commitment, they will find themselves feeling internal pressure to consent to larger requests to justify their acceptance of the smaller requests. Over time, their attitudes will reflect those of someone who has taken a strong stance on the issue, in order to justify all the steps that they have taken.

Cognitive Dissonance Theory

When considering how behaviors can shape attitudes, self-justification plays an important part. In role-playing, public declarations, justification of effort, and foot-in-the-door scenarios, individuals justify their actions (including language) through beliefs. The theory that seeks to explain why self-justification is such a powerful influence on attitude modification is cognitive dissonance theory.

Cognitive dissonance theory explains that we feel tension ("dissonance") whenever we hold two thoughts or beliefs ("cognitions") that are incompatible, or when attitudes and behaviors don't match. When this occurs, we may feel like hypocrites or feel confused as to where we stand. The theory explains that in order to reduce this unpleasant feeling of tension, we make our views of the world match how we feel or what we've done.

Cognitive dissonance theory can explain people's reactions to situations in which there is insufficient justification for actions that were taken. Without sufficient justification for an action, people are likely to experience dissonance, and thus adjust their beliefs to match what they have done. For example, consider two parents trying to motivate their respective children to study and earn good grades. To accomplish this, one parent institutes a reward system in which the child gets $100 for every A. The second parent rewards their child with $5 for every A. In the first situation, the child may feel coerced into earning good grades. Thus, although he or she may study hard for the reward and earn a lot of money, the child will be less likely to have an internal belief that the grades themselves are important. The behavior of studying hard is easily justified by the reward. In the second situation, the child may work to receive As but have insufficient external justification for having done so, because the reward is insufficient. In cases of insufficient justification, cognitive dissonance theory indicates that there will be some tension that needs to be resolved. The child has earned some As (behavior) but does not have a supporting attitude available to explain the behavior. Thus, the child is likely to adopt the attitude that grades are important to him or her. Consider how cognitive dissonance theory can similarly be used to explain why mild punishment of appropriate severity is more effective at creating internal attitude change than unjustifiably harsh punishment.

Cognitive dissonance can also be used to explain the way people react after they make decisions. Imagine that a woman is trying to decide between two men who have expressed their romantic interest in her. One is exciting and passionate, but utterly undependable and irresponsible. The other is somewhat subdued, but very considerate and dependable. After making her decision, no matter which way she decides, she is sure to experience some dissonant thoughts about the man she rejected. If she chooses the exciting man, she may miss the dependability and consideration of the subdued man; if she chooses the subdued man, she may lament the lack of excitement and passion. According to cognitive dissonance theory, she will tend to change her attitudes to accentuate the positive qualities of her choice and the negative qualities of the alternative. Thus, if she chooses the exciting man, she may internalize beliefs that excitement and passion are important to a relationship and that dependability is overrated. If she chooses the subdued man, she may instead espouse the belief that it is consideration and dependability that are the centerpieces of a relationship and that passion and excitement are fleeting. The important point is that her endorsement of either of these beliefs will come after she makes her decision in order to alleviate the tension of losing what she turned down.

7.4 EMOTION

You walk through your front door, set your keys down, and turn on the light just like you always do when, "Surprise!" Balloons fall from the ceiling, friends jump out of their hiding places, and a cake is brought out. Without any conscious effort, you scream, cover your mouth with your hands, and explode into a giant grin. You feel a pang as your heart skips a beat and then feel a warm glow as you look around at the smiling faces. The thought pops into your head, "A surprise party! How exciting!"

Emotion is quite an interesting phenomenon. It blurs the arbitrary boundary between what we consider mental and what we consider physical. What is really going on when an emotional state arises?

Three Components of Emotion

Emotion is complex and consists of three components: a physiological (body) component, a behavioral (action) component, and a cognitive (mind) component. The physical aspect of emotion is one of **physiological arousal**, or an excitation of the body's internal state. For example, when being startled at a surprise party, you may feel your heart pounding, your breathing becoming shallow and rapid, and your palms becoming sweaty. These are the sensations that accompany emotion (in this instance, surprise).

7.4

The behavioral aspect of emotion includes some kind of expressive behavior; for example, spontaneously screaming and bringing your hands over your mouth. The cognitive aspect of emotion involves an appraisal or interpretation of the situation. Initially upon being startled, the thought "dangerous situation" or "fear" may arise, only to be reassessed as "surprise" and "excitement" after recognizing the circumstances as a surprise party. This describes how the situation is interpreted or labeled. Interestingly, many emotions share the same or very similar physiological and behavioral responses; it is the mind that interprets one situation that evokes a quickened heart rate and tears as "joyful" and another with the same responses as "fearful."

Universal Emotions

Darwin assumed that emotions had a strong biological basis. If this is true, then emotions should be experienced and expressed in similar ways across cultures, and in fact, this has been found to be the case. There are six major universal emotions: happiness, sadness, surprise, fear, disgust, and anger. Regardless of culture, most people can readily identify these emotions simply by observing facial expressions. Further supporting the idea that emotions have an innate basis is the finding that children's capacities for emotional expression and recognition appear to develop along similar timelines, regardless of their environments. However, environmental factors like culture do play a role in how emotion is expressed.

| Happiness | Sadness | Surprise | Fear | Disgust | Anger |

Courtesy Wikimedia Commons

Figure 5   Universal emotions

Adaptive Role of Emotion

The relationship between performance and emotional arousal is a U-shaped correlation: people perform best when they are moderately aroused. This is known as the **Yerkes-Dodson law** (often referred to as Optimal Arousal theory). A student will perform best when neither too complacent nor too overwhelmed, but rather in a "sweet spot" of optimum arousal (though this "sweet spot" can vary greatly from person to person and from task to task). The **optimal-arousal theory**, based on the Yerkes-Dodson law, further predicts that, while moderate arousal is ideal for optimum success, a higher level of arousal is better for easier tasks than for harder ones. For example, the Yerkes-Dodson law has been used to understand the social facilitation effect (see Chapter 6): performing difficult tasks that haven't been practiced sufficiently in front of others makes us overly nervous, beyond the optimal level of arousal for performance, whereas simple, well-practiced tasks move closer to optimal arousal with the presence of others and increased emotional activation.

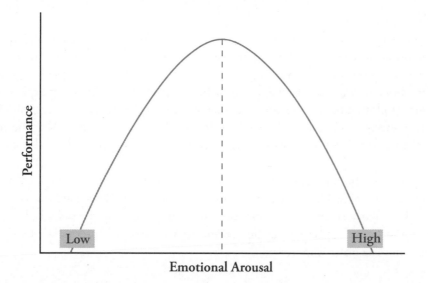

Figure 6   Yerkes-Dodson law regarding the relationship between arousal and performance

In addition to moderating performance, emotion has several other adaptive roles. It enhances survival by serving as a useful guide for quick decisions. A feeling of fear when walking alone down a dark alley while a shadowy figure approaches can be a valuable tool to indicate that the situation may be dangerous. A feeling of anger may enhance survival by encouraging attack on an intruder. The MCAT exam often emphasizes the adaptive benefits of emotional arousal. The most intensely unpleasant negative emotions, such as rage and terror, enhance survival by restricting the individual's attention and focusing it upon whatever is causing the emotional response.

Other emotions may have a role in influencing individual behaviors within a social context. For example, embarrassment may encourage social conformity. Additionally, in social contexts, emotions provide a means for nonverbal communication and empathy, allowing for cooperative interactions.

On a more subtle level, emotions are a large influence on our everyday lives. Our choices often require consideration of our emotions. A person with a brain injury to their prefrontal cortex (which plays a role in processing emotion) has trouble imagining their own emotional responses to the possible outcomes of decisions. This can lead to inappropriate decisions that can cost someone a job, a marriage, or his or her savings. Imagine how difficult it would be to refrain from risky behaviors, such as gambling or spending huge sums of money, without the ability to imagine your emotional response to the possible outcomes.

Theories of Emotion

The most commonsense way to think about emotion is that something happens (a stimulus), then you experience the emotion, and then you have a physiological and behavioral response. For example, you're walking down the street and a scary dog starts chasing you (stimulus), you first experience the emotion (fear), then the physiological response (your heart begins to race) and behavioral response (you run away). Indeed, this commonsense logic was how emotions were assumed to operate until the late 1800s, when scientists began proposing very different theories. There are three predominant theories that attempt to explain how the components of emotion—the physiological, the behavioral, and the cognitive—are interconnected.

7.4

James-Lange Theory

The James-Lange theory of emotion was proposed in the late 1800s and basically flips the commonsense notion of how emotion is experienced: instead of first experiencing the emotion and then the physiological reaction, the James-Lange theory proposes that first we experience the physiological response and then we experience the emotion. In other words, if a scary dog begins to chase you, first you experience an increased heart rate and this is followed by the conscious labeling of the experience as "fear." This may seem counterintuitive; it implies you feel afraid because your heart is racing. This theory suggests that the emotional experience (the brain labeling the situation as fear-inducing) is the result of the physiological response.

We frequently experience situations and events (stimuli) that result in various physiological reactions like increased muscle tension, increased heart rate, sweating, and many others, which are caused by the autonomic nervous system. This theory suggests that emotions are a result of these physiological responses, and not their cause. James and Lange suggested that autonomic activity induced by emotional stimuli generate the feeling of emotion, not the other way around.

There is some evidence in support of the James-Lange theory. For example, breathing patterns can also lead to certain emotions; short, shallow breathing creates a feeling of panic, while long, deep breathing creates a feeling of calm. People with cervical spine damage often experience less arousal and reduced emotions, because they no longer perceive physiological arousal from their bodies. However, the theory does not explain all scenarios and makes two assumptions that may be problematic. First, it assumes that each emotion originates from a distinctive physiological state. However, many emotions share very similar if not identical physiological profiles; for example, fear and sexual arousal involve very similar physiological patterns. Second, the theory assumes that we possess the ability to label these physiological states accurately. However, there is some evidence that the same physiological state can be interpreted differently based on context. For example, a physiological state similar to fear can be interpreted as excitement at a surprise party.

Cannon-Bard Theory

Walter Cannon, a critic of the James-Lange theory, suggested (1) that in order for the James-Lange theory to adequately describe the process of emotion, there must be different physiological responses corresponding to each distinct emotion; and (2) that physiological experiences do not appear to differ from one another to the extent that would be essential to discriminate one emotion from another based only on our bodily reactions. Cannon also conducted a series of experiments in the early 1900s on cats whereby he severed the afferent nerves of the sympathetic branch of the autonomic nervous system (thereby preventing the cats from receiving any physiological input from their bodies) and exposed them to emotion-inducing stimuli. Cannon (and his grad student, Philip Bard) found that the cats still experienced emotion, even in the absence of physiological input from their bodies, thus casting significant doubt on the James-Lange theory. Therefore, the Cannon-Bard theory of emotion suggests that after a stimulus, the physiological response and the experience of emotion occur simultaneously and independently of each other. For example, a scary dog comes running after you (stimulus) and you then experience fear (emotion) and an increased heart rate (physiological response) at the same time; the fear does not cause the increased heart rate and the increased heart rate does not cause the fear. The Cannon-Bard theory is able to explain the overlap in physiological states between emotions like fear and sexual arousal, because the cognitive labeling is independent from the physiological reaction, rather than directly caused by it. However, it struggles to explain phenomena in which controlling the physiological response influences the experience of emotion (e.g., deep breathing causes us to feel more calm).

Schachter-Singer Theory

According to the **Schachter-Singer theory** of emotion, once we experience physiological arousal, we make a conscious cognitive interpretation based on our circumstances, which allows us to identify the emotion that we are experiencing. Thus, like the James-Lange theory, this suggests that each emotional experience begins with an assessment of our physiological reactions. Unlike James-Lange, however, it suggests that the cognitive label is given based on the situation, rather than being a one-to-one correlate of the physiological experience. Therefore, as with this Cannon-Bard theory, physiological states can be similar but cognitively labeled differently (for example, fear and sexual arousal). Therefore, the sight of the scary dog would cause the physiological change of an increased heart rate, which would be interpreted as the result of fearing the dog because of the situation. This would then inspire a behavioral response (running away). This theory accounts for several situations, but suffers from the same shortcoming as the Cannon-Bard theory in that it does not explain how physiological responses influence cognitive aspects of emotion.

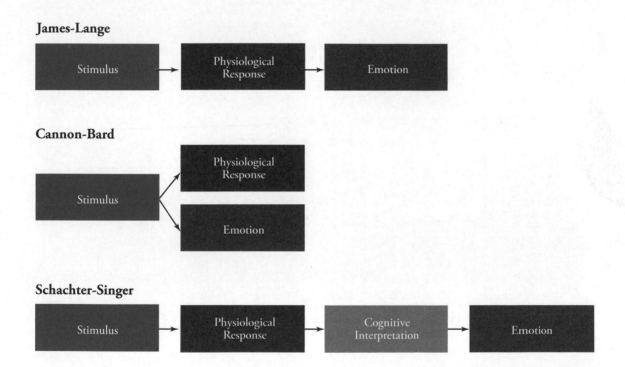

Figure 7 Schematic comparison of the theories of emotion

Chapter 7 Summary

- Personality is defined as the individual pattern of thinking, feeling, and behavior associated with each person.

- Sigmund Freud pioneered psychoanalytic theory, which proposes that personality is the result of an individual's unconscious thoughts, feelings, and memories.

- The id is ruled by the pleasure principle and is unconscious, the ego is ruled by the reality principle and uses logical thinking and planning to control consciousness and the id, and the superego inhibits the id and influences the ego to follow moralistic, rather than realistic, goals.

- According to Freud, people develop through five psychosexual stages: the oral stage, the anal stage, the phallic stage, the latent stage, and the genital stage; failure to resolve developmental conflicts within each stage leads to fixation.

- Erik Erikson added social and interpersonal factors to supplement Freud's theory; Erikson's developmental stages involve the resolution of the following crises: trust vs. mistrust, autonomy vs. shame, initiative vs. guilt, industry vs. inferiority, identity vs. role confusion, intimacy vs. isolation, generativity vs. stagnation, and integrity vs. despair.

- Carl Rogers pioneered the humanistic perspective in psychology and believed that incongruence between behavior and self-concept causes psychopathology.

- Behaviorists believe that personality is determined by conditioning; environmental reinforcements and punishments determine an individual's personality and behaviors.

- The social cognitive perspective suggests that personality is formed by a reciprocal interaction among behavioral, cognitive, and environmental factors.

- The Five-Factor Model describes five major personality traits: extroversion, neuroticism, openness to experience, agreeableness, and conscientiousness.

- Motivation is influenced by drives, instincts, feedback, arousal, and needs.

- The drive-reduction theory suggests that individuals engage in certain behavior in an attempt to alleviate physiological states of discomfort.

CHAPTER 7 FREESTANDING PRACTICE QUESTIONS

1. Which of the following is a universal emotion likely to occur with learned helplessness?

   A) Guilt
   B) Disgust
   C) Sadness
   D) Hopelessness

2. Research shows that emotions with salient labels are easier to remember, and when the recall state is similar to the initial state. This is most consistent with the:

   A) dual coding hypothesis and the Optimal Arousal theory.
   B) depth of processing model and the Optimal Arousal theory.
   C) method of loci and the self-reference effect.
   D) the self-reference effect and the dual coding hypothesis.

3. Psychoanalytic psychotherapy is a long-term therapeutic approach in which the therapist and client engage in deep analysis of the client's dreams, childhood, and life experiences in an attempt to gain insight into the unconscious. One important process in this type of therapy is known as transference, in which the client associates feelings with the therapist that originated in feelings for another person, in many cases a parent. If this resulted in the client accusing the therapist of angry feelings she herself held, this would be most reminiscent of the ego defense mechanism of:

   A) repression.
   B) reaction formation.
   C) projection.
   D) displacement.

4. According to the James-Lange theory:

   A) motivation follows action.
   B) emotion follows physiologic arousal.
   C) physiologic arousal follows emotion.
   D) emotions are validated by inner dialogue.

5. Pooja is hungry and buys a sandwich at the nearby sandwich shop. According to drive-reduction theory, she:

   A) has returned her body to homeostasis.
   B) has raised her glucose levels to an unhealthy level.
   C) will have created another imbalance and feel thirsty.
   D) will continue to feel hungry.

6. An individual despairs because she senses a lack of purpose in her work. Although she is considered successful within her career and earns enough to support her family, she feels as though her work has lacked purpose and has not benefited society as much as she would like. As her first grandchild is born, she reflects on whether she wants to consider a radical career change to a more fulfilling career that she believes does more social good and allows her to feel a greater sense of purpose. Which Erikson stage is she likely in, paired with the correct Maslow need she is striving to fulfill?

   A) Integrity vs. despair seeking self-actualization needs
   B) Generativity vs. stagnation seeking esteem needs
   C) Integrity vs. despair seeking esteem needs
   D) Generativity vs. stagnation seeking self-actualization needs

7. Rafael walks into a dark room, turns on the light, and his friends yell "surprise." Rafael's racing heartbeat is interpreted as surprise and joy instead of fear. Which theory of emotion is supported by his reaction?

   A) Optimal arousal
   B) Schachter-Singer
   C) Cannon-Bard
   D) James-Lange

8. A married couple has gone camping with their son and are discussing site protocol with a park ranger when suddenly a bear appears from the woods. Which sympathetic response is most consistent with the Schachter-Singer theory of emotion?

A) The park ranger feels an increased heart rate, then connects the event with several past experiences, and feels a sense of anxious alertness while holding bear spray to use in the event of an emergency.

B) The mother feels intense fear as she tries to catch her breath, which has instantly increased.

C) The father clutches his wife's wrist as he goes into shock, realizing when he is unable to move his hand that he is paralyzed with fear.

D) The son feels a rush of adrenaline and runs immediately into the tent, realizing once he is inside that he is in a state of panic.

9. Which of the following best summarizes Carl Rogers' view of personality?

A) Personality traits such as inhibition, extroversion, and conscientiousness are constant over time.

B) Individual, adult personalities are the result of repressed childhood memories.

C) People's personality traits are overwhelmingly positive and goal-directed.

D) Personality is mainly formed by behavioral expectations.

CHAPTER 7 PRACTICE PASSAGE

Maslow's hierarchy of needs is a well-established model of motivation within the humanistic framework. Maslow asserted that the ultimate goal of the individual is self-actualization, to become the best version of oneself, or who one was meant to be. However, many obstacles stand in the way of this path to self-actualization.

One method researchers have used to model self-actualization is to measure degree of convergence between the real and ideal selves. In humanistic psychology, the gap between these two aspects of self-concept is a predictor of psychopathology, on the one hand, and degree of life satisfaction on the other. Researchers created an instrument to measure this convergence, the Self Perceived Actualization Index (SPAI). The SPAI began as a 103-item questionnaire, but factor analysis showed that certain clusters of questions correlated with one another, and researchers were able to narrow the number of questions down to 34. The final version of the SPAI contained questions such as "In an ideal world, I would love to have more education" and "I sometimes wish I could start over in a new career and get back the time I lost" rated on a Likert Scale from 1 to 7. The SPAI was then checked against similar instruments for reliability and consistency.

A group of researchers in the field of clinical psychology created a study to explore how self-perceived actualization was related to motivation from the perspective of a Maslowian hierarchy. They created a study with three groups: high actualization, low actualization, and control. The researchers then checked for interactions between self-actualization and motivation, and how they affected mood and altruistic behavior. Each group was told not to eat before coming to the research laboratory then given a small meal before participating in the study. Over time, as hunger increased, the researchers wanted to see the extent to which participants were willing to engage in altruistic behaviors, modeled by the extent to which they were willing to share their winnings from a game. The researchers found that as participants became hungrier, they were less likely to share their winnings with other participants. There was also a mediating effect of actualization, such that individuals who scored higher on the SPAI were less susceptible to hunger effects on their altruism and mood.

In a follow-up study, the same team of researchers conducted a personality assessment and found significant correlations with certain personality characteristics and positive affect and altruistic behavior.

1. The checks in the research methodology were to check for

   I. internal validity.
   II. external validity.
   III. construct validity.

   A) I only
   B) I and III only
   C) II and III only
   D) I, II, and III

2. Which of the following conclusions is best supported by the research?

   A) Altruism is a surface trait dependent on context.
   B) Altruism is a source trait that is relatively stable.
   C) Altruism is a surface trait that is relatively stable.
   D) Altruism is a source trait that is dependent on context.

3. Which of the following is the most likely connection the researchers were trying to establish with respect to the Maslowian hierarchy?

   A) Meeting love and belonging needs plays a stabilizing role in the effects of not getting esteem needs met.
   B) Meeting self-actualization needs plays a stabilizing role in the effects of not getting physiological needs met.
   C) Meeting esteem needs plays a stabilizing role in the effects of not getting safety needs met.
   D) Meeting physiological needs plays a stabilizing role in the effects of not getting esteem needs met.

4. A low rating on which of the following items is most likely to be interpreted as having high self-actualization?

   A) Love and belonging needs
   B) Integrity
   C) Conscientiousness
   D) Neuroticism

5. Which of the following pairs of correlations did researchers most likely find in the follow-up study?

A) A positive correlation between neuroticism and positive affect and a positive correlation between conscientiousness and altruistic behavior

B) A positive correlation between neuroticism and positive affect and a negative correlation between conscientiousness and altruistic behavior

C) A negative correlation between neuroticism and positive affect and a positive correlation between conscientiousness and altruistic behavior

D) A negative correlation between neuroticism and positive affect and a negative correlation between conscientiousness and altruistic behavior

6. Which of the following is likely to lead to convergence similar to the type mentioned in the passage between real and ideal self?

A) Unconditional positive regard and successful resolution during the autonomy vs. shame and doubt phase

B) High self-concept and successful resolution during the latency phase

C) Strong emotional regulation due to positive cognitive appraisals of potentially threatening stimuli

D) Unstable source traits that are congruent with an idealized self-concept

SOLUTIONS TO CHAPTER 7 FREESTANDING PRACTICE QUESTIONS

1. **C** Learned helplessness occurs when an organism learns through experience that it has no control over a situation and gives up, despite the fact that the environment has changed in such a way that it now has autonomy. Among the answer choices, this is closest to sadness, which is characterized by low energy and feelings of being unable to change the environment, and often results in decreased activity (choice C is correct). Guilt is not one of the six universal emotions (choice A is wrong). The expression of disgust originates in the reaction often displayed when one consumes disagreeable food, and now includes situations where we observe someone else acting in a way with which we strongly disagree. The phenomenon of learned helplessness is not associated with a negative judgement of another person's actions (choice B is wrong). Hopelessness is not one of the six universal emotions (choice D is wrong).

2. **B** The depth-of-processing model states that experiences which receive a greater depth of neural and cognitive processing are more likely to be remembered. This is consistent with deep emotions with salient labels leading to greater recall. Optimal Arousal theory states that there is an optimal level of emotional arousal, consistent with the emotional arousal implied in the recall state, which the question stem suggests is like the initial state (choice B is correct). The dual-coding hypothesis refers to the fact that it is easier to remember words when they are related to images and is not related to emotions (choice A is wrong). The method of loci is a recall strategy in which an individual imagines that she is moving through a space and connects images with the objects or ideas that she is trying to remember. This is unrelated to emotional arousal (choice C is wrong). The self-reference effect refers to the fact that it is easier to recall events that have personal relevance. This can connect to greater emotional salience, but this is not necessarily so (choice D is wrong).

3. **C** Projection involves an attempt to disown one's own unacceptable feelings or characteristics by falsely attributing them to others. The question stem describes such a situation, in which the patient projects her feelings onto the therapist (choice C is correct). Repression is an attempt to ignore or forget strong emotional memories, often related to childhood. No repression of memories is mentioned in the question stem (choice A is wrong). Reaction formation is characterized by behaving in a manner that is actually the opposite of one's true feelings. The question stem does not indicate that the client acts in a way that is the opposite of her feelings, rather that she attributes her own feelings to the therapist (choice B is wrong). Displacement involves shifting a forbidden desire or impulse onto another object of desire or interest that is more acceptable (choice D is wrong).

4. **B** The James-Lange theory of emotion posits that emotion is experienced after the body's physiological response to a stimulus (choice B is correct; choice C is wrong). Motivation is not part of the James-Lange theory (choice A is wrong), and neither is inner dialogue (choice D is wrong).

5. **A** According to drive-reduction theory, the drive is hunger in this case; to reduce the need, Pooja needs to eat something. Since she does this, theoretically she will return to homeostasis (choice A is correct). The sandwich could conceivably increase glucose levels in the body, but it is not certain that they will be raised to unhealthy levels (choice B is incorrect). Yes,

she may be thirsty as well, but that is not stated in the question, nor will a sandwich necessarily make one thirsty (choice C is incorrect). Lastly, as the sandwich will likely satiate the hunger, there is not enough evidence to support the idea that she might remain hungry (choice D is incorrect).

6. **D** This is a two-by-two question; approach one part of the answer choice at a time and use Process of Elimination. For the Erikson phase, the question stem states that the individual is experiencing doubt about the impact of her career. This is connected with the phase of generativity vs. stagnation. Integrity vs. despair involves reflecting back on one's life and evaluating whether it was a life worth living (choices A and C are wrong). The question stem states that the individual was already successful in her career, so it is unlikely that she is striving for esteem needs (choice B is wrong). The question also states that she would like to feel a greater sense of purpose, which corresponds closely to self-actualization (choice D is correct).

7. **B** Rafael can cognitively appraise the situation to know he is not in danger. Thus, while he is experiencing a physiological response to a stimulus, he is ultimately demonstrating cognitive interpretation of that physiological response, which is consistent with the two-factor theory of Schachter and Singer (choice B is correct). The Optimal Arousal theory (often referred to as the Yerkes-Dodson law) is not a theory of emotion (choice A is incorrect). The Cannon-Bard theory does not connect the cognitive interpretation of the physiological response (choice C is incorrect). The James-Lange theory also does not work here because the physiological response would only lead to one emotional output, most likely fear (choice D is incorrect).

8. **A** The Schachter-Singer theory of emotion is characterized by the role of cognitive evaluation and context. Emotions with identical physiological markers can be experienced differently based on the interpretation of the situation. A park ranger who experiences a sympathetic response but experiences alertness instead of fear because of memories and experiences is an example of the Schacter-Singer theory (choice A is correct). The mother's experience is consistent with Canon-Bard because the emotion and physiological responses occur simultaneously (choice B is wrong). The father's shock does not specify any sympathetic response, as indicated by the answer choice (choice C is wrong). The son realizes his emotion after the physiological response. This is consistent with the James-Lange theory (choice D is wrong).

9. **C** Rogers believed in the intrinsic goodness of the humans, hence why he belongs to the humanistic school of psychology; choice C most mirrors his views (choice C is correct). Choice A is somewhat extreme in claiming personality traits are "constant over time," they are not; nonetheless, this is not Rogers' perspective (choice A is incorrect). Choice B is the psychoanalytic perspective of personality (choice B is incorrect), and choice D is the behavioral explanation of personality (choice D is incorrect).

SOLUTIONS TO CHAPTER 7 PRACTICE PASSAGE

1. **B** The passage states that the researchers checked for reliability and consistency, and these are both attributes related to the validity of psychometric instruments: whether they measure what they purport to, and whether repeated assessments lead to similar results. The validity of a measurement tool is related to internal validity, so Item I is true (choice C is wrong). Neither of the checks made by researchers for reliability and consistency is related to whether the research applies to real world situations in the greater population, so Item II is not true (choice D is wrong). Construct validity is specifically related to how well-designed an instrument is, which is exactly what the researchers checked for. Therefore, Item III is true (choice B is correct, and choice A is wrong).

2. **A** This question can be answered more quickly by dividing it into two parts. First, note that altruism in the passage is dependent on context. Individuals became less altruistic as they got hungrier. Source traits tend to be largely stable across situations, whereas surface traits are largely dependent on context so can vary widely depending on the situation. The fact that altruism tends to change for participants in the study suggests that it is a surface trait (choices B and D are wrong). Surface traits tend to be more dependent on context and are not stable because they can vary widely from situation to situation (choice A is correct, and choice C is wrong).

3. **B** The passage indicates that individuals who scored high on the SPAI, a measure of self-actualization, were more stable and saw less of a decline in altruism when they were hungry. Since hunger is a physiological need, this suggests that self-actualization played a stabilizing role on not getting physiological needs met (choice B is correct). The SPAI measures self-actualization, how much individuals feel that they are leading the life they want, not love and belonging, the extent to which they feel loved and cared for (choice A is wrong). Esteem needs refer to a sense of accomplishment and high self-esteem, not self-actualization, and safety needs refer to the absence of threat, as opposed to not having a physiological need (hunger) met (choice C is wrong). Physiological needs are the needs that were tested in the passage, as individuals became more hungry. Therefore, this is not the need that played a stabilizing role (choice D is wrong).

4. **D** Neuroticism is associated with negative emotions and difficulty dealing with stress. Low levels of neuroticism would indicate a more positive emotional experience and better stress management. This is likely to be associated with self-actualization (choice D is correct). Love and belonging needs would need to be met first, according to Maslow, before achieving self-actualization. Therefore, high levels of love and belonging, not low levels, would be associated with self-actualization (choice A is wrong). Integrity would result in positive resolution of Erikson's last stage of development, integrity vs. despair. This positive resolution would be associated with a sense of a life well-lived, which is a sense of self-actualization. Therefore, high levels, not low levels, of integrity would be associated with self-actualization (choice B is wrong). Conscientiousness is associated with awareness of others' conditions, thoughtfulness, and responsibility. It is not clear that this attribute is directly related to self-actualization, but conscientiousness is generally considered to be socially desirable, so it is more likely that high levels are associated with self-actualization than low levels (choice C is wrong).

5. **C** For two-by-two question types, evaluate one part of the answer choice at a time and use POE. Neuroticism is associated with negative emotions, so a negative correlation is expected between neuroticism and positive emotions (choices A and B are wrong). Conscientiousness is related to thoughtfulness and consideration for others' states, so a positive correlation is expected between conscientiousness and altruistic behavior (choice C is correct, and choice D is wrong).

6. **A** Unconditional positive regard is a concept in humanistic psychology that, when provided by parents, caregivers, therapists, or other significant figures provides an individual the best chance at reaching self-actualization. Also, successful resolution of the autonomy vs. shame and doubt phase would lead to a sense of independence and autonomy that would make it more likely that an individual could lead a life congruent with his or her ideals (choice A is correct). Self-concept is not conceptualized as being high or low, like perhaps self-esteem would be. It is more likely to be referred to in terms of how integrated or differentiated it is. Also, the latency phase in Freud's stage theory is not associated with psychosexual conflict, so successful resolution here would lead to minimal benefits. Freud considered the first three stages directly before the latency phase to be far more important (choice B is wrong). Resilient response to potentially threatening stimuli is a positive attribute that would probably be associated with greater life satisfaction, but how this would be related to real and ideal selves and their convergence is not clear (choice C is wrong). Source traits are considered the more stable traits, as opposed to surface traits, which vary more from situation to situation (choice D is wrong).

EXPLORING THE RELATIONSHIP BETWEEN FREQUENCY OF INSTAGRAM USE, EXPOSURE TO IDEALIZED IMAGES, AND PSYCHOLOGICAL WELL-BEING IN WOMEN

Sherlock, Mary; Wagstaff, Danielle L.

Psychology of popular media culture Vol. 8, Iss. 4, (Oct 2019): 482-490. DOI:10.1037/ppm0000182

The appealing features of social networking sites (SNSs), such as the ability to communicate with others despite geographical distance, have attracted billions of users worldwide, with many incorporating social networking into their daily routine (Boyd & Ellison, 2007). Between 2014 and 2015, 72% of Australians accessed the Internet for social networking purposes, with younger age groups (<35 years) being the heaviest Internet users (Australian Bureau of Statistics, 2016). Indeed, 80% of university students use their devices (i.e., laptops, tablets, and mobile phones) for social networking purposes.

METHOD

Participants were 129 women, ranging in age from 18 to 35 years ($M = 24.60$ years, $SD = 4.54$), who indicated they currently used Instagram. Participants were recruited from the authors' university's undergraduate psychology participant pool, as well as volunteers recruited via SNSs and flyer advertisements on university campuses. The research was approved by the institutional human ethics research committee, and all participants provided their informed consent. The study was hosted on SurveyMonkey and included two parts. Participation took approximately 30 to 40 min, and upon completion, participants were presented with a debriefing statement regarding the nature of the manipulation.

Materials and Procedure

Participants completed a survey containing the following scales presented in random order:

The 20-item Centre for Epidemiologic Studies Depression Scale (Radloff, 1977) was used to measure depressive symptoms. Participants were asked to answer a number of questions relating to how they felt or behaved in the week prior, including "I felt depressed" and "I had crying spells," on a scale from 1 (*rarely or none of the time*) to 4 (*all of the time*). Higher scores indicate higher depressive symptoms.

The Centre for Epidemiologic Studies Depression Scale had high internal reliability ($\alpha = .93$).

The Heatherton Self-Esteem Scale (Heatherton & Polivy, 1991) measures state self-esteem across three domains: performance, social interaction, and appearance. Participants respond to 20 items such as "I feel self-conscious" and "I feel as smart as others," on a 5-point scale from 1 (*not at all*) to 5 (*extremely*). Higher scores indicate higher self-esteem. The Heatherton Self-Esteem Scale had high internal reliability ($\alpha = .96$).

The State-Trait Anxiety Inventory (Spielberger, Gorsuch, Lushene, Vagg, & Jacobs, 1983) is a commonly used measure of general anxiety and contains 20 items for assessing state anxiety and 20 for trait anxiety. Items include "I am tense" and "I am a steady person," which participants answer on a 4-point scale from 1 (*almost never*) to 4 (*almost always*). Higher scores indicate greater anxiety. The State-Trait Anxiety Inventory had high internal reliability ($\alpha = .96$).

The Physical Appearance State and Trait Anxiety Scale (PASTAS; Reed, Thompson, Brannick, & Sacco, 1991) measures an individual's body image anxiety as they generally feel (trait) and as they currently feel (state). The trait scale asks participants to best indicate the extent to which they generally feel anxious, tense, or nervous about specific body parts such as "my hips" and "my buttocks" on a 5-point scale from 1 (*never*) to 5 (*always*). The state scale asks how they feel about the same body parts "right now" on a scale from 1 (*not at all*) to 5 (*exceptionally so*). Higher scores indicate higher physical appearance anxiety. The scale had high internal reliability ($\alpha = .91$).

Self-rated physical attractiveness was measured by two questions: "Rate what you perceive to be your own physical attractiveness compared to your same sex friends" and "Rate what you perceive to be your own physical attractiveness compared to the general population," on a scale from 1 (*extremely less attractive*) to 9 (*extremely more attractive*). Scores were summed to create a single value for self-rated attractiveness. The items correlated strongly (*r* = .72).

The Body Image Disturbance Questionnaire (BIDQ; Cash, Phillips, Santos, & Hrabosky, 2004) assesses concerns about physical appearance. The Body Image Disturbance Questionnaire consists of seven items such as "Are you concerned about the appearance of some part(s) of your body, which you consider especially unattractive?" which participants answer on a scale from 1 (*not at all concerned*) to 5 (extremely *concerned*). Higher scores indicate higher body image disturbance. The scale showed high internal consistency (α = .93).

Social comparison was measured using the Iowa-Netherlands Comparison Orientation Scale (INCOM; Gibbons & Buunk, 1999), with 11 items measuring how frequently individuals compare themselves with others. Items include "I always like to know what others in a similar situation would do," measured on a 5-point scale from 1 (*disagree strongly*) to 5 (*agree strongly*). Higher scores indicate higher frequency of social comparison. The Iowa-Netherlands Comparison Orientation Scale showed high internal reliability (α = .83).

Instagram use was measured using questions derived by the researchers. Items related to frequency of use. That is, "how many followers do you have on Instagram?" from 1 (*1–10*) to 11 (*1,000+*), "How many accounts do you follow on Instagram?" from 1 (*1–10*) to 11 (*1,000+*), and "In the past week, on average, approximately how much time per day have you spent actively using Instagram," from 1 (*less than 10 min*) to 6 (*more than 3 hr*).

Design

Part 1 consisted of a correlational design in which we correlated Instagram use with each of the psychological well-being variables, and with age. Because Lup et al. (2015) found that the relationship between Instagram use and depression was mediated by social comparison, we attempted to replicate these findings, as well as explore the mediation by social comparison of the relationship between Instagram use and other psychological well-being variables.

RESULTS

Instagram Use and Psychological Well-being

As shown in Table 1, the average time spent on Instagram correlated positively with depressive symptoms, trait anxiety, social comparison orientation, physical appearance anxiety, and body image disturbance. The time spent on Instagram also correlated negatively with self-esteem, and thus findings are consistent with the hypothesis. Exploring the other Instagram measures taken, we found that number of followers correlated positively with depression and trait anxiety, and negatively with self-esteem. The number of accounts followed correlated positively with depression and negatively with self-esteem. Additionally, age correlated negatively with Instagram use, $r = -0.36$, $p < .001$, and negatively with social comparison, $r = -0.21$, $p = .019$.

Descriptive Statistics for Each Scale, Plus Correlations Between Scales

Table 1   Descriptive Statistics for Each Scale, Plus Correlations Between Scales

Variable	Descriptive statistics		Pearson's correlation coefficients								
	M	*SD*	1	2	3	4	5	6	7	8	9
1. Time spent on Instagram	2.65	1.65									
2. Number of accounts followed	7.06	2.69	.58**								
3. Number of followers	6.97	2.43	.53**	.77**							
4. Depressive symptoms	22.65	12.77	.49**	.21*	.22*						
5. Trait anxiety	49.88	11.93	.42**	.30**	.28**	.81**					
6. Physical appearance anxiety	41.55	13.47	.47**	.29**	.16	.48**	.59**				
7. Body image disturbance	16.91	6.62	.33**	.26*	.16	.48**	.63**	.64**			
8. Self-rated attractiveness	8.21	2.91	−.11	−.05	.11	−.26**	−.49**	−.48**	−.56**		
9. Self-esteem	59.91	17.77	−.47**	−.24**	−.18*	−.74**	−.84**	−.75**	−.65**	.55**	
10. Social comparison	40.17	7.22	.42**	.25**	.15	.43**	.59**	.57**	.43**	−.28**	−.62**

* *p* < .05   ** *p* < .01

DISCUSSION

Instagram Use and Psychological Well-being

There is an array of evidence demonstrating excessive Facebook use is related to negative mental health outcomes (Błachnio et al., 2013, 2015; Fardouly et al., 2014; Haferkamp & Krämer, 2011; Labrague, 2014). In this study, we demonstrated that heavier Instagram use (as well as number of followers and number of people followed) correlated with a range of psychological well-being outcomes, including depressive symptoms, general anxiety, physical appearance anxiety, self-esteem, and body image disturbance. Previously, Lup et al. (2015) showed that the relationship between Instagram use and depressive symptoms was mediated by social comparison. Here, we discovered a similar relationship, with social comparison having a significant mediating effect on the relationship between Instagram use and depressive symptoms, as well as general anxiety, physical appearance anxiety, self-esteem, and body image disturbance. These results are also in line with previous research demonstrating that social comparison behavior after exposure to social media has a negative effect on mental health (Feinstein et al., 2013; Labrague, 2014; Vogel et al., 2014). Similarly, Hendrickse et al. (2017) found that appearance-related comparisons on Instagram mediated the relationship between Instagram photo activity and the drive for thinness and body dissatisfaction.

This research is important, as Instagram has some distinguishing features that set it apart from Facebook and relatively fewer studies have focused on Instagram. Importantly, Instagram is associated with a range of social trends, such as "fitspiration," which can lead to negative body image outcomes (Tiggemann & Zaccardo, 2015). Thus, excessive Instagram exposure may have an effect on other aspects of psychological well-being that extend beyond depressive symptoms to self-esteem and body image (e.g., Hendrickse et al., 2017). Although Facebook use is linked to negative outcomes, our assertion that exposure to visual media, specifically, can lead to negative outcomes is complemented by research by Meier and Gray (2014). Meier and Gray showed that Facebook photo activity, rather than total Facebook activity, correlated positively with body dissatisfaction. Therefore, based on our findings, increased use of the image-based platform Instagram, in which users post idealized images, is likely putting users at higher risk of negative outcomes than the users of other forms of social media.

In our sample, younger participants spent more time on Instagram, and engaged in higher levels of social comparison. Although our sample was restricted to a young adult to adult demographic (i.e., age 18–35 years), these findings suggest that Instagram use could pose an even higher risk to psychological well-being in adolescents.

In this study, we showed that the number of followers also correlated with the range of psychological well-being variables. Because Facebook and Instagram users are likely to share positive and idealistic portrayals of themselves, teenagers may feel they are "missing out" or "everyone is doing better" than themselves when making social comparisons online. This seems to relate to the extent to which individuals follow others who are unknown to them, with Chou and Edge (2012) showing that those who used Facebook for longer, and who followed more strangers, agreed more that others had better lives. These negative outcomes may be larger for teenagers who are less popular than their peers (Nesi & Prinstein, 2015).

Finally, although the aim of this research was to explore the effects of Instagram use on female psychological well-being, men are also prone to body dissatisfaction after exposure to idealized images (Galioto & Crowther, 2013; Hargreaves & Tiggemann, 2004), and social comparison can also mediate the link between social media use and depressive symptoms in men (Steers et al., 2014). Hence, it is worthwhile for future research to address the outcomes of excessive Instagram use in both adolescent samples and in men, including long-term impact.

JOURNAL ARTICLE EXERCISE 2

Remember that the science sections on the MCAT include a significant number of passages with experiments. You'll need to be able to extract information efficiently and analyze data effectively in order to do well on these passages.

This is the second of three "Journal Article Exercises" in this book. In the first exercise, we showed you the type of information you should be able to extract from the article and the sorts of things to pay attention to in the data. In this exercise, you'll do more of that on your own, and in the final exercise we'll show you how that article might get turned into an MCAT-style passage.

As a reminder, when analyzing an experiment, you should be able to:

- identify the control group(s)
- extract information from graphs and data tables
- determine how the experimental group(s) change relative to the control
- determine if the results are statistically significant
- come to a reasonable conclusion about WHY the results were observed
- consider potential weaknesses in the study
- determine how to increase the power of the study
- decide what the next most logical experiment or study should be

Again, the goal of these exercises is NOT to learn content from the articles, just to get a little more comfortable reading and extracting information from them.

For the (abridged) article on pages 203–205, try to summarize the purpose of the experiment and the methods in 4–5 sentences. Consider the following mnemonic: Oh ouR Car Won't Start (ORCWS).

- **O = Organism and Organization**: Is the research being conducted on humans or on animals or on bacteria in a petri dish, or something else? What is being done to these organisms? Are there any unique qualities to these organisms? Are there multiple groups? Is the study conducted over a long period of time with multiple data points, or is it a short-term study? Does it have a large or small n?

- **R = Results**: Where and how are the results presented? Is it a graph? A data table? Figures and images? What is/are the independent variable(s)? What is/are the dependent variable(s)? What are the results? Do the results show correlation or cause and effect, or both? Describe.

- **C = Control and Comparison**: Is there a control group? How does it differ from the experimental group? Is it given a placebo or nothing at all? Is it held under different conditions? If there are multiple experimental groups, how do they differ from one another? Is it a blinded study? If so, double-blind or single-blind?

- **W = Weirdness**: Does anything or do any of the results stand out as unexpected?

- **S = Statistics**: Was any sort of statistical analysis done? How is it presented? Are there error bars on a graph? Standard errors around a mean? Are there p-values? Is there an asterisk indicating statistical significance? Is there any data that is not statistically significant?

Try interpreting the data on your own before reading the results/discussion section. When you do read the discussion, consider:

- What are the conclusions of the study?
- How are the conclusions supported by the data?
- What potential weaknesses or flaws do you see in the experimental design? Are these addressed in the discussion section?
- How might this study be potentially biased?
- How might this study be improved?
- What would be the next most logical experiment?

Let's answer the above questions for the article on pages 203–205.

Write brief responses to the questions below:

1. **O = Organism and Organization:**
   - Is the research being conducted on humans or on animals or on bacteria in a petri dish, or something else?

     _____

     _____

   - What is being done to these organisms?

     _____

     _____

   - Are there any unique qualities to these organisms?

     _____

     _____

   - Are there multiple groups?

     _____

     _____

   - Is the study conducted over a long period of time with multiple data points, or is it a short-term study?

     _____

     _____

   - Does it have a large or small n?

     _____

     _____

2. **R = Results:**
   - Where and how are the results presented? Is it a graph? A data table? Figures and images?

     _____

     _____

   - What is/are the independent variable(s)?

     _____

     _____

   - What is/are the dependent variable(s)?

     _____

     _____

   - What are the results of the study?

     _____

     _____

- Do the results show correlation or cause and effect, or both? Describe.

  _____

  _____

3. **C = Control and Comparison:**
   - Is there a control group?

     _____

     _____

   - How does it differ from the experimental group? Is it given a placebo or nothing at all? Is it held under different conditions?

     _____

     _____

   - If there are multiple experimental groups, how do they differ from one another?

     _____

     _____

   - Is it a blinded study? If so, double-blind or single-blind?

     _____

     _____

4. **W = Weirdness:**
   - Does anything or do any of the results stand out as unexpected?

     _____

     _____

5. **S = Statistics:**
   - Was any sort of statistical analysis done?

     _____

     _____

   - How is it presented? Are there error bars on a graph? Standard errors around a mean? Are there p-values? Is there an asterisk indicating statistical significance?

     _____

     _____

   - Is there any data that is not statistically significant?

     _____

     _____

6. **Interpreting the data:**
   - What are the conclusions of the study?

     _____

     _____

- How are the conclusions supported by the data?

  _____

  _____

- What potential weaknesses or flaws do you see in the experimental design? Are these addressed in the discussion section?

  _____

  _____

- How might this study be potentially biased?

  _____

  _____

- How might this study be improved?

  _____

  _____

- What would be the next most logical experiment?

  _____

  _____

7. **Final Summary of Experiment and Results:**

   _____

   _____

   _____

   _____

   _____

   _____

SOLUTIONS TO JOURNAL ARTICLE EXERCISE 2

1. **O = Organism and Organization:**
   - Is the research being conducted on humans or on animals or on bacteria in a petri dish, or something else? *Humans*
   - What is being done to these organisms? *Participants filled out surveys*
   - Are there any unique qualities to these organisms? *All participants were women, all 18-35*
   - Are there multiple groups? *No*
   - Is the study conducted over a long period of time with multiple data points, or is it a short-term study? *Very short, 30–40 minutes*
   - Does it have a large or small *n*? *Relatively small: 129 participants*

2. **R = Results:**
   - Where and how are the results presented? Is it a graph? A data table? Figures and images? *Data table*
   - What is/are the independent variable(s)? *None, this is a correlational study.*
   - What is/are the dependent variable(s)? *None, this is a correlational study.*
   - What are the results of the study? *The average time spent on Instagram correlated positively with depressive symptoms, trait anxiety, social comparison orientation, physical appearance anxiety, and body image disturbance. The time spent on Instagram also correlated negatively with self-esteem. The number of followers also correlated positively with depression and trait anxiety, and negatively with self-esteem. The number of accounts followed correlated positively with depression and negatively with self-esteem. Additionally, age correlated negatively with Instagram use and negatively with social comparison.*
   - Do the results show correlation or cause and effect, or both? Describe. *The study is correlational and thus does not allow us to infer a cause and effect relationship.*

3. **C = Control and Comparison:**
   - Is there a control group? *No*
   - How does it differ from the experimental group? Is it given a placebo or nothing at all? Is it held under different conditions? *N/A*
   - If there are multiple experimental groups, how do they differ from one another? *N/A*
   - Is it a blinded study? If so, double-blind or single-blind? *Not a blinded study*

4. **W = Weirdness:**
   - Does anything or do any of the results stand out as unexpected? *No.*

5. **S = Statistics:**
   - Was any sort of statistical analysis done? *Yes*
   - How is it presented? Are there error bars on a graph? Standard errors around a mean? Are there *p*-values? Is there an asterisk indicating statistical significance? *R-values, standard deviation around the mean, asterisks*
   - Is there any data that is not statistically significant? *There are a few measures that are not statistically significant (e.g., self-rated attractiveness is not significant for low amount of time spent on Instagram).*

6. **Interpreting the data:**
   - What are the conclusions of the study? *Authors demonstrated that heavier Instagram use (as well as number of followers and number of people followed) correlated with a range of psychological well-being outcomes, including depressive symptoms, general anxiety, physical appearance anxiety, self-esteem, and body image disturbance.*
   - How are the conclusions supported by the data? *R-values are used to indicate both the direction and the strength of a correlation.*
   - What potential weaknesses or flaws do you see in the experimental design? Are these addressed in the discussion section? *Relatively small sample size, largely university students (who might react differently than those not in university), men were not included in the study.*
   - How might this study be potentially biased? *By the limited (mostly university student, all female) sample.*
   - How might this study be improved? *A wider participant pool, including men*
   - What would be the next most logical experiment? *Repeat the study, with a larger n, but also potentially with males, or participants from various countries/cultures.*

7. **Final Summary of Experiment and Results:**
   - *This correlational research implies that excessive exposure to Instagram can be damaging to users, especially when they engage in negative social comparisons. Exposure to content of idealistic beauty and fitness standards could be harmful in the long-term, considering the achievement of many of these ideals is unrealistic. This may be of particular importance in adolescents, who are heavy users of social media and engage in more social comparisons than do older adults.*

Chapter 8
Psychological Disorders and Stress

Psychological disorders affect personality, motivation, and attitude. The study and treatment of psychological disorders is an important field of psychology. Not only do the disorders help us understand how our minds and bodies function properly (by understanding what happens when something goes awry), but they also constitute a huge area of clinical practice.

8.1 PSYCHOLOGICAL DISORDERS

It is estimated that, in America, roughly one in every four adults (ages 18 and over) meets the diagnostic criteria for a psychological disorder. Psychological disorders are therefore an important part of our culture and comprise a significant component of our health care system. Psychological disorders, particularly when they go untreated, also affect our economy by impacting our social welfare and criminal justice systems.

Understanding Psychological Disorders

Although psychological disorders affect about one-quarter of the population, serious psychological disorders are less common, affecting roughly one in 17 people, or 6% of the U.S. population. A **psychological disorder** is a set of behavioral and/or psychological symptoms that are not in keeping with cultural norms, and that are severe enough to cause significant personal distress and/or significant impairment to social, occupational, or personal functioning. Sometimes cultural norms can be ruled out as a source of behavior; for example, when what appears to be a delusion or even a hallucination can be better understood in terms of religious or spiritual practice, that belief or experience would not count as a symptom of a psychological disorder. When cultural norms cannot explain behavior, the core components of diagnosis for a psychological disorder are *symptom quantity and severity*, and *impact on functioning*. A psychological disorder is *diagnosable* based on specific symptoms and symptom thresholds, and *treatable* (or at least *manageable*) with various types of medication and/or therapy.

Biopsychosocial Approach to Mental Health

As the three parts of the term indicate, the bio-psycho-social approach recognizes the interaction between nature (the biological, such as genetic predispositions) and nurture (the psychological, such as individual environmental forces), as well as the social (including cultural forces). For example, while not exclusive to Western cultures, eating disorders appear to be far more common in wealthier countries that espouse a thin ideal (like the United States) than they are in other parts of the world. It is also possible, for a given psychological disorder, that the underlying genetic and physiological dynamics are similar, but that the manifestation of the disorder for a particular person is influenced by cultural or social factors. Figure 1 presents the separate and overlapping influences that have been shown to correlate with psychological disorders.

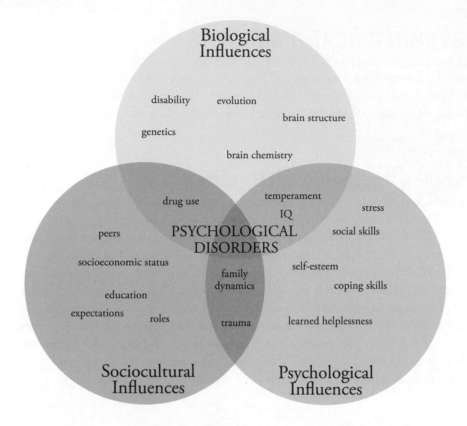

Figure 1   Biopsychosocial model of psychological disorders

Classifying Psychological Disorders

It is important to understand the classification of psychological disorders in order to understand the symptoms and prevalence of each. Without classification, it would be impossible to know what the biological and genetic risk factors are, which treatments work the best, and so on. In the United States and elsewhere in the world, current standards for classification and diagnosis are gathered in the **Diagnostical and Statistical Manual of Mental Disorders, Fifth edition (DSM-5)**, published in May 2013. Each new edition of the DSM reflects changes in research and clinical perspectives. For example, since the publication of the fourth edition in 1994, research findings and clinical experience prompted the publishers of the DSM-5 to combine the four separate autism disorders into one—Autism Spectrum Disorder—and to change the symptom categories from three to two areas. In several areas, in fact, the newest version of the DSM emphasizes the existence of a spectrum of behavior ranging from normal to disordered. Accurate diagnosis is critical; most insurance companies require a diagnosis based on DSM criteria before they will cover the cost of therapy.

For the purposes of the MCAT, familiarize yourself with the categories of disorders presented on the following pages in Table 1. Note that this list is not all-inclusive but instead presents the psychological disorders that are most likely to be tested.

Table 1 Categories of Psychological Disorders

Broad Category	Description	Specific Psychological Disorders
Anxiety Disorders	Anxiety disorders are characterized by excessive fear (of specific real things or more generally) and/or anxiety (of real or imagined *future* things or events) with both physiological and psychological symptoms.	• Separation Anxiety Disorder • Specific Phobia(s) • Social Anxiety Disorder • Panic Disorder • Generalized Anxiety Disorder
Obsessive-Compulsive and Related Disorders	Disorders in this category are distinct from anxiety disorders in that they involve a pattern of obsessive thoughts or urges that are coupled with maladaptive behavioral compulsions; the compulsions are experienced as a necessary/urgent response to the obsessive thoughts/urges, creating rigid, anxiety-filled routines.	• Obsessive-Compulsive Disorder • Body Dysmorphic Disorder • Hoarding Disorder
Trauma- and Stressor-Related Disorders	Traumas and stressors are central to the definition of these disorders, which involve unhealthy or pathological responses to one or more harmful or life-threatening events, including witnessing such an event. Subsequent symptoms include patterns of anxiety, depression, depersonalization, nightmares, insomnia, and/or a heightened startle response.	• Posttraumatic Stress Disorder • Acute Stress Disorder • Adjustment Disorders
Somatic Symptom Disorders	Somatic symptom disorders are characterized by physical symptoms that cannot be explained by a medical condition or substance use, and are not attributable to another psychological disorder, but that nonetheless cause emotional distress.	• Somatic Symptom Disorder • Illness Anxiety Disorder • Conversion Disorder • Factitious Disorder (imposed on self or another)
Bipolar and Related Disorders	Bipolar and related disorders involve mood swings or cycles (called episodes) ranging from manic to depressive, in which manic episodes tend to be followed by depressive episodes, and vice versa.	• Bipolar I Disorder • Bipolar II Disorder • Cyclothymic Disorder
Depressive Disorders	Depressive disorders are characterized by a disturbance in mood or affect. Specific symptoms include difficulties in sleep, concentration, and/or appetite; fatigue; and inability to experience pleasure (anhedonia).	• Major Depressive Disorder • Persistent Depressive Disorder (dysthymia) • Premenstrual Dysphoric Disorder

Broad Category	Description	Specific Psychological Disorders
Schizophrenia Spectrum and Other Psychotic Disorders	Psychotic disorders are characterized by a general "loss of contact with reality" which can include "positive" symptoms, such as delusions and hallucinations, and/or "negative" symptoms, such as flattened affect (e.g., monotone vocal expression).	• Delusional Disorder • Brief Psychotic Disorder • Schizophreniform Disorder • Schizophrenia • Schizoaffective Disorder
Dissociative Disorders	Dissociative disorders are characterized by disruptions in memory, awareness, identity, or perception. Many dissociative disorders are thought to be caused by psychological trauma.	• Dissociative Identity Disorder • Dissociative Amnesia • Depersonalization/Derealization Disorder

Personality Disorders	Personality disorders are characterized by enduring maladaptive patterns of behavior and cognition that depart from social norms, present across a variety of contexts, and cause significant dysfunction and distress. These patterns permeate the broader personality of the person and typically solidify during late adolescence or early adulthood.	Cluster A:
		  • Paranoid
		  • Schizoid
		  • Schizotypal
		Cluster B:
		  • Antisocial
		  • Borderline
		  • Histrionic
		  • Narcissistic
		Cluster C:
		  • Avoidant
		  • Dependent
		  • Obsessive-compulsive

Neurodevelopmental Disorders	Neurodevelopmental disorders are characterized by developmental deficits varying from specific learning impairments to global impairments of social skills or intelligence.	• Intellectual Disability • Attention-Deficit/Hyperactivity Disorder (ADHD) • Autism Spectrum Disorder (ASD)
Neurocognitive Disorders	Neurocognitive disorders are characterized by cognitive abnormalities or general decline in memory, problem-solving, and/or perception.	• Major and Mild Neurocognitive Disorders (MMND) • MMND Due to Alzheimer's Disease • MMND Due to Parkinson's Disease • Major or Mild Vascular Neurocognitive Disorder
Feeding and Eating Disorders	Feeding and eating disorders are characterized by abnormal eating behaviors such as severe undereating (anorexia nervosa) and purging to maintain unhealthy weight (bulimia nervosa).	• Anorexia Nervosa • Bulimia Nervosa • Pica • Binge Eating Disorder

Types of Psychological Disorders

The nine categories of psychological disorders discussed in this section correspond to the nine categories of disorders listed by the AAMC that you should be familiar with for the MCAT: Anxiety Disorders, Obsessive-Compulsive and Related Disorders, Trauma- and Stressor-Related Disorders, Somatic Symptom and Related Disorders, Bipolar and Related Disorders, Depressive Disorders, Schizophrenia Spectrum and Other Psychotic Disorders, Dissociative Disorders, and Personality Disorders. The following section discusses neurodevelopmental and neurocognitive disorders.

1. Anxiety Disorders

Anxiety is an emotional state of unpleasant physical and mental arousal—a preparation to fight or flee. For a person with an anxiety disorder, the anxiety is intense, frequent, irrational (out of proportion), and uncontrollable; it causes significant distress or impairment of normal functioning (at-work productivity, success in intimate relationships, and so on). Four types of anxiety disorders are discussed here: panic disorder, generalized anxiety disorder, specific phobia, and social phobia (now called "Social Anxiety Disorder").

Symptoms mimicking an anxiety disorder can also be caused by general medical conditions, alcohol, certain recreational drugs, or medication use or withdrawal. If a person has a medical condition or uses substances that are likely to be causing the symptoms, the diagnosis is "anxiety disorder due to a general medical condition" or "substance-induced anxiety disorder." This approach to specifying non-psychological causes applies to the other sections of the DSM-5 as well.

Panic Disorder A person with **panic disorder** has suffered at least one **panic attack** and is worried about having more of them. The panic attacks can be triggered by certain situations, but they are more often uncued or "spontaneous," occurring unexpectedly and with sometimes unpredictable frequency.

During a **panic attack**, a person commonly experiences intense dread, along with shortness of breath, chest pain, a choking sensation, and cardiac symptoms such as a rapid heartbeat or palpitations. There may also be trembling, sweating, lightheadedness, or chills. Many fear they are dying of a heart attack or stroke during a panic attack. One danger of panic attacks is that they can mask other illnesses, such as heart attacks and **mood disorders**. Although panic attacks are brief (often less than 30 minutes in duration), they can be excruciating, and people with panic disorder live in fear of having more panic attacks. Panic disorder can be debilitating if left untreated, but people with this disorder do respond well to treatment.

Generalized Anxiety Disorder A person with **generalized anxiety disorder** (GAD) feels tense or anxious much of the time about many issues, but does not experience panic attacks. The source of this underlying, chronic nervousness can seem like a moving target, shifting from one situation to another, or there may be no identifiable source. The distress and impairment associated with GAD is not often severe; it may include restlessness, tiring easily, poor concentration, irritability, muscle tension, and insomnia or restless sleep.

Specific Phobia and Social Phobia There are several types of **phobias**. In specific and social phobias, the sufferer feels a strong fear that he or she recognizes as unreasonable. He or she nevertheless almost always experiences either general anxiety or a full panic attack when confronted with the feared object or situation. People with phobias often go to great lengths to avoid the triggers they fear, and this avoidance itself is part of the symptom profile.

Specific phobia is a persistent, strong, and unreasonable fear of a certain object or situation. Specific phobias are classified into four types (plus "other") depending on the types of triggers they involve (see Table 2).

Table 2 Types of Specific Phobias

Type of Specific Phobia	Example of Triggers
Situational	Flying, elevators, bridges, crowds (in agoraphobia)
Natural Environment	Thunderstorms, heights, water, lightning
Blood-Injection-Injury	Injections, blood, surgical procedures
Animal	Spiders, snakes, dogs

Social Anxiety Disorder, or **Social Phobia**, is an unreasonable, paralyzing fear of feeling embarrassed or humiliated while one is seen or watched by others, even while performing routine activities such as eating in public or using a public restroom. Here too a prominent symptom is avoidance, which can lead to social isolation.

2. Obsessive-Compulsive and Related Disorders

Separated now from anxiety disorders, these disorders feature at least one pronounced repetitive behavior that exceeds cultural norms and rituals such as grooming practices or maintaining a healthy body weight. Unsuccessful attempts to decrease or otherwise manage these behaviors are also central to the diagnosis. Without therapeutic intervention, these conditions tend to increase over time in terms of severity or level of self-harm, or both.

Obsessive-Compulsive Disorder A person with **obsessive-compulsive disorder (OCD)** has obsessions, compulsions, or both. **Obsessions** are repeated, intrusive, uncontrollable thoughts or impulses that cause distress or anxiety. The person knows the thoughts are irrational, and despite attempts to disregard or suppress them, typically resorts to responding to them through a compulsive behavior. **Compulsions** are repeated physical or mental behaviors (e.g., counting) that are performed in response to an obsession or in accordance with a set of strict rules, in order to reduce distress or prevent something dreaded from occurring. The person realizes that the compulsive behavior is not rational, being either unrelated to the dreaded event, or related but clearly excessive. Nevertheless, if the person does not perform the behavior, he or she feels intense anxiety and a conviction that the terrible event will happen. Some common obsessions and compulsions are listed in Table 3.

Table 3 Common Obsessions and Compulsions

Obsessions (Thoughts)	Compulsions (Actions)
• Irrational fear of contamination by dirt, germs, or toxins • Pathological doubt that a task was done, or fear of having inadvertently harmed someone or violated a law • Fear of harming someone violently or sexually, or otherwise behaving in an unacceptable way	• Washing self (often hands) or surroundings repeatedly, sometimes with a lengthy ritual • Checking repeatedly that a task was done, sometimes with a lengthy ritual • Counting to a certain number before certain tasks, or performing a behavior a certain number of times (such as folding a shirt) • Arranging objects or performing actions with perfect symmetry or precision

3. Trauma- and Stressor-Related Disorders

Like the disorders in the previous section, these were also separated in the DSM-5 from what used to be a much broader category of anxiety disorders. Although anxiety can accompany a response to a traumatic or stressful event, many people who have been exposed to such an event display primarily symptoms other than anxiety (such as dysphoria, aggression, and/or dissociation).

Posttraumatic Stress Disorder **Posttraumatic stress disorder (PTSD)** can arise when a person feels intense fear, horror, or helplessness after experiencing, witnessing, or otherwise confronting an extremely traumatic event that involves actual or threatened death, serious injury, or sexual violence to the self or others. It is estimated that most people (more than half) will experience at least one traumatic event in their lifetime, but only a small subset of those will develop PTSD. Approximately 8% of men and 20% of women develop PTSD after a trauma. Rates of PTSD are higher in males of Latino heritage and males who have served in active combat, for whom the estimated prevalence reaches 20%.

The traumatic event is often *relived* (not just remembered) through dreams and flashbacks in which the person feels as though the event is currently happening, and which can include multisensory reprocessing, such as the intrusion of smells and sounds from the original event context. Some experience mental or physiological distress (e.g., elevated heart rate or blood pressure) when reminded of the event, however indirectly. A person with PTSD tries to avoid people, places, feelings, thoughts, or conversations that are reminders of the event, or even avoids people and feelings in general. The person may also be chronically physiologically hyperaroused, with symptoms such as an increased startle response, insomnia, angry outbursts, poor concentration, and extreme alertness (called **hypervigilance**). For a diagnosis of PTSD, these symptoms must have been present for more than a month. Symptoms may not begin until months or even years after the trauma.

Acute stress disorder Similar to PTSD, but its symptoms last between 3 days and 1 month. Indeed, some instances of PTSD begin as acute distress disorder.

Adjustment disorders In adjustment disorders, the maladaptive response is to a stressor (a romantic break-up, job issues, marital issues) rather than a trauma. This response may last between 3 and 6 months. The diagnosis also applies in cases where the subsequent distress appears in some way to be disproportionate to the cause.

For all three conditions, it is noteworthy that individuals from low-SES communities, or who are otherwise disadvantaged, encounter more stressors in their everyday lives and are thus at increased risk for a disorder in this category.

4. Somatic Symptom and Related Disorders

A **somatic symptom disorder** is a psychological disorder characterized primarily by distress and decreased functioning due to persistent physical symptoms and concerns, which may mimic physical (somatic) disease but generally are not rooted in any detectable pathophysiology. Further, the somatic symptoms do not improve with medical treatment. This symptom/behavior pattern is commonly referred to as "hypochondriasis," but as the differences between these disorders should make clear, that term lacks precision.

Though they are often treated with skepticism even by physicians (a large majority of these diagnoses occur in the primary care setting), most people with somatic symptom disorders—the exception being factitious disorders—genuinely experience their symptoms and/or believe that there is something physically wrong with them. The DSM-5 accounts for this complexity with streamlined presentation of four subtypes: somatic symptom disorder, illness anxiety disorder, conversion disorder, and factitious disorder.

Somatic Symptom Disorder For someone with **somatic symptom disorder**, the central complaint is one or more somatic symptoms—such as chronic pain or headaches or fatigue—and diagnosis also requires evidence of diminished functioning stemming from excessive preoccupation with and/or anxiety about the symptoms. Whether the symptoms in any way coincide with a related medical problem or illness, the distress and/or disruption of daily life caused by the symptoms warrants at least consideration of the diagnosis.

Illness Anxiety Disorder One reason **"hypochondriasis"** can be considered imprecise is that it refers to concern about both illness and somatic symptoms. **Illness anxiety disorder** differs from somatic symptom disorder insofar as the somatic aspect of the illness is not as central or can even be nonexistent. In illness anxiety disorder, the distress is predominantly psychological, with people experiencing persistent preoccupation with both their health condition and health-related behaviors, including seeking treatment.

Conversion Disorder A person with **conversion disorder** experiences a change in sensory or motor function—such as weakness, tremors, seizures, or difficulty talking or eating—that has no discernible physical or physiological cause and that seems to be significantly affected by psychological factors. The symptoms of conversion disorder typically begin or worsen after an emotional conflict or other stressor. As the terminology suggests, the emotion or anxiety is "converted" into a physical symptom. The change in function is severe enough to warrant medical attention, or to cause significant distress or impairment in work, social, or personal functioning. Diagnosis of conversion disorder is possible, for example, when a person suddenly experiences blindness but his or her blink reflex remains intact.

Factitious Disorder This disorder is colloquially referred to as "Münchhausen Syndrome" (when imposed on oneself) or "Münchhausen by proxy" (when imposed on someone else). In **factitious disorder imposed on self**, a person has not just fabricated an illness but has gone the further step of either falsifying evidence or symptoms of the illness or inflicting harm to him- or herself to induce injury or illness. Though the person presents the illness to others and thus attracts interpersonal and/or medical attention, diagnosis requires evidence that the person behaves this way even without obvious benefit. When someone induces physical or psychological symptoms in someone else, often a child—and then presents the other person as ill or injured—the perpetrator of the deception is diagnosed with **factitious disorder imposed on another**.

5. Bipolar and Related Disorders

Bipolar Disorders Most people with a **bipolar disorder** (formerly called manic depression) experience cyclic mood episodes oscillating between the extremes or 'poles' of depression and mania.

Table 4 Diagnostic Criteria for Bipolar and Related Disorders and Depressive Disorders

	Manic Episode	Hypomanic Episode	Major Depressive Episode
Duration	At least one week, nearly every day	At least four consecutive days	At least two weeks
Mood	Elevated, expansive, or irritable mood	Elevated, expansive, or irritable mood	Depressed; diminished interest or pleasure in almost all activities
Self-image	Inflated, grandiose	Inflated, grandiose	Feelings of worthlessness or excessive guilt
Appetite/weight	May show diminished appetite or interest in food	May show diminished appetite or interest in food	Increase or decrease in body weight by 5% or more in a month
Sleep need	Decreased	Decreased	Insomnia or hypersomnia
Cognition	Flight of ideas or racing thoughts; distractibility	Flight of ideas or racing thoughts; distractibility	Diminished ability to think or concentrate; recurrent thoughts of death or suicide
Speech	Rapid, pressured	Rapid, pressured	May manifest muted or flat affect in speech
Energy/behavior	Increased energy and goal-directed activity and/or psychomotor agitation	Increased energy and goal-directed activity and/or psychomotor agitation	Fatigue or loss of energy; psychomotor agitation or slowness
Judgment	Lack of consequential thinking	Lack of consequential thinking	May include suicide attempt or a specific plan for committing suicide
Impairment in functioning	Severe, marked impairment; may require hospitalization (to prevent harm to self or others); may include psychotic features	Unequivocal, observable change that is not typical of the individual; not severe enough to cause marked impairment or to necessitate hospitalization	Clinically significant distress or marked impairment in one or more areas of functioning

In a **manic episode**, a person has experienced an abnormal euphoric, unrestrained, or irritable mood for at least one week, as well as a marked increase in either goal-directed activity (e.g., increased energy and productivity at work) or in psychomotor agitation, which stems from an urge to be engaged in goal-directed activity but without the focus necessary to do so. (Hence, the "surplus" energy causes agitation and irritability.) For example, someone experiencing a manic episode may feel compelled to spend hours shopping online or looking for an activity to absorb the energy. These symptoms are severe enough to cause psychotic features, hospitalization, or impairment of work, social, or personal function.

Bipolar I disorder is diagnosed only if there has been a spontaneous manic episode not triggered by treatment for depression or caused by another medical condition or medication. The disorder may include a swing to a full depressive episode, or only to partial or moderate depression (dysthymic symptoms), or no depression at all (although this is rare). In a **mixed episode**, a person has met the symptoms for both major depressive and manic episodes nearly every day for at least a week, and the symptoms are severe enough to cause psychotic features, hospitalization, or impaired work, social, or personal functioning. In the simplest terms, the only requirement for a diagnosis of **bipolar I disorder** is that the person has experienced at least one manic or mixed episode.

In a person with **bipolar II disorder**, the manic phases are less extreme. A person with bipolar II disorder has experienced cyclic moods, including at least one major depressive episode and one hypomanic episode, but has not met the criteria for a manic or mixed episode. In a **hypomanic episode**, for at least four days a person has experienced an abnormally euphoric or irritable mood, with at least three of the symptoms for a manic episode, but at a less severe level. With hypomania, the impairment or distress is less serious, and there is no psychosis or hospitalization. In a **major depressive episode**, a person has felt worse than usual for most of the day, nearly every day, for at least two weeks. The individual also has at least five of the following emotional, behavioral, cognitive, and physical symptoms: depressed mood or decreased interest in activities, significant increase or decrease in weight or appetite, excessive or insufficient sleep, agitated or slowed psychomotor activity, fatigue or loss of energy, feelings of low self-worth or excessive guilt, impaired concentration or decision-making, and thoughts of death or suicide. The diagnosis of bipolar II disorder requires both types of episodes.

Cyclothymic Disorder **Cyclothymic disorder** is similar to the bipolar disorders, but the moods are less extreme, with symptoms not meeting the criteria for either a manic or a major depressive episode. A person with cyclothymic disorder has experienced cyclic moods, including multiple hypomanic episodes, as well as episodes of depressed mood that are milder than a major depressive episode, for at least two years. These mood swings have never been absent for more than two months.

6. Depressive Disorders

A **depressive disorder** is more than acute moodiness; it is a persistent pattern of abnormal and often painful mood symptoms severe enough to cause significant personal distress and/or impairment to social, occupational, or personal functioning. While **emotions** or **feelings** are measurable in terms of seconds, minutes, or hours, **mood** describes a baseline of weeks or months; mood is a person's sustained internal emotion that colors his or her view of life. Three depressive disorders are discussed in this section: major depressive disorder, persistent depressive disorder (dysthymia), and premenstrual dysphoric disorder (this last condition is new in DSM-5).

Major Depressive Disorder A person with **major depressive disorder** (MDD) has suffered one or more major depressive episodes (as discussed in the previous section). Ten percent of people with major depressive disorder attempt suicide and many more contemplate it or devise a suicide plan. These symptoms do not indicate major depression if they occur within two months of bereavement, as they may be part of a normal grieving reaction. In seasonal affective disorder (or what DSM-5 refers to as MDD "with seasonal pattern"), episodes of depression occur during certain seasons, usually fall and winter.

Persistent Depressive Disorder (Dysthymia) **Persistent depressive disorder** (PDD), also called **dysthymic disorder** or **dysthymia**, is a less intense, but typically more chronic form of depression. A person with PDD has experienced milder symptoms of depression most days for at least two years, with symptoms never absent for more than two months, but without a major depressive episode. Onset is typically adolescence or early adulthood, and the persistence of the condition often leaves people feeling like they've "always felt this way" or as if they are a "depressed person" to their core.

Premenstrual Dysphoric Disorder In **premenstrual dysphoric disorder**, which is diagnosed only in women, many of the symptoms of a major depressive episode are present, with the caveat that they intensify in the final week before the onset of menses and then improve, and in many cases disappear, in the week after menstruation has ended. There are a few symptoms that distinguish the illness from the other two depressive disorders discussed here: feeling keyed up or on edge, specific food cravings, a sense of being overwhelmed or out of control, as well as the physical symptoms of the body's preparation for menstruation: tenderness or swelling in the breasts, joint or muscle pain, and bloating.

Figure 2 compares the various mood states or episodes for depressive disorders and bipolar and related disorders. Persistent depressive disorder is thus a milder (though often more persistent) form of major depressive disorder, whereas bipolar disorder I, bipolar disorder II, and cyclothymia generally involve cycling through either manic or hypomanic episodes, and dysthymic or depressed episodes.

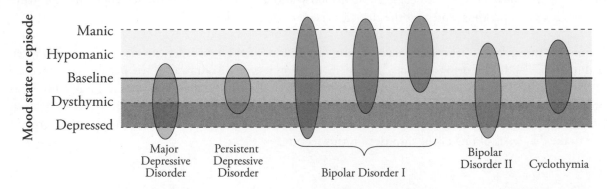

Figure 2 Depressive disorders and bipolar (and related) disorders based on diagnostic criteria for mood state or episode

7. Schizophrenia Spectrum and Other Psychotic Disorders

Schizophrenia spectrum and other psychotic disorders are diagnosed when someone has been experiencing one or more of the following **positive symptoms**: delusions, hallucinations, disorganized thinking (as manifested in disorganized speech), disorganized or abnormal motor behavior, and/or one or more **negative symptoms**, such as decreased emotional expression (presentation of "flat" **affect**), *avolition* (lack of motivation or purpose), and/or *alogia* (decreased or absent speech). Positive symptoms indicate the presence of an atypical behavior or other characteristic. Negative symptoms indicate a decrease in, or lack of, a typical behavior or other characteristic. The general profile of the disorders in this section is that they involve some sort of splitting off or distancing of the person from aspects of his or her everyday reality.

Although schizophrenia literally means "split mind," the term refers to a split in mental functions, or a split from reality; it does not indicate a split in identity. Many people incorrectly use the term schizophrenia to mean "multiple personality disorder" (a condition now called dissociative identity disorder).

A **delusion** is a false belief that is not due to culture, and is not relinquished despite evidence that it is false. For example, a person might believe that he or she is a certain movie star. Delusions are different from strongly held non-psychotic beliefs, both in intensity and plausibility. For someone with **delusional disorder**, one or more delusions have been present for at least a month, and counterevidence is generally denied or distorted to keep the delusion intact. Common delusions include erotomania (the belief that someone is in love with you), grandiosity (the belief that you have a special talent or insight), and persecution (the belief that you are being followed, drugged, harassed, and so on).

A **hallucination** is a false sensory perception that occurs while a person is conscious (not during sleep or delirium). It is important to distinguish between true hallucinations, which occur in the absence of related sensory stimuli, and illusions, which are misperceptions of actual sensory stimuli (which may occur in low light). The most common hallucinations are auditory and visual.

Schizophrenia is diagnosed when someone has been experiencing positive, and sometimes negative, symptoms for longer than six months. Here the impact on functioning is greatest, with impairment in work, relationships, and/or self-care. Though the symptoms may subside at times to a prodromal level (just below the diagnostic threshold), there is no complete remission without medication. On the schizophrenia spectrum, schizophrenia proper thus represents the chronic version of the disorder.

Symptoms mimicking a schizophrenia spectrum (or other psychotic) disorder can also be caused by a general medical condition, or by alcohol, drug, or medication use or withdrawal. If the person has a medical condition or uses substances that could be causing the symptoms, the diagnosis should be psychotic disorder due to a general medical condition or substance-induced psychotic disorder. Symptoms of psychosis can also occur with mood or developmental disorders. All of these disorders must be ruled out before one can make diagnosis of one of the disorders in this section.

8. Dissociative Disorders

During a dissociative experience, some of a person's thoughts, feelings, perceptions, memories, or behaviors are separated from conscious awareness and control, in a way that is not explainable as mere forgetfulness. This separation sometimes occurs as a defense against a traumatic situation that is too overwhelming to hold in awareness. In a **dissociative disorder**, the disruptions in awareness, memory, and identity are extreme and/or frequent, and they cause distress or impair the person's functioning. Dissociative disorders can be triggered by severe stress or psychological conflicts, and they usually begin and end suddenly.

Dissociative Identity Disorder A person with **dissociative identity disorder** alternates among two or more distinct personality states (or identities), only one of which interacts with other people at a given time. The condition may be experienced as a "possession" by another personality or identity, as it involves amnesia—loss of awareness or memory—for one or more of the personality states. These distinct identities may vary widely in age, gender, and personality traits, and they may or may not be aware of one another. This disorder was previously known as multiple personality disorder.

Dissociative Amnesia A person with **dissociative amnesia** has had at least one episode of forgetting some important personal information, creating gaps in memory that are usually related to severe stress or trauma. The person may wander aimlessly during the episode or experience it as a kind of journey, in what is called a **dissociative fugue**. Most often, the amnesia is localized, meaning that everything that happened during a particular time frame is forgotten, but it can also be selective (only some events during a particular time frame are forgotten), generalized (the person's whole lifetime is forgotten), continuous (everything since a certain time is forgotten), or systematized (only particular categories of information are forgotten, such as everything relating to the person's family). The disorder usually begins and ends suddenly, with full recovery of memory, though it may also linger with some information only gradually, if ever, fully coming back to consciousness. Unfortunately, when remission means recovery of disturbing memories, amnesia may give way to suicidal ideation or behavior, or to PTSD or another condition.

Depersonalization/Derealization Disorder A person with **depersonalization disorder** has a recurring or persistent feeling of being cut off or detached from his or her body or mental processes, as if observing themselves from the outside, in something like an out-of-body experience. In a **derealization disorder**, on the other hand, a person experiences a feeling that people or objects in the external world are unreal. In both cases, the person knows that the feeling is not accurate—his or her "reality testing" remains intact—and the depersonalization and/or derealization, plus awareness of this incongruity, causes distress or impairs functioning. The disorder usually first occurs in late adolescence, with almost all cases having a first onset before the person is 25 years old. Onset and remission can be sudden or gradual, with stress or novel situations often playing an exacerbating role.

9. Personality Disorders

Personality traits are stable patterns of thought, feeling, and behavior that influence how a person experiences, thinks about, and interacts with the people and events in his or her life. A **personality disorder** is an enduring, rigid set of personality traits that deviates from cultural norms, impairs functioning, and causes distress either to the person with the disorder or to those in his or her life. The symptom profile therefore involves a list of the prominent traits that characterize each "disordered" personality. Because many personality disorders are **egosyntonic**—generally in harmony with a person's ego or self-image—it is usually the consequences of the personality disorder, such as depression, rather than its symptom structure, that cause a person to seek treatment.

The degree of distress or impairment is important. Because personality traits are not simply binary—"normal" versus "pathological"—but instead represent a continuum (for example, from independent to nonconforming to antisocial), the same constellations of traits that are found in personality disorders can also be present to varying degrees in normal people. A difficult or rigid personality becomes a personality disorder when the pattern causes significant distress or impairment, has been present since adolescence or young adulthood, affects nearly all personal and social situations, and creates dysfunction in two or more of the following areas: affect, cognition, impulse control, and interpersonal functioning.

In the DSM-5, the personality disorders have been organized, or "clustered," into three categories. **Cluster A** includes the paranoid, schizoid, and schizotypal personality disorders associated with irrational, withdrawn, odd, or suspicious behaviors. **Cluster B** includes the antisocial, borderline, histrionic, and narcissistic personality disorders associated with emotional, dramatic, and self-centered behaviors, and intense interpersonal conflict. **Cluster C** includes the avoidant, dependent, and obsessive-compulsive personality disorders, associated with fearful, anxious, over-controlled behaviors.

Table 5 Personality Disorders

Category	Personality Disorder	Traits
Cluster A	Paranoid Schizoid Schizotypal	Irrational, Withdrawn, Odd, Suspicious
Cluster B	Antisocial Borderline Histrionic Narcissistic	Emotional, Dramatic, Self-centered, Intense
Cluster C	Avoidant Dependent Obsessive-Compulsive	Fearful, Anxious, Over-controlled

Cluster A

Paranoid Personality Disorder A person with **paranoid personality disorder** mistrusts and misinterprets others' motives and actions without sufficient cause, suspecting them of deceiving, harming, betraying, or attacking him or her. The person tends to be guarded, tense, and self-sufficient, generally in counterproductive/maladaptive ways.

Schizoid Personality Disorder A person with **schizoid personality disorder** is a loner with little interest or involvement in close relationships, even those with family members. The person seems unaffected emotionally by interactions with other people, appearing instead detached or cold. This disorder is thus characterized by one of the negative symptoms of schizophrenia.

Schizotypal Personality Disorder A person with **schizotypal personality disorder** has several traits that cause problems interpersonally, including limited or inappropriate affect; magical or paranoid thinking; and odd beliefs, speech, behavior, appearance, and perceptions. This disorder is thus characterized by some of the positive symptoms of schizophrenia. The person tends to have no confidantes other than close relatives. Many cases eventually develop into schizophrenia (the disorder is cross-listed in the DSM-5 in the section on Schizophrenia Spectrum and Other Psychotic Disorders).

Cluster B

Antisocial Personality Disorder A person with **antisocial personality disorder** has a history of serious behavior problems beginning as a young teen (often even younger), including significant aggression against people or animals, deliberate property destruction, lying or theft, and serious rule violation. In addition, the person must have a history (since age 15) of repeatedly disregarding the rights of others in various ways without remorse, through illegal activities, dishonesty, impulsiveness, physical fights, disregard for safety, and financial irresponsibility. This disorder is cross-listed in the DSM-5 in the section on Disruptive, Impulse-Control, and Conduct Disorders. It is more frequently encountered in men and specifically in incarcerated men.

Borderline Personality Disorder A person with **borderline personality disorder** suffers from enduring or recurrent instability in his or her impulse control, mood, and image of self and others. Impulsive and reckless behavior, together with extreme mood swings, reactivity, and anger, can lead to unstable relationships and to damage, both to the person with the disorder and to others in his or her life. Feeling empty, with an unstable sense of self, the person is terrified of abandonment by others, whom the person may first idealize and then devalue or demonize. Self-harming and suicidal behaviors may also occur. There is some evidence that this disorder is a generalized and more severe form of a bipolar disorder and/or that it is linked to childhood sexual abuse. It is more frequently encountered in women.

Histrionic Personality Disorder A person with **histrionic personality disorder** strongly desires to be the center of attention, and often seeks to attract attention through personal appearance and seductive behavior. The person's expressions of emotion are dramatic, yet the emotions themselves are often shallow and shifting, and the person may believe that his or her relationships are more intimate than they are. The person may also be suggestible, and vague in his or her speech.

Narcissistic Personality Disorder A person with **narcissistic personality disorder** feels grandiosely self-important, with fantasies of beauty, brilliance, and power. The person feels a desperate need for admiration in a variety of contexts and may be intensely envious. Lacking empathy, he or she may continually exploit others and behave in an arrogant, haughty, and entitled manner.

Cluster C

Avoidant Personality Disorder A person with **avoidant personality disorder** feels inadequate, inferior, and undesirable and is preoccupied with fears of criticism and conflict. The person feels ashamed, and avoids interpersonal contact and new activities, unless he or she is certain of being liked. The person is also restrained and inhibited in relationships.

Dependent Personality Disorder A person with **dependent personality disorder** feels a need to be taken care of by others and an unrealistic fear of being unable to take care of him- or herself. The person also has trouble assuming responsibility and making decisions, preferring to gain approval by making others responsible and seeking others' advice and reassurance regarding decisions. In relationships, he or she is clingy, submissive, and afraid to express disagreement. Others often take advantage of the person because he or she is willing to do or tolerate almost anything, even abuse, in order to gain support and nurturing, and to avoid abandonment. He or she urgently seeks another relationship if one is lost.

Obsessive-Compulsive Personality Disorder A person with **obsessive-compulsive personality disorder** (OCPD) may be perfectionistic, rigid, and stubborn, with a strong need for control. The person resists others' authority, and will not cooperate with or delegate to others unless things are done his or her way. Often workaholic and moralistic beyond the level of the surrounding culture or religion, the person also may be depressed and have trouble expressing affection. A preoccupation with orderliness and list-making across a variety of situations can interfere with effectiveness and efficiency. OCPD is cross-listed in the DSM-5 in the section on Obsessive-Compulsive and Related Disorders.

Biological Bases of Nervous System Disorders

Schizophrenia

Recall that schizophrenia is a disorder characterized by positive symptoms, such as delusions, hallucinations, and disorganized speech, as well as negative ones, such as flat affect, decreased or absent speech, and avolition. Although schizophrenia presents as a thought disorder, it is important to remember that psychological characteristics have a physical or neurological basis; the division between these two is largely a conceptual one (based on an outdated **mind-body dualism** framework). Schizophrenia is a neurological disorder with a strong genetic basis. Studies have found that in identical twins, if one twin has schizophrenia, the other has about a 50% chance of also having it; if the second twin does not have schizophrenia, the first twin is likely to have a lesser form of it (e.g., schizophreniform disorder). The onset of schizophrenia happens around adolescence. The **stress-diathesis theory** suggests that while genetic inheritance provides a biological predisposition for schizophrenia, stressors elicit the onset of the disease.

There are numerous brain changes that have been noted in people with schizophrenia. One idea formed from observations is the **dopamine hypothesis**, which suggests that the pathway for the neurotransmitter dopamine is hyperactive in people with schizophrenia. This is due both to an overabundance of dopamine and to hypersensitive dopamine receptors. This finding, along with evidence of hyperactivation of the temporal lobes in people with this condition, may explain the presence of the positive signs of schizophrenia (like auditory hallucinations). Dopamine antagonist medications have been found to be helpful as antipsychotics.

Additionally, *hypo*activation of the frontal lobes may be responsible for the negative signs of schizophrenia, creating a kind of pseudo-depression, flat affect, and impaired speech. Individuals with schizophrenia have also been found to have smaller brains due to atrophy: schizophrenic individuals display increased ventricles (cavities in the brain), and enlarged sulci and fissures (less folding).

Depression

Depression also appears to have a strong genetic basis—there is increased risk of developing depression when a first-degree family member has it. Depression has been linked to diminished functioning in pathways in the brain that involve the neurotransmitters dopamine, serotonin, and norepinephrine. Antidepressants thus target and try to stimulate these pathways. Depression can often accompany other neurological diseases, such as Parkinson's and traumatic brain injury, due to damage to similar or overlapping areas of the brain.

Neurodevelopmental Disorders

As the name "neurodevelopmental" implies, something abnormal occurred to the brain during early development, whether *in utero* or shortly after birth. While **intellectual disability** can have several causes, a notable one is Down syndrome (trisomy 21) in which a third copy of chromosome 21 is present in the genome. In the case of **attention-deficit/hyperactivity disorder (ADHD)**, PET scans have suggested a general understimulation of the brain, which helps explain why stimulants may alleviate some of the behavioral symptoms. In the case of **autism spectrum disorder (ASD)**, brain structure and chemistry are still being studied; one leading hypothesis involves the underformation of mirror neurons.

Neurocognitive Disorders

Dementia (the general term for what is called a neurocognitive disorder in DSM-5) is a severe loss of cognitive ability beyond what would be expected from normal aging. **Alzheimer's disease** ("major or minor neurocognitive disorder due to Alzheimer's disease") is the most prevalent form of dementia, affecting a large number of people who reach their 80s and especially their 90s (over 50% for this latter group, according to some estimates). It is a disease that is characterized by **anterograde amnesia**, the inability to form new memories, as well as stepwise **retrograde amnesia**, with more recent memories degrading first, such that the last memories to fade are typically the oldest. Alzheimer's patients may thus be able to recall events from decades earlier but forget people and events that were encountered recently. Their visual memory will be impaired as well, such that they may get lost and confused. Needless to say, living with Alzheimer's disease can be very confusing, frustrating, and emotionally painful both for the patient and for family members and friends.

Alzheimer's disease is a cortical disease, meaning that it affects the cortex, the outermost tissue of the brain. It is caused by the formation of **neuritic plaques**, hard formations of beta-amyloid protein and **neurofibrillary tangles** (clumps of tau protein). It is unclear why these plaques and tangles form, though there is some evidence of at least partial genetic susceptibility. Some theories suggest that when these plaques build up, they reach a critical mass and then begin to cause cell death by "gunking up" neuronal connections, preventing nutrients and waste from traveling to and from some neurons. Currently, there is no cure for Alzheimer's, and treatments are directed at slowing the progress of the illness rather than reversing it.

Finally, there is some evidence of abnormalities in the activity of the neurotransmitter acetylcholine in the hippocampus. It should be no surprise that the hippocampus could be involved, because this is the area of the brain that plays a major role in the formation of new memories. As mentioned above, the disease tends to progress in a predictable pattern: as it progresses, the patient loses increasingly older memories, as well as language function and spatial coordination. Eventually, patients are not able to perform daily functions without assistance.

Parkinson's disease ("major or mild neurocognitive disorder due to Parkinson's disease" in the DSM-5) is a movement disorder caused by the death of cells that generate dopamine in the **basal ganglia** and **substantia nigra**, two subcortical structures in the brain. Among the symptoms are a resting tremor (shaking), slowed movement, rigidity of movements and facial expressions, and a shuffling gait. As the disease progresses, language is typically spared. However, depression and visual-spatial problems may arise. It is estimated that 50% to 80% of Parkinson's patients eventually experience dementia as their disease progresses. In order to treat Parkinson's, patients are given L-dopa treatments. L-dopa is a precursor to dopamine and is used because it is able to pass the blood-brain barrier, entering the brain's blood supply (dopamine is not able to cross the blood-brain barrier).

8.2 STRESS

The Nature of Stress

Stress is a great reminder that often what is considered to be psychological is simultaneously physiological. Under acute conditions of stress, such as while giving a formal presentation, it is common to feel physical symptoms such as increased heart rate and sweating. Prolonged periods of stress can have negative consequences, including immunosuppression, infertility, and hypertension. However, stress is not a simple stimulus-response phenomenon. How a stimulus is perceived plays a large role in how much stress is experienced.

Appraisal

Not everyone responds the same way to events that can trigger a stressful reaction. For example, imagine that a couple is at home in bed when suddenly they hear a creaking sound in another room. One person may assume that the sound is due to the age of the house or the steps of a pet, while the other may attribute the sound to a possible burglar sneaking around the house. Obviously, though the stimulus is the same, one person is going to become much more stressed than the other. What is most important for determining the stressful nature of an event is its **appraisal**, or how it is interpreted by the individual. When stressors are appraised as being challenges, as one may perceive the MCAT, they can actually be motivating. On the other hand, when they are perceived as threatening aspects of our identity, well-being, or safety, they may cause severe stress. Additionally, events that are considered negative and uncontrollable produce a greater stress response than those that are perceived as negative but controllable.

Different Types of Stressors

There are three main types of stressors, which differ in terms of their severity: catastrophes, significant life changes, and daily hassles.

1) **Catastrophes** are unpredictable, large-scale events that include natural disasters and war. They are events that almost everyone would appraise as dangerous and stress-inducing. The repercussions of a catastrophic event are often felt for years after the event. In the months following 9/11, many people developed psychological disorders including anxiety, depression, and posttraumatic stress disorder (PTSD). Health consequences can also follow prolonged periods of stress, as may be common in refugee camps or shelters.

2) **Significant life changes** include events such as moving, leaving home, losing a job, marriage, divorce, death of a loved one, and other such changes. The frequency of these events during young adulthood may explain the high degree of stress during this time. These events can be risk factors for disease and death, with several concurrent events creating greater risk than single stressful events would.

3) **Daily hassles** are the everyday irritations of life including bills, traffic jams, misplacing belongings, and scheduling activities. These things are fairly universal events, but some people take them lightly, while others may become overwhelmed. These little stressors can accumulate and lead to health problems such as hypertension and immunosuppression.

Effects of Stress on Psychological Functions

Moderate amounts of stress can actually improve psychological functioning by providing more energy and motivation for cognitive activities (for example, cramming the day before a final exam). However, when stress is not at an optimal level, it can impair psychological functioning by leading to fatigue, decreased ability to concentrate, and irritability. In addition, when stress is accompanied by a perceived lack of control over the stress-inducing events, over time someone may develop **learned helplessness**, which is a sense of exhaustion and lack of belief in one's ability to manage situations. With severe or prolonged stress, some people may develop PTSD. This disorder is characterized by symptoms of re-experiencing the traumatic event through flashbacks or nightmares, hypervigilance to one's surroundings, and avoidance of situations related to the stressful event.

Stress Outcomes/Response to Stressors

Physiological

Our bodies respond to stress by activating two parallel systems. The first is the **sympathetic nervous system**, the "fight or flight" response. This system responds to acute stress situations; it releases the stress hormones epinephrine (adrenaline) and norepinephrine (noradrenaline) into the bloodstream from the adrenal glands. This response causes increased heart and respiratory rates, directs blood flow toward the skeletal muscles rather than the digestive system, releases sugar into the bloodstream, and dulls pain. It is a fast-acting response.

The second is a cognitive system initiated by the hypothalamus, located just above the brainstem. The hypothalamus releases corticotropin-releasing hormone (CRH), a messenger that stimulates the pituitary gland to release **adrenocorticotropic hormone (ACTH)**. ACTH then signals the adrenal glands to release cortisol into the bloodstream. **Cortisol** is a glucocorticoid, a hormone that shifts the body from using sugar (glucose) as an energy source toward using fat as an energy source. This "glucose-sparing" effect keeps blood sugar levels high during stress situations (important because the only energy source the brain can use is glucose), thus ensuring that the brain will have enough fuel to stay active. This chain of events is a slower process than the near-instantaneous fight or flight response, and it is primarily triggered during long-term stress.

While short-term cortisol release can be helpful, prolonged release due to chronic stressors is harmful. Most notably, prolonged cortisol release inhibits the activity of white blood cells and other functions of the immune system. Thus, stress itself does not make us sick but rather increases the vulnerability to illness. It has been shown that stress can exacerbate the course of diseases including AIDS, cancer, and heart disease.

Emotional

Emotional stresses can be correlated with worse medical outcomes. For example, anger can trigger cardiac events such as heart attacks, arrhythmias, and even sudden death in people who already have heart disease. High levels of stress can contribute to the development of anxiety and depressive disorders, which are characterized by negative mood and irritability.

Behavioral

People respond in many different ways to stress, and an individual may respond differently to the same stressor depending on the circumstances. Sometimes we confront stressful situations, while at other times we avoid uncomfortable situations or emotions. Avoidance can be accompanied by habits such as cigarette smoking, consuming alcohol, or eating as a means of temporary physical comfort. In response to high stress situations, some people develop PTSD, which involves three clusters of symptoms: avoidance, hyperarousal, and re-experiencing. Avoidance involves avoiding both circumstances that remind one of the trauma and emotions associated with the trauma. Thus, someone with PTSD may tell a horrific story of personal trauma in a flat tone that is disconnected from the associated emotion. Hyperarousal involves heightened sensitivity (making a person easily startled) and hypervigilance to surroundings due to fear of danger. Re-experiencing symptoms are responses to triggers related to the traumatic event, such as flashbacks and nightmares. Sleep disturbances are common side effects of stress.

Managing Stress

There is an optimal level of stress that is motivating and invigorating. Too little stress can lead to complacency, while too much can be overwhelming and debilitating. However, stress is largely a personal experience based on an appraisal of situations. People vary in their ability to modulate their stress levels to remain close to the optimum.

One effective way of coping with stress is aerobic exercise. Exercise has been shown to be a useful adjunct to antidepressant drugs and psychotherapy, and is about as effective as these treatments in reducing depression. In addition to lowering blood pressure, aerobic exercise may help by increasing the production of neurotransmitters that boost mood, including norepinephrine, serotonin, and endorphins.

A second means for managing stress is through the use of biofeedback and relaxation. **Biofeedback** is a means of recording and feeding back information about subtle autonomic responses in an attempt to train the individual to control those involuntary responses. For example, people can be trained to adjust their muscle tension, heartbeats, and respiratory rates. This has been a particularly effective means of treating tension headaches. Many of the same benefits can occur through relaxation training, including meditation, progressive muscle relaxation, visual imagery, and yoga.

A third means of effectively managing stress is through the utilization of social support. Stronger social support has been associated with lower blood pressure, lower stress hormones, and stronger immune system function. The impact of stressful events can be mediated when individuals can express their emotional reactions and recollection of traumatic events through talking about them, writing in journals, or other means best suited to those individuals.

There is an unclear relationship between spirituality and health. Many studies have established that religious activity is associated with longer life expectancy and healthier immune functioning; however, it is unclear whether this is a causal relationship. Those who are more involved religiously also tend to have healthier diets and are less likely to smoke or drink. They also tend to have stronger social support systems within the religious community of which they are part. Thus, it is unclear whether other variables explain the improvement in health. Regardless, there may be important aspects inherent in or associated with spirituality and religion that can promote health.

Chapter 8 Summary

- Psychological disorders are sets of symptoms at odds with societal norms that are severe enough to cause personal distress or significantly impair functioning.

- The DSM-5 categorizes disorders according to symptoms and offers research-based treatments.

- Anxiety disorders, including panic disorders and phobias, involve an unpleasant and unwanted fight-or-flight-like response in situations where there is no immediate threat or danger and are not related to acute trauma.

- Obsessive-compulsive disorders are characterized by uncontrollable thoughts or behaviors that are often repeated as rituals and interrupt normal functioning.

- Trauma-or-stressor-related disorders include posttraumatic stress disorder, a disorder caused by a stressful life event that leads to a fear response in the presence of triggering stimuli.

- Somatic symptom disorders mimic the symptoms of some physical disorder in the absence of a diagnosable condition.

- Bipolar disorders are characterized by a fluctuation between a depressive state and a manic state.

- Depressive disorders involve a lowered mood and feelings of dejection or worthlessness.

- Schizophrenic disorders often include delusions, disorganized and abnormal behavior, hallucinations, and impaired social functioning.

- Dissociative identity disorder, previously known as multiple personality disorder, involves a disintegrated identity in which individuals can appear to assume different personalities in different states.

- Personality disorders are inflexible patterns of thought and behavior that create problems in day-to-day functioning and well-being.

CHAPTER 8 FREESTANDING PRACTICE QUESTIONS

1. A patient suffering from social anxiety disorder has been referred to two different therapists with different approaches. The first therapist uses the psychoanalytic approach, while the second therapist uses a cognitive-behavioral approach. Which answer choice most accurately reflects the beliefs and goals of these two therapists, respectively?

A) The first therapist will focus his efforts on analyzing and interpreting the patient's behaviors and interactions, with the end goal of helping his patient reach insight into their unconscious desires. The second therapist will focus on identifying and subsequently replacing her patient's learned behaviors with new, healthier behaviors.
B) The first therapist will focus on identifying and subsequently replacing his patient's unhealthy habits and cognitive processes. The second therapist will focus her efforts on analyzing and interpreting the patient's behaviors and interactions, with the end goal of helping her patient reach insight into their unconscious desires.
C) The first therapist will focus his efforts on analyzing and interpreting the patient's behaviors and interactions, with the end goal of helping his patient reach insight into their unconscious desires. The second therapist will focus on identifying and subsequently replacing her patient's unhealthy habits and distorted cognitive processes.
D) The first therapist will focus his efforts on exploring his patient's childhood experiences, to uncover any psychosexual fixation that they may have developed. The second therapist will focus on showing her patients unconditional positive regard and helping them remove barriers toward self-actualization.

2. Conversion disorder is characterized by:

A) a constant fear of being ill.
B) panic attacks and severe anxiety.
C) frequent vague complaints about a physical symptom.
D) functional impairment of a limb or sensory ability with no apparent physical cause.

3. All the following are Cluster B personality disorders EXCEPT:

A) histrionic behavior disorder.
B) schizoid personality disorder.
C) narcissistic personality disorder.
D) borderline personality disorder.

4. A child shows difficulty engaging with other children and needs to follow a very strict routine every day to function properly. If the routine is broken, he cries and has a very difficult time adjusting. These symptoms may satisfy which of the following diagnoses?

A) Attention-deficit hyperactivity disorder
B) Obsessive-compulsive personality disorder
C) Obsessive-compulsive disorder
D) Autism spectrum disorder

5. Parkinson's disease involves:

   I.   overstimulation of dopamine-producing neurons in the peripheral nervous system.
   II. cell death in the basal ganglia and substantia nigra.
   III. neurofibrillary tangles and neuritic plaques in the brain.

A) I only
B) II only
C) I and II
D) II and III

6. Which of the following represents a stressor that would be considered a "catastrophe?"

   I.   A terrorist attack that kills hundreds of people
   II. Divorce
   III. Death of a child

A) I only
B) III only
C) I and III
D) I, II, and III

CHAPTER 8 PRACTICE PASSAGE

In the late 1800s, psychiatrist William Gull described one of his patients as suffering from a "perversion of the will" that resulted in "simple starvation." Today, Gull's patient would likely be diagnosed with *anorexia nervosa* (AN), which is characterized by a dramatic distortion of perceived body image and dangerously low weight achieved through food restriction, excessive exercise, or other extreme means (abuse of diet pills, laxatives, etc.). According to multiple studies, AN has the highest mortality rate of all mental illnesses. This finding is likely due to the severe health consequences associated with AN, including cardiovascular stress, gastrointestinal dysfunction, and malnutrition.

Several theories have been advanced to explain the etiology or risk factors of AN and other eating disorders. Some researchers posit that AN is primarily a sociocultural phenomenon rooted in Western culture's espousal of a thin body ideal. According to these theorists, the disorder initially progresses through three stages: exposure to the thin ideal, internalization of the thin ideal, and perceived discrepancy between oneself and the thin ideal. In an effort to conform to the thin ideal, individuals who have AN employ extreme behaviors to reduce their weight. Other researchers point to personality traits or family dynamics as the primary sources of AN pathology. Finally, some theorists prefer to view AN from an addiction perspective.

In an effort to determine best treatment practices for AN and other eating disorders, some studies have compared treatment results of various clinical interventions. For example, Britain's National Institute for Clinical Excellence (NICE) conducted a comprehensive review of both inpatient and outpatient interventions for all of the AN treatment centers in the United Kingdom, collecting data on psychoanalytic therapy, behavioral therapy (BT), cognitive behavioral therapy (CBT), and family-based treatment (FBT). Published in 2004, the NICE study concluded that no particular treatment approach was significantly superior to any other particular approach in terms of treatment outcome. In another study conducted in 2010, researchers examined treatment outcome differences between FBT and ego-oriented individual therapy (EOIT) with adolescent patients. Selection criteria required a diagnosis of AN between twelve and eighteen months prior to therapy, as well as therapy duration between twelve and twenty sessions.

The FBT group contained fifty-two subjects, while the EOIT group contained fifty subjects. Figure 1 displays the results of this study.

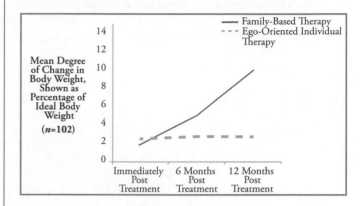

Figure 1   Treatment outcome results for FBT and EOIT

Material used in this passage was adapted from the following sources:

Risk Factors for Eating Disorders, R. H. Striegel-Moore and C.M. Bulik, in *American Psychologist*. © 2007 by the American Psychological Association.

Eating Disorders: Core interventions in the treatment and management of anorexia nervosa, bulimia nervosa, and related eating disorders. © 2004 by the British Psychological Society and the Royal College of Psychiatrists.

Randomized clinical trial comparing family-based treatment with adolescent-focused individual therapy for adolescents with anorexia nervosa. J. Lock, D. Le Grange, W. S. Agras, A. Moye, S. W. Bryson, and B. Jo, in the Archives of General Psychiatry. © 2010 by the American Medical Association.

1. Most AN sufferers demonstrate largely consistent eating patterns marked by some sporadic binging; AN sufferers generally stick to a very specific restrictive diet, eating only "safe foods" a majority of the time, but binging occasionally on other foods. Despite this irregularity in behavior, AN sufferers' attitudes about food remain consistent. What concept best describes this behavior, in terms of AN sufferers maintaining a specific attitude about food, but demonstrating slightly inconsistent eating behavior?

A)   The reality principle
B)   The principle of aggregation
C)   The self-actualizing tendency
D)   Vicarious learning

2. Heather was recently diagnosed with anorexia nervosa, and she has experienced continued weight loss and severe stomach pain. According to learning theory, for Heather, her physical symptoms would be considered:

   I. positive reinforcement.
   II. extinction.
   III. punishment.

   A) I only
   B) III only
   C) I and III only
   D) I, II, and III

3. An empirical basis for the addiction model of AN would most likely come from research that:

   A) discovers that a majority of those diagnosed with AN have at least one parent who is alcohol dependent.
   B) identifies high comorbidity of AN and tobacco dependence.
   C) proves that there is an inverse relationship between dopamine production in the brain and the activity of the satiety center controlled by the hypothalamus in individuals with AN.
   D) shows that those with AN have a higher mortality rate than individuals dependent on methamphetamines.

4. Which of the following scenarios best reflects how a psychoanalytic therapist would treat a patient with AN?

   A) The therapist would make sure to establish a relationship with the client based on rapport and mutual trust, and would always provide unconditional positive regard to the client.
   B) The therapist would help the patient gain awareness of his or her unconscious motives for AN-related behavior, and help the patient to transition from self-loathing and guilt to reality.
   C) The therapist would attempt to recondition negative behaviors.
   D) The therapist would help the patient pinpoint negative thoughts and feelings, and help the patient learn positive self-talk and healthier behaviors.

5. Noreen, who was diagnosed with AN, now participates in family therapy. Based on the chart in Figure 1, what should the therapist expect?

   A) Noreen will gain approximately 10% of her ideal body weight by the end of 12 months.
   B) Noreen will gain approximately five pounds by the end of six months.
   C) Noreen's weight will double halfway through the treatment.
   D) Noreen will gain ten pounds by the end of treatment.

6. Which of the following conclusions can be inferred from the results displayed in Figure 1?

   A) Family-based therapy is superior to ego-oriented individual therapy in reducing the negative thought processes associated with AN.
   B) The distortions in self-image characteristic of those with AN derive from an underdeveloped ego.
   C) Attachment theory is relevant to treating AN.
   D) AN typically derives from poor parenting.

SOLUTIONS TO CHAPTER 8 FREESTANDING PRACTICE QUESTIONS

1. **C**   In choice C, the first therapist focuses on uncovering unconscious desires, which is consistent with the psychoanalytic method, and the second therapist is concerned with correcting maladaptive patterns, consistent with the cognitive behavioral method. In choice A, the second therapist does not seem to focus on any cognitive influences. Based on the description, the second therapist is taking a behavioral approach, not a cognitive-behavioral approach (choice A is incorrect). In choice B, the approach of the first therapist is consistent with cognitive-behavioral therapy, and the second therapist's approach is consistent with psychoanalytic therapy. This is the opposite of the question stem (choice B is incorrect). In choice D, the first therapist's goals are consistent with psychoanalysis, but the second therapist is using a humanist perspective, rather than cognitive behavioral therapy (choice D is incorrect).

2. **D**   Conversion disorder is a somatoform disorder in which a person displays blindness, deafness, or other symptoms of sensory or motor failure without a physical cause (choice D is correct). A constant fear of illness refers to illness anxiety disorder (hypochondriasis), not conversion disorder (choice A is wrong). Panic attacks and severe anxiety are symptoms of anxiety disorders, while conversion disorder is a type of somatoform disorder (choice B is wrong). Frequent vague complaints about physical symptoms are characteristic of somatization disorder, not conversion disorder (choice C is wrong).

3. **B**   Schizoid personality disorder is classified under Cluster A personality disorders, not Cluster B (choice B is correct). This person will likely be markedly detached from friends and family members and have a flat affect, whereas Cluster B disorders are more emotional and dramatic (choices A, C, and D are incorrect).

4. **D**   Many diagnoses like obsessive-compulsive disorder and personality disorders are diagnosed only in adolescence/adulthood. This is a child, so this must be a neurodevelopmental disorder (choices B and C can be eliminated). The child is not exhibiting impulsivity/hyperactivity nor inattention (choice A can be eliminated), but rather restrictive behavior and difficulty in social situations, since he is having difficulty engaging with peers. This is descriptive of autism spectrum disorder (ASD, choice D is correct).

5. **B**   Item I is false: Parkinson's disease is the result of the death of dopamine-producing neurons in the brain; furthermore, while there are *some* dopamine-producing neurons in the peripheral nervous system, the primary neurotransmitter responsible for muscle movement is acetylcholine, not dopamine (choices A and C can be eliminated). Note that both remaining answer choices include Item II, so it must be true: Parkinson's is primarily caused by cellular death of neurons in the basal ganglia and substantia nigra of the brain; these neurons are dopamine-producing and inhibitory, connecting with the motor cortices in the brain and help to smooth out movement and inhibit excessive movement. Death of neurons in these areas results in the characteristic shaking, rigidity, and slowness of movement initiation. Item III is false: neurofibrillary tangles and neuritic plaques in the brain are characteristic of Alzheimer's disease, not Parkinson's disease (choice D can be eliminated, and choice B is correct).

6.   **A**   Item I is true: catastrophes are unpredictable, large-scale events that include natural disasters and wartime devastation. Catastrophes are events that almost everyone would appraise as dangerous and stress-inducing (choice B can be eliminated). Item II is false: divorce is considered a significant life change, not a catastrophe (choice D can be eliminated). Item III is false: while emotionally devastating, the death of a child would be considered a significant life change, not a catastrophe, because it is not a large-scale event affecting many people (choice C can be eliminated, and choice A is correct).

SOLUTIONS TO CHAPTER 8 PRACTICE PASSAGE

1. **B** The principle of aggregation explains how attitudes are better at predicting general patterns of behavior, but cannot always account for specific behaviors. The principle of aggregation best explains the periodically inconsistent behavior of binging, despite the fact that the attitude of AN sufferers toward food remains consistent (choice B is correct). According to Freud, the ego is ruled by the reality principle, which employs logical thinking to control consciousness and the id; while the reality principle may be involved in the choices AN sufferers make about eating, it does not explain the inconsistent behavior in light of a consistent attitude (choice A is wrong). The self-actualizing tendency is an innate drive toward recognizing one's full potential; it does not explain the scenario described in the question stem (choice C is wrong). Vicarious learning involves an individual learning by observing another individual; this does not explain the scenario described in the question stem (choice D is wrong).

2. **C** Item I is true: according to learning theory, positive reinforcement is an operant conditioning term that refers to a favorable consequence that reinforces a particular behavior. In Heather's case, the physical symptom of weight loss is considered a reward for her eating behavior (because she has AN and weight loss is desirable for her) and is thus a positive reinforcement (choice B can be eliminated). Item II is false: extinction is the process by which the behavior in question ceases due to the absence of a favorable consequence; since the question stem makes no mention of Heather ceasing her behavior, extinction does not explain her physical symptoms (choice D can be eliminated). Item III is true: punishment refers to a negative consequence experienced as a result of the behavior; Heather's stomach pain is a punishment for her eating behaviors (choice A can be eliminated, and choice C is correct).

3. **C** The hypothalamus is the brain structure associated with appetite regulation, while dopamine is the neurotransmitter associated with the pleasure pathways of the brain. Many illicit and addictive substances manipulate the dopamine system in some fashion, either by stimulating the release of dopamine or by inhibiting its absorption. If AN is a form of addiction, there would likely be an inverse relationship between the brain region that communicates satiety and the pleasure center of the brain; in other words, when the satiety center is not active (an individual with AN is not sated or full), dopamine is produced. This would indicate that the pleasure center of the brain is triggered when an individual with AN starves him- or herself, thus establishing a biochemical basis for the addiction model (choice C is correct). It is important to recognize that the context in which the passage mentions an addictions model suggests that AN is itself a type of addiction. It does not refer to mere correlations with addiction, such as family members with addictions (choice A is wrong) or comorbidity with other addictions (choice B is wrong). Finally, the possibility that AN is more lethal than substance abuse does not logically yield the conclusion that AN is also an addiction (choice D is wrong).

4. **B** Psychoanalytic therapy focuses on helping the patient gain awareness of his or her unconscious motives, and then make choices that are based on reality rather than on drives (id) or guilt (superego; choice B is correct). Humanistic therapy is more concerned with establishing a relationship between the therapist and the "client" based on mutual trust and unconditional positive regard (choice A is wrong). Behavioral therapy might involve reconditioning of negative behaviors (choice C is wrong) and cognitive-behavioral therapy best describes targeting negative thoughts/feelings and learning positive self-talk and healthier behaviors (choice D is wrong).

5. **A** The vertical axis of the chart in Figure 1 reflects the percentage of ideal body weight. Therefore, Figure 1 demonstrates that those in family-based therapy will gain 10% of their ideal body weight by the end of 12 months (choice A is correct). The vertical axis of Figure 1 does not represent pounds gained (choices B and D are wrong). Additionally, although the percentage of ideal body weight doubles six months post-treatment, weight gained during treatment is not depicted in Figure 1. Further, the six-month marker shows a doubling of *percentage* of ideal body weight rather than a doubling of total baseline weight (choice C is wrong).

6. **C** The chart in Figure 1 suggests that family-based therapy is superior to ego-oriented individual therapy in helping those with AN to gain weight post-treatment; but it does not suggest that family-based therapy is superior to individual therapy at reducing the negative thought processes associated with AN (choice A is wrong). However, it does imply that family relationships play a key role in AN pathology, which is consistent with attachment theory (choice C is correct). Attachment theory maintains that parent-child relationships strongly influence the child's attitudes about the self and the world. Nevertheless, a relevance of attachment and relationships to successful treatment of the disorder does not automatically imply that the disorder was caused by poor parenting. It may simply mean that familial relationships can help the patient to develop more positive self-images or become more aware of unhealthy behavior (choice D is wrong). Although psychodynamic theory may view distorted body image as a function of poor reality-testing, which is the domain of the ego, this focus would not be supported (or contradicted) by the relative superiority of family-based therapy to individual therapy (choice B is wrong).

A RANDOMIZED CONTROLLED TRIAL OF EMOTION REGULATION THERAPY FOR GENERALIZED ANXIETY DISORDER WITH AND WITHOUT CO-OCCURRING DEPRESSION

Mennin, Douglas S; Fresco, David M; O'Toole, Mia Skytte; Heimberg, Richard G.
Journal of Consulting and Clinical Psychology Vol. 86, Iss. 3, (Mar 2018): 268-281. DOI:10.1037/ccp0000289

Generalized anxiety disorder (GAD) is a burdensome condition marked by chronic and excessive worry (American Psychiatric Association, 2013) and considerable suffering. Highly impairing when occurring alone, GAD is especially impacting when it co-occurs with major depressive disorder (MDD; e.g., Whisman, Sheldon, & Goering, 2000; Henning, Turk, Mennin, Fresco, & Heimberg, 2007). Given high rates of comorbidity and overlapping symptoms, GAD and MDD are often regarded as "distress disorders" (e.g., Watson, 2005; also "emotional disorders"; Barlow, Sauer-Zavala, Carl, Bullis, & Ellard, 2014). Despite the availability of efficacious treatments, GAD and MDD frequently exhibit suboptimal long-term treatment response (e.g., Farabaugh et al., 2012; Newman, Przeworski, Fisher, & Borkovec, 2010).

EMOTION REGULATION THERAPY

In an effort to integrate and synthesize theory and findings from traditional cognitive behavior therapy and affect science, Mennin and Fresco (2013, 2014) have advanced an emotion dysregulation model that characterizes distress disorders as marked by heightened emotional experience (i.e., motivational intensity) coupled with NSRP, which functions as a compensatory strategy to manage the experience of strongly felt emotional and somatic experiences. Building on this framework, Emotion Regulation Therapy (ERT; e.g., Fresco, Mennin, Heimberg, & Ritter, 2013; Mennin & Fresco, 2014) represents a mechanism-targeted intervention that integrates findings from affect science with principles from cognitive–behavioral therapy (CBT; see Mennin, Ellard, Fresco, & Gross, 2013). This model posits that dysfunction in distress disorders can best be understood by (a) motivational mechanisms, reflecting the functional and directional properties of an emotional response tendency; (b) regulatory mechanisms, reflecting the alteration of emotional response trajectories utilizing less (i.e., attentional) and more (i.e., metacognitive) cognitively elaborative systems; and (c) contextual learning consequences, reflecting the promotion of broad and flexible behavioral repertoires (Renna, Quintero, Fresco, & Mennin, 2017). With respect to GAD, dysfunction results from a failure in each of these normative systems of functioning. Specifically, GAD is characterized by heightened emotional experience (i.e., motivational intensity) coupled with negative self-referential processing, which functions as compensatory strategy to manage the experience of strongly felt emotional and somatic experiences. Using a motivational framework (i.e., identifying reward- and risk-based impulses), ERT instructs patients to engage in mindful emotion regulation skills to counteract negative self-referential processing (e.g., worry, rumination, and self-criticism) in service of pursuing intrinsically rewarding and goal-directed actions in their lives.

Building on these encouraging findings, the present study sought to further examine the efficacy of ERT using a controlled research design. Consistent with the stage model of psychosocial intervention development (e.g., Onken, Carroll, Shoham, Cuthbert, & Riddle, 2014), the current study utilized a randomized controlled trial (RCT) design comparing patients randomly allocated to immediate ERT with patients assigned to a modified attention control condition (MAC), wherein patients received periodic contact from study therapists to assess clinical status and offer encouragement while they completed assessments and then awaited their turn to receive open label ERT following their participation in the MAC. We hypothesized that ERT would demonstrate superiority to the MAC in reducing symptoms associated with anxiety, depression, and disability, while increasing quality of life. We further hypothesized that ERT would exceed the MAC in ameliorating deficits in hypothesized mechanisms reflecting mindful attention and metacognitive regulation (i.e., trait mindfulness, decentering, cognitive reappraisal, and trait emotion dysregulation). We also examined long-term outcome (at 3- and 9-month following treatment) of both acutely and post-MAC treated patients to determine the enduring effects of ERT on all study outcomes. Here, we expected the largest change to be found in the acute phase after which trajectories would maintain effects into the follow-up periods.

Importantly, given the deliberate focus in ERT on the development of adaptive regulatory skills and the successful probing and improvement of these regulation-related variables in our prior OT (Mennin et al., 2015), we also hypothesized that improvements in less and more elaborative regulatory abilities (i.e., trait mindfulness, decentering, cognitive reappraisal, and trait emotion dysregulation) would mediate primary outcomes (i.e., GAD severity, worry, depression, disability, and life satisfaction) of those treated with ERT compared with the MAC condition. Finally, we examined indices of clinical significance in GAD- and MDD-related outcomes to show that improvements reflect gains of considerable magnitude beyond mere statistical change (Kazdin, 1999).

METHOD

Participants

One Hundred Thirty-Four individuals sought treatment both as part of routine care or specifically in response to directed recruitment efforts for the study (e.g., fliers). All individuals were assessed for general eligibility for clinical care using diagnostic assessment (see below). Fifty-three adults at two psychology training clinic sites in the Northeastern United States (Site 1 was located in Philadelphia, PA, $n = 28$; Site 2 was located in New Haven, CT, $n = 25$) ultimately expressed interest in the study and consented to be randomized. Institutional Review Boards approved procedures for the study at both sites, and all patients provided informed consent. The targeted sample size was based on a power analysis proposed in the NIMH funded R34 to enroll 34 patients drawing on meta-analytic effect sizes comparing an active treatment to WL control. This proposed sample size also anticipated expected attrition during the RCT of 4 patients leaving 30 completers. As such we would be powered to detect group by time interaction effect sizes ranging from Cohen's $d = .44$ (no attrition) to 48 (with expected attrition). Seeing as we successfully enrolled 53 patients with 44 completers, our study was actually powered to detect group by time interaction effect sizes ranging from $d = .36$ (full sample) to .38 (completers).

Interviewers at both sites were clinical psychologists or doctoral students in clinical psychology trained according to the guidelines of the ADIS or SCID. Patients were required to have a primary or coprimary diagnosis (based on clinical severity) of GAD to be admitted into the study. In addition, an independent assessor also administered the GAD module at pre-, mid-, posttreatment, and at the follow-up assessments. Further, modules with positive diagnoses at pretreatment were readministered at posttreatment and into the follow-up periods. Diagnostic agreement (in diagnosis and CSR within 1 point; ADIS CSR was used at both sites) for GAD between the intake clinician and the independent assessor at pretreatment was necessary for study inclusion. Agreement rate was 100% across both sites.

Additional inclusion criteria consisted of fluency in spoken and written English; and willing and able to give informed written consent.

The sample was mostly women (75%), with a mean age of 39 ($SD = 14.5$), primarily White (87%; Asian American/Pacific Islander 2%; African American 6%; other 6%), non-Hispanic (91%), and well-educated (64% had at least a college education). Twenty-five patients were employed full time followed by working part-time ($n = 7$), being full-time students ($n = 5$), unemployed ($n = 10$), a homemaker ($n = 4$), or retired ($n = 2$). Median annual family income for the sample was $48,819 (Range = $0 to $176,000). Twenty-three patients had a concurrent MDD diagnosis. Thirty-one patients had at least one additional current diagnosis (Range: 1–5) including obsessive–compulsive disorder ($n = 7$), panic disorder ($n = 10$), posttraumatic stress disorder ($n = 4$), social phobia ($n = 17$), specific phobia ($n = 7$), dysthymic disorder ($n = 5$), and eating disorder ($n = 1$). Thirteen patients participated while receiving concurrent antidepressant medication; 7 patients enrolled receiving benzodiazepines. Of the 53 consented patients, 28 were randomized to treatment and 25 were randomized to the MAC condition. Group assignment was determined by a random-number generator at the outset of the trial. Patients and clinicians remained unaware of randomization condition until after the signing of informed consent.

Twenty-five patients in the immediate treatment condition (89%) and 20 in the MAC condition (80%) completed the acute phase of the study. Reasons for attrition from acute ERT included a patient's mother had a major mental health issue that required leaving the area, a patient decided to leave the area to transfer to another university, a patient did not return after reporting an abuse history, a patient began taking psychotropic medication, and divorce proceedings made it difficult for another patient to regularly attend sessions. Twenty MAC completers initiated open-label ERT and 15 completed treatment (75%). Three- and 9-month follow-up assessments were conducted for all patients who completed the treatment. There were no demographic differences across the two sites, and no baseline clinical and demographic differences associated with treatment response (analyses available upon request). Thus, analyses were conducted on the full sample aggregated across sites. RCT analyses compared ERT with MAC patients at pre-, mid-, and postacute treatment. Follow-up analyses were conducted on all patients who received ERT (immediate ERT + MAC patients who received open-label ERT).

Treatment

ERT consisted of 20 weekly sessions of 60-min duration except for Sessions 11–16 which lasted 90 min to accommodate exposure exercises. In the first half, sessions focused on teaching emotion regulation strategies via attention regulation and more verbally elaborate metacognitive regulation. In the second half of ERT, patients were encouraged to deploy regulation skills during in-session and out-of-session exposures that simultaneously invoked both engagement of a context that is both rewarding and threatening. The final sessions focused on consolidating gains and preparing for termination (Fresco et al., 2013; Mennin & Fresco, 2014).

Ten clinical psychology doctoral students trained to administer ERT by the first and second authors served as protocol therapists, and received 2 hours of weekly group supervision to discuss active cases. All therapists reviewed their session video to generate a detailed timestamped and annotated note detailing how each intervention was received and what issues arose in implementation. Every video and accompanying note was reviewed by the first and second authors prior to supervision. Each case was discussed for approximately 20 min with additional time provided when emergent clinical management issues came to light.

Measures

Patients completed clinician-assessed and self-report measures of anxiety, depression, worry, disability, and quality of life as well as hypothesized mechanisms. The assessment schedule for these measures was pretreatment, midtreatment, postacute treatment, and three- and 9-month follow-up. Intake interviewers and independent assessors (all assessment points) were blind to patients' assignment in the RCT.

Clinician and diagnostic assessment

Independent assessors provided clinical assessment of patients at all points utilizing the ADIS CSR and a modified version of the *Clinical Global Impression Rating Scales* (CGI; Guy, 1976). A version with anchor points developed specifically for rating improvement (CGI-I) in symptoms associated with GAD was utilized. Patients received a rating of 1 (very much improved) or 2 (much improved) were classified as responders.

Self-report symptom and severity measures

The *Penn State Worry Questionnaire* (PSWQ; Meyer, Miller, Metzger, & Borkovec, 1990) is a widely used 16-item measure of trait worry (α = .85). The 7-item *State–Trait Anxiety Inventory* (STAI; Bieling, Antony, & Swinson, 1998) is an abbreviated version of this frequently used measure, comprised of the seven items that loaded most highly on an anxiety factor (present sample α = .85). The *Mood and Anxiety Symptom Questionnaire-Short Form* (MASQ; Watson & Clark, 1991) is a 62-item instrument that comprises four subscales: General Distress Anxious Symptoms (GDA; present sample α = .79), General Distress Depressive Symptoms (GDD; present sample α = .92), Anxious Arousal (AA; present sample α α = .89), and Anhedonic Depression (AD; present sample α = .66). The *Beck Depression Inventory-II* (BDI–II; Beck, Steer, & Brown, 1996) is a 21-item self-report measure that assesses the affective, cognitive, behavioral, and somatic symptoms of depression (present sample α = .90). The Brooding subscale of *Rumination Scale*(RS; Treynor, Gonzalez, & Nolen-Hoeksema, 2003) is a five-item measure of self-reported rumination uncontaminated by depression symptom content (present sample α = .77; only given at Site 2). The Sheehan Disability Scale (SDS; Sheehan, 1983) is a commonly utilized measure assessing impairment at work, in social relationships, and in responsibilities at home and with family (present sample α = .60). The *Quality of Life Inventory* [QOLI; Frisch, Cornell, Villanueva, & Retzlaff, 1992] assesses the degree to which an individual is satisfied with 16 areas of his or her life (e.g., health, standard of living, friendships, relationship with family, community, etc.; present sample α = .81).

Hypothesized mechanism measures

The *Five Facet Mindfulness Questionnaire* (FFMQ; Baer, Smith, Hopkins, Krietemeyer, & Toney, 2006) is a 39-item self-report measure assessing trait mindfulness (present sample α = .90). The 11-item Decentering subscale of the *Experiences Questionnaire* (EQ; Fresco et al., 2007) assessed decentering (i.e., the metacognitive ability to observe items that arise in the mind with distance and perspective; present sample α = 71). The *Difficulties in Emotion Regulation Scale* (DERS; Gratz & Roemer, 2004) is a 36-item measure of the acceptance of emotions, ability to engage in goal-directed behavior when distressed, impulse control, awareness of emotions, access to strategies for regulation, and clarity of emotions (present sample α = .93). The Cognitive Reappraisal subscale of the *Emotion Regulation Questionnaire* (ERQ; Gross & John, 2003) is a 6-item measure of cognitive reappraisal (present sample α = .91).

The following measures were considered "primary outcomes" (given centrality to hypotheses and primary focus of other GAD trials) and only these measures were utilized in mediation analyses: GAD CSR, PSWQ, BDI, SDS, & QOLI. Although MDD CSR and the RSQ are centrally related to hypotheses, there were limitations in data collection of these latter two measures, and, thus, they were not suitable to examine as outcomes in mediation analyses (i.e., MDD CSR was only assessed at pre- and posttreatment; RSQ was only administered at site 2).

RESULTS

Acute Treatment Effects

Means and standard deviations for all outcomes at the three acute time points are reported in Table 1. There were no significant between-groups differences at pretreatment on any of the measures. The Time × Group interaction effects for all three of the diagnostic measures (GAD CSR and MDD CSR, and mean CSR of additional diagnoses) were significant and of moderate to large effect sizes (Hedge's gs ranging from .72 to .83). The Time × Group interaction effects for all self-reported anxiety outcomes (PSWQ, STAI-7, MASQ-AA, MASQ-GDA), self-reported depression outcomes (BDI, RSQ Brooding, MASQ-AD, MASQ-GDD), disability/quality of life outcomes (SDS, QOLI), and the hypothesized mechanism variables (FFMQ, EQ Decentering, ERQ Reappraisal, DERS) were significant in the expected direction, ranging in effect size from .51 to 1.50. All results survived the correction for multiple comparisons according to the Benjamini-Hochberg critical value. Result statistics can be found in Table 1.

Mediation Analyses

Mediation analyses were conducted on the six primary outcomes for the four hypothesized mechanisms utilized as mediators. Result statistics are reported in Table 2. All proposed mediators showed an indirect effect of group on the primary outcomes.

Table 1 Treatment Effects Presented as Means (*M*), Standard Deviations (*SD*), *Z* Statistics, and Hedge's *g* Effect Size

Measure	Emotion regulation therapy (*n* = 28)			Modified attention control (*n* = 25)			Time × Group interaction effect		
	Pre	Mid	Post	Pre	Mid	Post	*z*	*p*	*g*
Diagnostic measure									
GAD CSR[a]	5.6 (.6)	4.1 (1.1)	3.0 (1.3)	5.9 (.6)	5.4 (1.2)	5.5 (.9)	−6.5	<.001	.83
MDD CSR[b]	4.3 (.5)	—	1.4 (2.0)	4.7 (.5)	—	3.5 (1.9)	−2.2	.030	.82
Mean CSR of additional diagnoses other than GAD[b]	4.3 (.4)	—	1.1 (1.3)	4.4 (.6)	—	2.5 (2.0)	−2.9	.004	.72
Self-reported anxiety									
PSWQ[a]	67.5 (7.3)	55.3 (10.2)	44.0 (9.9)	68.1 (11.8)	68.6 (10.3)	67.2 (10.9)	−6.9	<.001	1.50
STAI-7	18.6 (4.2)	15.3 (3.1)	12.3 (2.6)	19.7 (3.9)	19.9 (4.3)	19.7 (4.2)	−5.3	<.001	1.22
MASQ AA	29.1 (10.7)	24.0 (6.4)	21.0 (3.8)	33.0 (10.6)	32.2 (10.5)	31.0 (11.3)	−2.1	.037	.51
MASQ GDA	30.2 (9.6)	25.1 (5.2)	21.3 (4.7)	30.8 (7.8)	29.5 (7.6)	29.0 (7.2)	−4.1	<.001	.87
Self-reported depression									
BDI[a]	19.8 (9.9)	11.3 (7.7)	5.8 (5.8)	21.2 (10.7)	19.9 (10.3)	18.7 (11.3)	−4.2	<.001	.93
RSQ Brooding[a,b]	12.5 (2.4)	12.9 (3.0)	10.3 (2.3)	13.6 (2.9)	15.0 (3.4)	14.0 (3.2)	−3.7	<.001	.74
MASQ AD	69.6 (12.3)	61.0 (812.8)	53.0 (811.4)	74.8 (13.6)	76.5 (10.1)	73.1 (15.6)	−3.0	.002	.62
MASQ GDD	32.6 (8.8)	27.4 (5.2)	20.5 (5.3)	36.5 (10.9)	29.5 (7.6)	34.4 (12.5)	−3.1	.002	.69
Disability/quality of life									
SDS[a]	15.1 (6.2)	10.6 (5.7)	7.3 (5.4)	15.4 (5.8)	16.4 (6.5)	14.7 (7.2)	−3.8	<.001	.87
QOLI[a]	.7 (1.8)	1.2 (1.5)	2.2 (1.2)	−.1 (1.9)	.2 (1.7)	−.1 (1.8)	2.6	.009	.48
Proposed mediators									
FFMQ total	109.8 (15.5)	122.2 (20.7)	131.6 (17.7)	107.9 (23.6)	109.0 (20.9)	112.6 (23.0)	3.6	<.001	.83
ERQ Reappraisal	22.6 (6.2)	26.4 (5.2)	29.7 (4.4)	21.6 (9.2)	21.6 (9.7)	24.0 (9.9)	2.2	.031	.54
EQ Decentering	29.5 (6.7)	33.7 (7.0)	39.2 (5.1)	29.6 (5.2)	29.4 (5.1)	30.4 (6.5)	4.5	<.001	1.00
DERS total	98.2 (23.1)	82.3 (20.3)	74.6 (19.0)	104.8 (22.4)	102.2 (23.2)	96.0 (22.0)	−3.4	.001	.80

Note. *g* = Hedge's *g* Effect size; GAD = Generalized Anxiety disorder; CSR = Clinician's Severity Rating from the Anxiety Disorders Interview Schedule for *DSM-IV*, Lifetime Version; PSWQ = Penn State Worry Questionnaire; STAI = State Trait Anxiety Inventory; MASQ = Mood and Anxiety Symptom Questionnaire; AA = Anxious Arousal; GDA = General Distress Anxiousness; MDD = Major Depressive Disorder; BDI-II = Beck Depression Inventory II; RSQ = Response Style Questionnaire; AD = Anhedonic Depression; GDD = General Distress Depression; SDS = Sheehan Disability Scale; QOLI = Quality of Life Inventory; FFMQ = Five Facet Mindfulness Questionnaire; ERQ = Emotion Regulation Questionnaire; EQ = Experiences Questionnaire; DERS = Difficulties in Emotion Regulation Scale.
[a] Primary outcomes. [b] Clinician assessment not conducted at midtreatment.

Table 2 Indirect Effects of Proposed Mediators on Primary Outcomes

Mediator	*B*	BSSE	BCLL	BCUL
GAD CSR mediated by:				
FFMQ total Score	−.30	.18	**−.73**	**−.01**
DERS total score	−.39	.18	**−.81**	**−.10**
ERQ Reappraisal	−.27	.13	**−.67**	**−.07**
EQ Decentering	−.41	.19	**−.87**	**−.10**
PSWQ mediated by:				
FFMQ total score	−2.76	1.36	**−6.33**	**−.40**
DERS total score	−4.32	1.78	**−8.51**	**−1.23**
Reappraisal	−2.79	1.57	**−7.40**	**−.62**
EQ Decentering	−4.57	1.75	**−8.22**	**−1.36**
BDI mediated by:				
FFMQ total Score	−2.71	1.45	**−5.89**	**−.12**
DERS total score	−4.02	1.69	**−7.65**	**−.97**
ERQ Reappraisal	−2.34	1.18	**−5.04**	**−.34**
EQ Decentering	−3.12	1.26	**−5.86**	**−.87**
QOLI mediated by:				
FFMQ total Score	.29	.16	**.02**	**.64**
DERS total score	.42	.18	**.11**	**.83**
ERQ Reappraisal	.24	.13	**.04**	**.54**
EQ Decentering	.30	.13	**.09**	**.61**
SDS mediated by:				
FFMQ total Score	−1.58	.86	**−3.52**	**−.10**
DERS total score	−2.40	1.01	**−4.51**	**−.58**
ERQ Reappraisal	−1.48	.74	**−3.15**	**−.21**
EQ Decentering	−1.61	.69	**−3.17**	**−.47**

Note. BSSE = Bootstrapped standard error; BCLL = Bias-corrected lower level of 95% confidence interval; BCUL = Bias-corrected upper level of 95% confidence interval; GAD = generalized anxiety disorder; Schedule for DSM-IV, Lifetime Version; PSWQ = Penn State Worry Questionnaire; BDI-II = Beck Depression Inventory II; RSQ = Response Style Questionnaire; SDS = Sheehan Disability Scale; QOLI = Quality of Life Iventory; FFMQ = Five Facet Mindfulness Questionnaire; ERQ = Emotion Regulation Questionnaire; EQ = Experiences Questionnaire; DERS = Difficulties in Emotion Regulation Scale. Results refer to the indirect effect of the proposed mediators investigated separately. Significant (p < 0.05) indirect effects are in bold.

Follow-Up Effects and Clinical Response

Means and standard deviations from all patients who received ERT of all outcome variables at the five time points are reported in Table 3. All but one of the effect sizes was of a large magnitude, ranging from .70 to 1.77. Result statistics can be found in Table 3.

The proportion of participants meeting the criteria for treatment response is reported in Table 4. Employing both simple criteria and more stringent indices showed that participants continued to improve over the follow-up period on all the GAD-related response measures. Concerning the MDD-related response measures, the same pattern was detected although there was a slight decrease in response over the follow-up period on the two more stringent indices of clinical response (i.e., 30% improvement and high endstate functioning).

Further, although in the acute treatment phase, no patients initiated medication or additional psychotherapy, at the 3-month follow-up, 1 patient initiated antidepressant medication. At the 9-month follow-up, 2 additional patients initiated antidepressant medication and 1 patient initiated anxiolytic medication. With respect to psychotherapy, 1 patient at the 3-month follow-up and 4 patients at the 9-month follow-up initiated new psychological treatment.

DISCUSSION

The current study provides additional evidence for the efficacy of ERT following the promising findings of an earlier open label trial (Mennin et al., 2015). ERT was well tolerated as reflected in the high rate of treatment completion among all patients receiving ERT (83%) as well as among patients with comorbid MDD (83%). In terms of treatment efficacy, patients receiving immediate ERT versus the MAC demonstrated statistically and clinically meaningful improvement on measures of GAD and MDD symptoms, additional anxiety disorder severity, functional impairment, quality of life, worry, rumination, as well as theoretically consistent mechanism factors reflecting mindful attentional, metacognitive, and overall emotion dysregulation. This superiority of immediate ERT over MAC equaled or exceeded conventions for a medium effect size with many outcomes surpassing conventions for a large effect. Importantly, treatment effects attributable to ERT were largely maintained for nine months following the end of acute treatment.

Despite these promising findings, notable limitations must be considered that may also suggest directions for further investigation. First, the sample was relatively small and patients were only followed for nine months. Future studies would ideally treat and follow a larger sample for a longer period of time (~2 years) to better determine durability of treatment gains. Second, the sample was largely White and non-Hispanic. Future investigations with more racially and ethnically heterogeneous samples are needed to ideally show that ERT effects generalize to the full population of those suffering with distress disorders. Third, although the MAC included active attention from a clinician during the waitlist period and is appropriate for this stage of treatment development (e.g., Onken et al., 2014), the control comparison was relatively inert and not optimally equated against active treatment such as ERT.

In conclusion, the current findings provide considerable preliminary efficacy for ERT in treating GAD as well as associated MDD and other anxiety problems. Building on these encouraging findings, an important next step will be to determine the optimal duration and intensity of ERT (e.g., Renna, Quintero, et al., in press). On balance, the present results provide encouraging initial support for the efficacy and potential mechanisms of ERT in a sample of patients with GAD with and without comorbid MDD and suggest fruitful directions for improving our understanding and treatment of complicated clinical conditions such as the distress disorders.

Table 3   Long-Term Treatment Effects Presented as Means (*M*), Standard Deviations (*SD*), *Z* Statistics, and Hedge's *g* Effect Size

Measure	Time point *M* (*SD*)					Effect of time		
	Pre	Mid	Post	3-month follow-up	9-month follow-up	*z*	*p*	*g*
Diagnostic measure								
GAD CSR[a]	5.4 (.9)	4.3 (1.2)	2.9 (1.5)	2.9 (1.4)	2.6 (1.2)	−13.93	<.001	1.77
MDD CSR[b]	4.5 (.5)		2.8 (1.8)	2.8 (1.1)	2.1 (1.2)	−7.80	<.001	1.39
Mean CSR of additional diagnoses other than GAD[b]	4.4 (.6)		2.7 (1.4)	2.6 (1.1)	2.4 (1.1)	−11.81	<.001	1.47
Self-reported anxiety								
PSWQ[a]	67.9 (8.7)	57.3 (10.2)	47.4 (10.6)	48.0 (11.8)	49.9 (10.5)	−9.97	<.001	1.41
STAI-7	19.1 (4.2)	15.9 (3.3)	12.7 (3.3)	13.6 (3.9)	13.7 (3.7)	−8.64	<.001	1.28
MASQ AA	30.0 (6.9)	26.0 (8.4)	22.4 (5.7)	22.3 (5.4)	24.9 (6.1)	−4.53	<.001	.83
MASQ GDA	29.8 (6.9)	25.5 (6.0)	21.9 (4.9)	21.3 (5.1)	21.2 (5.7)	−8.77	<.001	1.34
Self-reported depression								
BDI[a]	19.2 (10.5)	11.7 (8.8)	6.4 (7.1)	8.8 (8.0)	9.4 (9.3)	−8.47	<.001	1.12
RSQ Brooding[a,c]	13.2 (2.9)	13.4 (2.5)	10.8 (2.5)	11.0 (2.8)	11.0 (2.5)	−4.46	<.001	1.04
MASQ AD	71.1 (13.9)	63.7 (13.8)	55.1 (12.0)	61.9 (13.7)	62.1 (13.9)	−5.43	<.001	.70
MASQ GDD	33.2 (10.5)	28.5 (9.6)	22.0 (7.1)	24.3 (7.7)	25.4 (9.4)	−6.71	<.001	.93
Disability/quality of life								
SDS[a]	15.1 (6.6)	12.6 (6.3)	7.5 (5.4)	7.3 (5.3)	7.3 (6.2)	−10.09	<.001	1.23
QOLI[a]	.2 (1.8)	.8 (1.7)	1.9 (1.4)	1.4 (1.4)	1.4 (1.5)	5.56	<.001	.81
Proposed mediators								
FFMQ total	111.2 (19.1)	118.0 (18.9)	130.6 (18.0)	131.4 (20.3)	130.8 (19.1)	9.03	<.001	1.30
ERQ Reappraisal	23.1 (8.1)	26.4 (6.1)	31.0 (5.8)	29.6 (5.3)	27.4 (5.9)	4.49	<.001	.80
EQ Decentering	29.9 (6.6)	32.9 (6.0)	38.5 (5.6)	36.8 (5.4)	36.5 (4.8)	8.62	<.001	1.17
DERS total	97.0 (22.6)	91.2 (20.5)	75.4 (20.8)	79.1 (19.8)	76.5 (18.9)	−9.72	<.001	1.24

Note. g = Hedge's *g* Effect size; GAD = Generalized Anxiety disorder; CSR = Clinician's Severity Rating from the Anxiety Disorders Interview Schedule for *DSM-IV*, Lifetime Version; PSWQ = Penn State Worry Questionnaire; STAI = State Trait Anxiety Inventory; MASQ = Mood and Anxiety Symptom Questionnaire; AA = Anxious Arousal; GDA = General Distress Anxiousness; MDD = Major Depressive Disorder; BDI-II = Beck Depression Inventory II; RSQ = Response Style Questionnaire; AD = Anhedonic Depression; GDD = General Distress Depression; SDS = Sheehan Disability Scale; QOLI = Quality of Life Inventory; FFMQ = Five Facet Mindfulness Questionnaire; ERQ = Emotion Regulation Questionnaire; EQ = Experiences Questionnaire; DERS = Difficulties in Emotion Regulation Scale.
[a] Primary outcomes. [b] Clinician assessment not conducted at midtreatment. [c] Only administered at Site 2.

Table 4   Percentages of Patients Receiving ERT Meeting Criteria for Treatment Response

Response	Posttreatment: No. responders (% ITT)	3-month follow-up: No. responders (% ITT)	9-month follow-up: No. responders (% ITT)
GAD clinical response			
ADIS GAD CSR <4	33/48 (69%)	29/40 (73%)	35/40 (88%)
CGI-improvement <3	37/48 (77%)	36/40 (90%)	39/40 (98%)
30% improvement (4+ of 6 criteria met)	36/48 (75%)	35/40 (88%)	36/40 (90%)
High endstate functioning (4+ of 6 criteria met)	32/48 (67%)	30/40 (75%)	32/40 (80%)
MDD clinical response			
ADIS MDD CSR <4	15/23 (65%)	15/19 (79%)	16/19 (84%)
CGI-improvement <3	16/23 (70%)	15/19 (79%)	17/19 (89%)
30% improvement (3+ of 4 criteria met)	13/23 (57%)	14/19 (74%)	12/19 (63%)
High endstate functioning (3+ of 4 criteria met)	14/23 (61%)	14/19 (74%)	12/19 (63%)

Note. ERT = Emotion Regulation Therapy; ITT = Intention to Treat: ITF = Intention to Follow; GAD = generalized anxiety disorder; ADIS = Anxiety Disorders Interview Schedule; CSR = Clinician's Severity Rating from the Anxiety Disorders Interview Schedule for *DSM-IV*, Lifetime Version; CGI = clinical global impression; MDD = major depressive disorder.

JOURNAL ARTICLE EXERCISE 3

The science sections on the MCAT include a significant number of passages with experiments. Questions for these passages often ask you to analyze data, read charts and graphs, and come to some reasonable conclusion based on the information they give you. If you don't know how to extract information efficiently and analyze data effectively, you will be at a distinct disadvantage.

There are three "Journal Article Exercises" in this book. In this final exercise, you'll read and extract information from the article, then complete an MCAT passage based on this article. After that, we'll show you the "correct" information to pull out and the answers to the passage.

As before, when analyzing an experiment, you should be able to:

- identify the control group(s)
- extract information from graphs and data tables
- determine how the experimental group(s) change relative to the control
- determine if the results are statistically significant
- come to a reasonable conclusion about WHY the results were observed
- consider potential weaknesses in the study
- determine how to increase the power of the study
- decide what the next most logical experiment or study should be

And, as before, the goal of these exercises is NOT to learn content from the articles, just to get a little more comfortable reading and extracting information from them.

For the (abridged) article on pages 243–249, try to summarize the purpose of the experiment and the methods in a few sentences. Remember the mnemonic: Oh ouR Car Won't Start (ORCWS).

- O = Organism and Organization
- R = Results
- C = Control and Comparison
- W = Weirdness
- S = Statistics

Try interpreting the data on your own before reading the results/discussion section. When you do read the discussion, consider:

- What are the conclusions of the study?
- How are the conclusions supported by the data?
- What potential weaknesses or flaws do you see in the experimental design? Are these addressed in the discussion section?
- How might this study be potentially biased?
- How might this study be improved?
- What would be the next most logical experiment?

Write brief responses to the questions below for the article on pages 243–249:

1. **O = Organism and Organization:**
   - Is the research being conducted on humans or on animals or on bacteria in a petri dish, or something else?

   _____

   _____

   - What is being done to these organisms?

   _____

   _____

   - Are there any unique qualities to these organisms?

   _____

   _____

   - Are there multiple groups?

   _____

   _____

   - Is the study conducted over a long period of time with multiple data points, or is it a short-term study?

   _____

   _____

   - Does it have a large or small *n*?

   _____

   _____

2. **R = Results:**
   - Where and how are the results presented? Is it a graph? A data table? Figures and images?

   _____

   _____

   - What is/are the independent variable(s)?

   _____

   _____

   - What is/are the dependent variable(s)?

   _____

   _____

   - What are the results of the study?

   _____

   _____

- Do the results show correlation or cause and effect, or both? Describe.

_____

_____

3. **C = Control and Comparison:**
   - Is there a control group?

   _____

   _____

   - How does it differ from the experimental group? Is it given a placebo or nothing at all? Is it held under different conditions?

   _____

   _____

   - If there are multiple experimental groups, how do they differ from one another?

   _____

   _____

   - Is it a blinded study? If so, double-blind or single-blind?

   _____

   _____

4. **W = Weirdness:**
   - Does anything or do any of the results stand out as unexpected?

   _____

   _____

5. **S = Statistics:**
   - Was any sort of statistical analysis done?

   _____

   _____

   - How is it presented? Are there error bars on a graph? Standard errors around a mean? Are there p-values? Is there an asterisk indicating statistical significance?

   _____

   _____

   - Is there any data that is not statistically significant?

   _____

   _____

6. **Interpreting the data:**
   - What are the conclusions of the study?

   _____

   _____

- How are the conclusions supported by the data?

  _____

  _____

- What potential weaknesses or flaws do you see in the experimental design? Are these addressed in the discussion section?

  _____

  _____

- How might this study be potentially biased?

  _____

  _____

- How might this study be improved?

  _____

  _____

- What would be the next most logical experiment?

  _____

  _____

7. **Final Summary of Experiment and Results:**

   _____

   _____

   _____

   _____

   _____

JOURNAL ARTICLE EXERCISE 3 PASSAGE

Generalized anxiety disorder (GAD) is marked by chronic and excessive worry and considerable suffering. Highly impairing when occurring alone, GAD is especially impacting when it co-occurs with major depressive disorder (MDD). Given high rates of comorbidity and overlapping symptoms, GAD and MDD are often regarded as "distress disorders". Despite the availability of efficacious treatments, GAD and MDD frequently exhibit suboptimal long-term treatment response.

A study randomly allocated participants to either an immediate Emotion Regulation Therapy (ERT) condition or to a modified attention control condition (MAC). ERT utilizes principles from cognitive–behavioral therapy, while the MAC condition participants received periodic contact from study therapists to assess clinical status and offer encouragement. Researchers hypothesized that ERT would demonstrate superiority to the MAC in reducing symptoms associated with anxiety, depression, and disability, while increasing quality of life. Participants were also examined in terms of their long-term outcomes (at 3- and 9-month intervals following treatment).

Overall, 53 adults at two psychology training clinic sites in the Northeastern United States expressed interest in the study and consented to be randomized. The participants with a primary diagnosis of GAD (43% with comorbid MDD) were randomly assigned to immediate treatment with ERT ($n = 28$) or a modified attention control condition (MAC, $n = 25$). The sample was mostly women (75%), with a mean age of 39, primarily White (87%), non-Hispanic (91%), and well-educated (64% college educated).

The study found that participants receiving immediate ERT versus the MAC demonstrated statistically and clinically meaningful improvement on measures of GAD and MDD symptoms, additional anxiety disorder severity, functional impairment, quality of life, worry, rumination, as well as theoretically consistent mechanism factors reflecting mindful attentional, metacognitive, and overall emotion dysregulation. Importantly, treatment effects attributable to ERT were largely maintained for nine months following the end of acute treatment. These findings provide encouraging support for the efficacy and hypothesized mechanisms underlying ERT and point to fruitful directions for improving our understanding and treatment of complex clinical conditions such as GAD with co-occurring MDD.

1. The researchers in the study utilized which of the following study designs?

A) Cross-sectional
B) Longitudinal
C) Historical research
D) Case study

2. Emotion Regulation Therapy, as defined in the passage, is based on which of the following psychological perspectives on personality?

A) Humanistic approach
B) Psychoanalytic approach
C) Social cognitive approach
D) Behavioralist approach

3. Which of the following can be concluded from the results of the study?

A) Participants in the Modified Attention Control demonstrated superior improvement on clinician rated and self-reported anxiety and depression, satisfaction with life, worrying and ruminating, and in self-perceived ability to manage emotions with mindfulness and perspective taking, relative to patients receiving immediate treatment.
B) Participants in the Emotion Regulation Therapy condition did not demonstrate long-term benefit from their assigned treatment condition.
C) Participants in the Modified Attention Control condition did not demonstrate long-term benefit from their assigned treatment condition.
D) Emotion Regulation Therapy participants demonstrated superior improvement on clinician rated and self-reported anxiety and depression, satisfaction with life, worrying and ruminating, and in self-perceived ability to manage emotions with mindfulness and perspective taking, relative to patients receiving delayed treatment.

4. Each of the following is a limitation of the study design EXCEPT:

A) the study only compared two types of treatment methods.
B) patients were only followed for nine months.
C) the sample was largely White and non-Hispanic.
D) the sample was largely female.

SOLUTIONS TO JOURNAL ARTICLE EXERCISE 3

1. **O = Organism and Organization:**
   - Is the research being conducted on humans or on animals or on bacteria in a petri dish, or something else? *Humans*
   - What is being done to these organisms? *They are subjected to two different types of treatment for GAD (generalized anxiety disorder) and MDD (major depressive disorder).*
   - Are there any unique qualities to these organisms? *The sample was mostly women (75%) with a mean age of 39 and also primarily white (87%).*
   - Are there multiple groups? *Yes, an ERT (emotion regulation therapy) treatment group, which is compared to the MAC (modified attention control) treatment group*
   - Is the study conducted over a long period of time with multiple data points, or is it a short-term study? *Long. The ERT group consisted of 20 weekly sessions of 60 to 90 minute durations. The MAC group received less contact, consisting of four 15-minute telephone contacts.*
   - Does it have a large or small *n*? *Small n: 28 in the ERT group and 25 in the MAC condition*

2. **R = Results:**
   - Where and how are the results presented? Is it a graph? A data table? Figures and images? *Data tables*
   - What is/are is the independent variable(s)? *Type of treatment received*
   - What is/are is the dependent variable(s)? *Clinical indicators of GAD and MDD (worry, rumination, disorder severity, functional impairment, and quality of life)*
   - What are the results of the study? *ERT patients evidenced statistically meaningful improvement in clinical indicators compared to the MAC group, even after the study concluded.*
   - Do the results show correlation or cause and effect, or both? Describe. *Cause and effect: the treatment group showed more improvement compared to the MAC group.*

3. **C = Control and Comparison:**
   - Is there a control group? *Yes (MAC group)*
   - How does it differ from the experimental group? Is it given a placebo or nothing at all? Is it held under different conditions? *The control group received a different type of treatment.*
   - If there are multiple experimental groups, how do they differ from one another? *Only one experimental group*
   - Is it a blinded study? If so, double-blind or single-blind? *Single-blind; the participants did not know the treatment method of the other group*

4. **W = Weirdness:**
   - Does anything or do any of the results stand out as unexpected? *No*

5. **S = Statistics:**
   - Was any sort of statistical analysis done? *Yes*
   - How is it presented? Are there error bars on a graph? Standard errors around a mean? Are there *p*-values? Is there an asterisk indicating statistical significance? *P values, standard deviations, Z-scores, and Hedge's g*
   - Is there any data that is not statistically significant? *No*

6. **Interpreting the data:**
   - What are the conclusions of the study? *Emotion Regulation Therapy (ERT) demonstrates superior improvement on clinician rated and self-reported anxiety and depression, satisfaction with life, worrying and ruminating, and in self-perceived ability to manage emotions with mindfulness and perspective taking, relative to patients receiving delayed treatment.*
   - How are the conclusions supported by the data? *Data shows significant differences between the ERT and MAC groups.*
   - What potential weaknesses or flaws do you see in the experimental design? Are these addressed in the discussion section? *Biased sample, mostly women and white*
   - How might this study be potentially biased? *Demographics of sample*
   - How might this study be improved? *More varied demographics (racially, sex, age, etc.)*
   - What would be the next most logical experiment? *Repeat the experiment with subjects in varying demographic groups.*

7. **Final Summary of Experiment and Results:**
   - *53 patients with a primary diagnosis of GAD (43% with comorbid MDD) were randomly assigned to immediate treatment with ERT (n = 28) or a modified attention control condition (MAC, n = 25). ERT patients, as compared with MAC patients, evidenced statistically and clinically meaningful improvement on clinical indicators of GAD and MDD. Treatment effects were maintained for nine months following the end of acute treatment. Overall, ERT resulted in high rates endstate functioning for both GAD and MDD that were maintained into the follow-up period.*

SOLUTIONS TO JOURNAL ARTICLE EXERCISE 3 PASSAGE

1. **B** The passage states that participants were examined in terms of their long-term outcomes (at 3- and 9-months following treatment). A study design that permits comparison of identical measures and groups at two or more points in time is known as a longitudinal study (choice B is correct). Cross-sectional designs measure at one specific point in time (choice A is incorrect), historical research focuses on examining past events, usually through primary or archival sources (choice C is incorrect), and a case study focuses on the examination of a single case (choice D is incorrect).

2. **C** Paragraph 2 states that ERT is based on the principles of cognitive-behavioral therapy (CBT). CBT, in turn, is based on the social cognitive perspective on personality, pioneered by psychologists such as Albert Bandura (choice C is correct). The humanistic approach lead to the creation of client-centered therapy, pioneered by Carl Rogers (choice A is incorrect). The psychoanalytic approach led to the creation of psychotherapy, pioneered by Sigmund Freud (choice B is incorrect). The behavioralist perspective on personality lead to behavioral therapy, pioneered by B.F. Skinner (choice D is incorrect).

3. **D** The final paragraph of the passage states that ERT participants had superior improvement, relative to the MAC condition, and displayed the beneficial treatment effects for nine months following the end of treatment (choice D is correct, and choice B is false). Choice A, which reverses the two participants groups, is incorrect. The results do not state that the MAC condition did not improve at all, only that their improvement was not as pronounced as that of the ERT condition (choice C is incorrect).

4. **A** Since this is an EXCEPT question, highlight the word "EXCEPT" and write "A B C D" on the noteboard. Then evaluate each answer choice, writing "Y" if it is a limitation of the study or "N" if it is not. Comparing two therapeutic approaches is not inherently a limitation in this study's design; while there certainly could be other, potentially more effective, methods of addressing either GAD or MDD in a therapeutic setting, this is not a limitation (write "N" next to "A" on the noteboard). Given that the paragraph 1 states GAD and MDD frequently exhibit suboptimal long-term treatment response, the fact that the patients were only followed for nine months could be a limitation. Future studies would ideally treat and follow a larger sample for a longer period (~2 years) to better determine durability of treatment gains (write "Y" next to "B" on the noteboard). The sample was largely white, non-Hispanic, and female. Future investigations with more racially and ethnically heterogeneous samples, in addition to being more diverse in terms of sex/gender, are needed to ideally show that ERT effects generalize to the full population of those experiencing distress disorders (write "Y" next to both "C" and "D" on the noteboard). Since choice A stands out with an "N" instead of a "Y," it is the correct answer choice.

Chapter 9
Learning, Memory, and Development

Learning is an important way that organisms interact with, are changed by, and change their environment. The basis of learning is that experiences can alter and change behavior, sometimes permanently. While learning occurs in many organisms, humans demonstrate the broadest range of different types of learning.

Human learning is influenced by many factors, including both innate and environmental variables. Learning and memory are intimately related and both play critical roles in human behavior, personality, attitudes, and development over the entire lifetime of an individual.

9.1 TYPES OF LEARNING

We have been learning since the day we were born. At times it comes more formally, like learning how to add and subtract in school, throw a baseball, or studying for the MCAT. Other times, learning occurs more informally, like learning how to walk, how to behave in certain social situations, or how to talk. Any way it happens, learning is an important part of how humans (and other animals) interact with one another and with the world around them.

Nonassociative Learning

Nonassociative learning occurs when an organism is repeatedly exposed to one type of stimulus. Two important types of nonassociative learning are habituation and sensitization. A **habit** is an action that is performed repeatedly until it becomes automatic, and **habituation** follows a very similar process. Essentially, a person learns to "tune out" the stimulus. For example, suppose you live near train tracks and trains pass by your house on a regular basis. When you first moved into the house, the sound of the trains passing by was annoying and loud, and it always made you cover your ears. However, after living in the house for a few months, you become used to the sound and stop covering your ears every time the trains pass. You may even become so accustomed to the sound that it becomes background noise and you don't even notice it anymore.

Dishabituation occurs when the previously habituated stimulus is removed. More specifically, after a person has been habituated to a given stimulus, and the stimulus is removed, this leads to dishabituation; the person is no longer accustomed to the stimulus. If the stimulus is then presented again, the person will react to it as if it were a new stimulus, and is likely to respond even more strongly to it than before. In the train example above, dishabituation could occur when you go away on vacation for a few weeks to a quiet beach resort. The train noise is no longer present, so you become dishabituated to that constant noise. Then, when you return to your home and the noisy train tracks, the first time you hear the train after you return, you notice it again. The noise may cause you to cover your ears again or react even more strongly because you have become dishabituated to the sound of the trains passing.

Sensitization is, in many ways, the opposite of habituation. During sensitization, there is an increase in responsiveness due to either a repeated application of a stimulus or a particularly aversive or noxious stimulus. Instead of being able to "tune out" or ignore the stimulus and avoid reacting at all (as in habituation), the stimulus actually produces a more exaggerated response. For example, suppose that instead of trains passing by outside your house, you attend a rock concert and sit near the stage. The feedback noise from the amplifier may at first be merely irritating, but as the aversive noise continues, instead of getting used to it, it actually becomes much more painful and you have to cover your ears and perhaps even eventually move. Sensitization may also cause you to respond more vigorously to other similar stimuli. For example, suppose that as you leave the rock concert, an ambulance passes. The siren noise, which usually doesn't bother you, seems particularly loud and abrasive after being sensitized to the noise of the rock concert. Sensitization is usually temporary and may not result in any type of long-term behavior change (you may or may not avoid rock concerts in the future and you are unlikely to respond so strongly to an ambulance siren when you hear one next week). Desensitization occurs when a stimulus that previously evoked an exaggerated response (something that we were sensitized to), no longer evokes an exaggerated response. Going back to the example of leaving a rock concert and being more sensitized to noise: at first the sound of the siren is very abrasive, but by the next morning loud noises no longer bother you—you have become desensitized.

Associative Learning

Associative learning describes a process of learning in which one event, object, or action is directly connected with another. There are two general categories of associative learning: classical conditioning and operant conditioning.

Classical Conditioning

Classical (or respondent) **conditioning** is a process in which two stimuli are paired in such a way that the response to one of the stimuli changes. The archetypal example of this is Pavlov's dogs. **Ivan Pavlov**, who first named and described the process of classical conditioning, did so by training his dogs to salivate at the sound of a ringing bell. Dogs naturally salivate at the sight and smell of food; it is a biological response that prepares the dogs for food consumption. The stimulus (food) naturally produces this response (salivating), however, dogs do not intrinsically react to the sound of a bell in any particular way. Pavlov's famous experiment paired the sound of a bell (an auditory stimulus) with the presentation of food to the dogs, and after a while, the dogs began to salivate to the sound of a bell even in the absence of food. The process of pairing the two initially unrelated stimuli changed the dogs' response to the sound of the bell over time; they became conditioned to salivate when they heard it. The dogs effectively learned that the sound of the bell was meant to announce food.

This example demonstrates a few key concepts about classical conditioning. This type of learning relies on specific stimuli and responses.

- A **neutral stimulus** is a stimulus that initially does not elicit any intrinsic response. For Pavlov's dogs, this was the sound of the bell prior to the experiment.
- An **unconditioned stimulus** (US) is a stimulus that elicits an **unconditioned response** (UR). Think of this response like a reflex. It is not a learned reaction, but a biological one: in this case, the presentation of food is the unconditioned stimulus and the salivation is the unconditioned response.
- A **conditioned stimulus** (CS) is an originally neutral stimulus (bell) that is paired with an unconditioned stimulus (food) until it can produce the conditioned response (salivation) without the unconditioned stimulus (food).
- Finally, the **conditioned response** (CR) is the learned response to the conditioned stimulus. It is the same as the unconditioned response, but now it occurs without the unconditioned stimulus. For the dogs, salivating at the sound of the bell is the conditioned response.

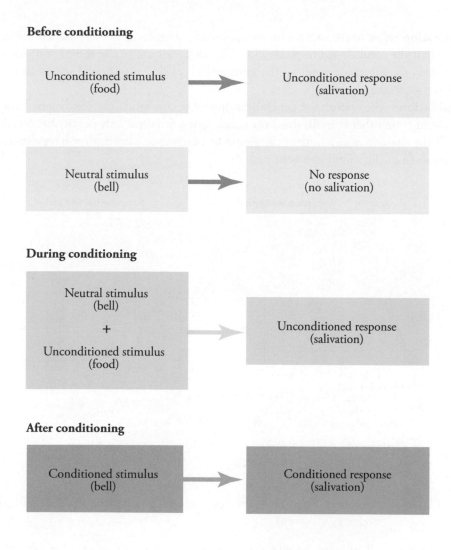

Figure 1   Conditioning in Pavlov's dogs

Acquisition, extinction, spontaneous recovery, generalization, and discrimination are the processes by which classically-conditioned responses are developed and maintained.

1) **Acquisition** refers to the process of learning the conditioned response. This is the time during the experiment when the bell and food are always paired.

2) **Extinction**, in classical conditioning, occurs when the conditioned and unconditioned stimuli are no longer paired, so the conditioned response eventually stops occurring. After the dogs have been conditioned to salivate at the sound of the bell, if the sound is presented to the dogs over and over without being paired with the food, then after some time the dogs will eventually stop salivating at the sound of the bell.

3) **Spontaneous recovery** happens when an extinct conditioned response occurs again when the conditioned stimulus is presented after some time. For example, if the behavior of salivating to the sound of the bell becomes extinct in a dog, and the paired stimuli are then presented to the dog again after some amount of lapsed time and the dog salivates, the conditioned response was spontaneously recovered.

4) **Generalization** refers to the process by which stimuli other than the original conditioned stimulus elicit the conditioned response. So, if the dogs salivate to the sound of a chime or a doorbell, even though those were not the same sounds as the conditioned stimulus, the behavior has been generalized.

5) **Discrimination** is the opposite of generalization and occurs when the conditioned stimulus is differentiated from other stimuli; thus, the conditioned response only occurs for conditioned stimuli. If the dogs do not salivate at the sound of a buzzer or a horn, they have differentiated those stimuli from the sound of a bell.

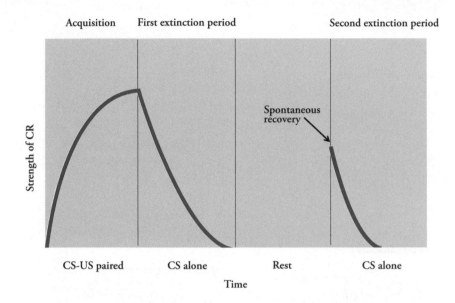

Figure 2   Curve of acquisition, extinction, and spontaneous recovery in classical conditioning

Organisms seem predisposed to learn associations that are adaptive in nature. One powerful and very long-lasting association in most animals (including humans) is **taste-aversion** caused by nausea and/or vomiting. An organism that eats a specific food and becomes ill a few hours later will generally develop a strong aversion to that food. Most organisms develop the aversion specifically to the smell or taste of the food (occurs in most mammals), but it is also possible to develop an aversion to the sight of the food (occurs in birds). The function of this quickly-learned response is to prevent an organism from consuming something that might be toxic or poisonous in the future. This response happens to be one that does not need a long acquisition phase (it is typically acquired after one exposure) and has a very long extinction phase; in fact for most organisms, it never extinguishes.

Operant Conditioning

The other category of associative learning is **operant** (or instrumental) **conditioning.** Whereas classical conditioning connects unconditioned and neutral stimuli to create conditioned responses, operant conditioning uses reinforcement (pleasant consequences) and punishment (unpleasant consequences) to mold behavior. However, just as with classical conditioning, timing is everything. In classical conditioning, it was important for the neutral stimulus to be paired with the unconditioned stimulus (that is, for them to occur together or very close together in time) in order for the neutral stimulus to become conditioned. In operant conditioning, it is just as important for the reinforcement or the punishment to occur around the same time as the behavior in order for learning to occur.

One of the most famous people to conduct research in the area of operant conditioning was **B.F. Skinner**. Skinner worked with animals and designed an operant conditioning chamber (later called a "Skinner box") that he used in a series of experiments to shape animal behavior. For example, in one series of experiments, a hungry rat would be placed inside a Skinner box that contained a lever. If the rat pressed the lever, a food pellet would drop into the box. Often the rat would first touch the lever by mistake, but after discovering that food would appear in response to pushing the lever, the rat would continue to do so until it was sated. In another series of experiments, the Skinner box would be wired to deliver a painful electric shock until a lever was pushed. In this example, the rat would run around trying to avoid the shock at first, until accidentally hitting the lever and causing the shock to stop. On repeated trials, the rat would quickly push the lever to end the painful shock.

Figure 3 Example of a "Skinner Box"

These examples demonstrate a few key concepts about operant conditioning.

> **Reinforcement**: A reinforcer is anything that will increase the likelihood that a preceding behavior will be repeated; the behavior is supported by reinforcement. There are two major types of reinforcement: positive and negative.
> - **Positive reinforcement** is the presentation of some sort of desirable stimulus that occurs immediately following a behavior. In the above experiments, the food pellet was a positive reinforcer for the hungry rat because it caused the rat to repeat the desired behavior (push the lever).
> - **Negative reinforcement** is the *removal* of some sort of undesirable stimulus immediately following a behavior. In the above experiments, the removal of the electric shock is negative reinforcement for the rat because it causes the rat to repeat the desired behavior (again, push the lever) to remove the undesirable stimulus (the painful shock).

Anything that *increases* a desired behavior is a reinforcer; both positive and negative reinforcements increase the desired behavior, but the process by which they do so is different. Positive reinforcement does it by adding a positive stimulus (something desirable) and negative reinforcement does it by removing a negative one (something undesirable). Positive reinforcement *adds* and negative reinforcement *subtracts* (this will be important when contrasted with punishment later). While several brain structures are involved in operant conditioning, the amygdala is understood to be particularly important in negative conditioning, while the hippocampus is believed to be particularly important in positive conditioning.

Another key distinction for reinforcement is between primary and secondary (or unconditioned and conditioned) reinforcers.

1) **Primary** (or unconditioned) **reinforcers** are somehow innately satisfying or desirable. These are reinforcers that we do not need to learn to see as reinforcers because they are integral to our survival. Food is a primary positive reinforcer for all organisms because it is required for survival. Avoiding pain and danger are primary negative reinforcers for the same reason; avoidance is important for survival.

2) **Secondary** (or conditioned) **reinforcers** are those that are learned to be reinforcers. These are neutral stimuli that are paired with primary reinforcers to make them conditioned. For example, suppose that every time a child reads a book, she receives a stamp. After accruing ten stamps, she can exchange these for a small pizza. The pizza, being food, is the primary reinforcer, and the stamps are a secondary reinforcer. The child learns to find the stamps desirable because they help her get something she wants—pizza. Secondary reinforcers can also be paired with other secondary reinforcers. For example, suppose that after collecting ten stamps, instead of receiving a pizza, the child receives a coupon that is good for one small pizza. In this example, both the stamps and the coupon are secondary reinforcers. Almost any stimulus can become a secondary reinforcer, but it must be paired with a primary reinforcer in order to produce learned behavior.

Operant conditioning relies on a **reinforcement schedule**. This schedule can be **continuous**, in which every occurrence of the behavior is reinforced, or it can be **intermittent**, in which occurrences are sometimes reinforced and sometimes not. Continuous reinforcement will result in rapid behavior **acquisition** (or rapid learning), but it will also result in rapid **extinction** when the reinforcement ceases. Intermittent reinforcement typically results in slower acquisition but great persistence (or resistance to extinction) of that behavior over time. Therefore, it is possible to initially condition a behavior using a continuous reinforcement schedule, and then **maintain** that behavior using an intermittent reinforcement schedule. For instance, a dog can be trained to sit in response to a hand motion on a continuous reinforcement schedule where a treat is given every time the dog sits; once the dog has sufficiently mastered this behavior, you can switch to an intermittent reinforcement schedule, where the dog receives a treat only occasionally when it sits in response to the hand motion.

There are four important intermittent reinforcement schedules: fixed-ratio, variable-ratio, fixed-interval, and variable-interval. Ratio schedules are based on the number of instances of a desired behavior required for the reward, and interval schedules are based on time.

1) A **fixed-ratio schedule** provides the reinforcement after a set number of instances of the behavior. Returning to the example of a hungry rat in a Skinner box, if the rat receives a food pellet every 10 times it pushes the lever after it has been conditioned, the rat will demonstrate a high rate of response (in other words, it will push the lever rapidly, many times to get the food).

2) A **variable-ratio schedule** provides the reinforcement after an unpredictable number of occurrences. A classic example of reinforcement provided on a variable-ratio schedule is gambling (e.g., a slot machine); the reinforcement may be unpredictable, but the behavior will be repeated with the hope of a reinforcement. Both fixed-ratio schedules and variable-ratio schedules produce high response rates; the chances that a behavior will produce the desired outcome (a treat or a jackpot or some other reinforcement) increases with the number responses (times the behavior is performed).

3) A **fixed-interval schedule** provides the reinforcement after an amount of time that is constant. The behavior will increase as the reinforcement interval comes to an end. For example, if an employee is reinforced by attention from the boss, the employee might work hard all the time, thinking the boss will walk by at any second and notice the hard work (and provide the positive reinforcement, attention). Once the employee learns that the boss only walks by at the top of the hour every hour, the employee may become an ineffective worker throughout the day, but be more effective as the top of the hour approaches.

4) A **variable-interval schedule** provides the reinforcement after an inconsistent amount of time. This schedule produces a slow, steady behavior response rate, because the amount of time it will take to get the reinforcement is unknown. In the employee-boss example, if the boss walks by at unpredictable times each day, the employee does not know when he or she might receive the desired reinforcement (attention). Thus, the employee will work in a steady, efficient manner throughout the day, but not very quickly. The employee knows it doesn't matter how quickly he works at any given time, because the potential reinforcement is tied to an unpredictable schedule.

Figure 4 demonstrates behavior response patterns to each of the four reinforcement schedules.

Figure 4 Behavior response patterns to each of the four reinforcement schedules

Table 1   Reinforcement Schedules: Response and Extinction Rates

	Definition	Response Rate	Extinction Rate	Notable Behavior Patterns
Continuous	Reinforcer given after every single response	SLOW	FAST	**Best way to teach new behavior,** but has the fastest rate of extinction
Fixed Ratio	Reinforcer given after set number of responses	FAST	MEDIUM	Post-reinforcement pause may be an analogue to procrastination
Fixed Interval	Reinforcer given after set amount of time	MEDIUM	MEDIUM	Long pause in responding following reinforcement, followed by accelerating rate
Variable Ratio	Reinforcer given after variable number of responses	FAST	SLOW	**Slowest rate of extinction** (behavior persists longest despite lack of reinforcer)
Variable Interval	Reinforcer given after variable amount of time	MEDUIM-FAST	SLOW	Tends to produce a low to moderate steady rate of responding

Note: these same schedules can also be used for punishments.

Reinforcement and reinforcement schedules explain how behaviors can be learned, but not every behavior is learned by simply providing a reinforcement. For example, think about how a baby learns to walk. Do babies spontaneously walk one day and then receive some sort of reinforcement from their parents for doing so? Of course not. Instead, parents **shape** the desired behavior by reinforcing the smaller intermediate behaviors necessary to achieve the final desired behavior, walking. Thus, parents will reinforce their child's attempts to pull herself up, so she will try again. Once she's mastered pulling herself up and standing while holding onto something, they will reinforce the child's attempts to stand while not holding anything. And so on until the child is able to walk on her own. Shaping is a way to learn more complex behaviors by breaking them down and reinforcing the "pieces of the puzzle" until the whole behavior is strung together.

Like reinforcement, punishment is also an important element of operant conditioning, but the effect is the opposite: reinforcement *increases* behavior, while punishment *decreases* it. **Punishment** is the process by which a behavior is followed by a consequence that decreases the likelihood that the behavior will be repeated. Like reinforcement, punishment can be both positive AND negative. **Positive punishment** involves presenting an undesirable stimulus after a behavior that one wishes to decrease. For example, if cadets speak out of turn in military boot camp, the drill sergeant makes them do twenty push-ups. Conversely, **negative punishment** involves the removal of a desirable stimulus after the **behavior has occurred.** For example, if a child breaks a window while throwing a baseball in the house, they lose TV privileges for a week. Positive punishment *adds* and negative punishment *subtracts*. Commonly, reinforcement and punishment are used in conjunction when shaping behaviors; however, it is uncommon for punishment to have as much of a lasting effect as reinforcement. Once the punishment has been removed, then it is no longer effective. Furthermore, punishment only instructs what *not* to do, whereas reinforcement instructs what *to* do. Reinforcement is therefore a better alternative to encourage behavior change and learning. Additionally, the processes described for classical conditioning (acquisition, extinction, spontaneous recovery, generalization, and discrimination) occur in operant conditioning, as well.

Note that the term "negative reinforcement" is often used incorrectly; colloquially, people use the term when they mean punishment.

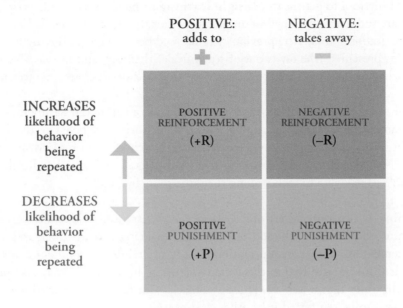

Figure 5   Schematic of positive and negative reinforcement and punishment

In conclusion, let's examine two specific types of operant learning: escape and avoidance. In **escape learning,** an individual learns how to get away from an aversive stimulus by engaging in a particular behavior. This helps negatively reinforce the behavior so that it is more likely to be repeated. For example, a child does not want to eat her vegetables (aversive stimulus) so she throws a temper tantrum. If the parents respond by not making the child eat the vegetables, then tantrums will be negatively reinforced, as they cause the removal of the aversive stimulus (the vegetables). On the other hand, **avoidance** occurs when a person performs a behavior to ensure an aversive stimulus is not presented. For example, a child notices Mom cooking vegetables for dinner and fakes an illness so Mom will send him to bed with ginger ale and crackers. The child has effectively avoided confronting the aversive stimulus (the offensive vegetables) altogether. As long as either of these techniques work (meaning the parents do not force the child to eat the vegetables), the child is reinforced to perform the escape and/or avoidance behaviors.

Cognitive Processes that Affect Associative Learning

Classical and operant conditioning fall under the behaviorist tradition of psychology, which is most strongly associated with Skinner. In **behaviorism,** all psychological phenomena are explained by describing the observable antecedents of behaviors and their consequences. Behaviorism is not concerned with the unobservable events occurring within the mind. This perspective views the brain as a "black box" which does not need to be incorporated into the discussion. While Skinner and other behaviorists contributed a great deal to science, this extreme form of behaviorism has lost favor. As a reaction to behaviorism, **cognitive psychology** emerged. In cognitive psychology, researchers began to focus on the brain, cognitions (thoughts), and their effects on how people navigate the world. Cognitive psychologists do not see learning as simply due to stimulus-pairing and reinforcement. Although its importance is acknowledged, cognitive psychologists do not believe that all learning can be explained in this way. For example, say a child learns that he can slide on his belly to reach a toy he wants under the bed. Then he learns that a grabbing tool can be used to pick up his toys from the ground. What will the child do when his toy is under the bed out of reach? He may figure out that he can combine the two behaviors: sliding on his belly and using the grabbing tool to get the toy. **Insight learning** is the term used to describe when previously learned behaviors are suddenly combined in unique ways. For the child, the two behaviors (sliding on the belly and using the grabbing tool) were previously reinforced because he got the toy he wanted each time. A new situation was presented (the toy is out of reach under the bed), and he was able to combine previously reinforced behavior in a novel way on his own to attain the desired outcome (retrieval of the toy).

This also works the other way around: previously unseen behavior can manifest quickly when required. In **latent learning**, something is learned but not expressed as an observable behavior until it is required. For instance, if a child in middle school always receives a ride to school from his dad, he may latently learn the route to school, even if he never demonstrates that knowledge. One day, when his dad is on a business trip, the child is able to navigate to school along the same route by bike.

Finally, conditioning is not only behavioral learning. For instance, in operant conditioning, certain behaviors are reinforced and the likelihood of that behavior being repeated increases as a result. Cognitively, the reinforcement establishes an expectation for a future reinforcer, so the process is not exclusively behavioral. There is thinking involved in this kind of learning. Expectations may also present themselves in stimulus generalization. If you were rewarded in one class for raising your hand before speaking, then you would expect that to be reinforced in another class as well.

Table 2 Comparison of Classical Conditioning and Operant Conditioning

	Classical Conditioning	**Operant Conditioning**
Defined	Organisms learn associations between stimuli that they don't control	Organisms learn associations between behaviors and resulting consequences
Response	Involuntary, automatic	Voluntary
Acquisition	Associating two stimuli	Associating response with consequence (reinforcement or punishment)
Extinction	Conditioned response decreases as the conditioned stimulus is continually presented alone	Response decreases without reinforcement
Spontaneous recovery	Reappearance, after a rest period, of a response	Reappearance, after a rest period, of a response
Generalization	Response to a stimulus similar (but not identical) to the conditioned stimulus	Response to a similar stimulus is also reinforced
Discrimination	Ability to distinguish between conditioned stimulus and other stimuli	Learning that certain responses, not others, will be reinforced

Biological Factors that Affect Nonassociative and Associative Learning

Learning is a change in behavior as a result of experience. While many extrinsic factors can influence learning, learning is also limited by biological constraints of organisms. For example, chimpanzees can learn to communicate using basic sign language, but they cannot learn to speak, in part because they are constrained by a lack of specialized vocal chords that would enable them to do so. It was long believed that learning could occur using any two stimuli or any response and any reinforcer. But again, biology serves as an important constraint. Associative learning is most easily achieved using stimuli that are somehow relevant to survival. Furthermore, not all reinforcers are equally effective. As previously discussed, a dramatic example of this is illustrated by food aversions. If an organism consumes something that tastes strongly of vanilla and becomes nauseated a few hours later (even if the nausea was not caused by the vanilla food), that organism will develop a strong aversion to both the taste and the smell of vanilla, even if the nausea occurred hours after consuming the food. This aversion defies many of the principles of associative learning previously discussed because it occurs after one instance, it can occur after a significant delay of hours, and it is often an aversion that can last for a very long time, sometimes indefinitely. In studies, researchers tried to condition organisms to associate the feeling of nausea with other stimuli, such as a sound or a light, but were unable to do so. Therefore, food aversions demonstrate another important facet of learning: learning occurs more quickly if it is biologically relevant.

The process of learning results in physical changes to the central nervous system (see Chapter 10). Different areas of the brain are involved with different types of learning. For example, the cerebellum is involved with learning how to complete motor tasks and the amygdala is involved with learning fear responses (brain lesion studies have helped scientists determine this).

Learning and memory are two processes that work together in shaping behavior, and it is impossible to discuss how learning is processed in the brain without discussing memory. Certain synaptic connections develop in the brain when a memory is formed. **Short-term memory** typically lasts only a matter of seconds, but can potentially be converted into **long-term memory** through a process called **consolidation**. Newly acquired information (such as the knowledge that a reward follows a certain behavior) is temporarily stored in short-term memory and can be transferred into long-term memory under the right conditions.

Long-term Potentiation

When something is learned, the synapses between neurons are strengthened and the process of long-term potentiation begins. **Long-term potentiation** occurs when, following brief periods of stimulation, an increase in the synaptic strength between two neurons leads to stronger electrochemical responses to a given stimulus. When long-term potentiation occurs, the neurons involved in the circuit develop an increased sensitivity (the sending neuron needs less prompting to fire its impulse and release its neurotransmitter, and/or the receiving neurons have more receptors for the neurotransmitter), which results in increased potential for neural firing after a connection has been stimulated. This increased potential can last for hours or even weeks. Synaptic strength is thought to be the process by which memories are consolidated for long-term memory (so learning can occur). At a given synapse, long-term potentiation involves both presynaptic and postsynaptic neurons. For example, dopamine is one of the neurotransmitters involved in pleasurable or rewarding actions. In operant conditioning, reinforcement activates the limbic circuits that involve memory, learning, and emotions. Since reinforcement of a desired behavior is pleasurable, the circuits are strengthened as dopamine floods the system, making it more likely the behavior will be repeated.

After long-term potentiation has occurred, passing an electrical current through the brain doesn't disrupt the memory associations between the neurons involved, although other memories will be wiped out. For example, when a person receives a blow to the head resulting in a concussion, he or she loses memory for events shortly preceding the concussion. This is due to the fact that long-term potentiation has not had a chance to occur (and leave traces of memory connections), while old memories, which were already potentiated, remain.

Long-term memory storage involves more permanent changes to the brain, including structural and functional connections between neurons. For example, long-term memory storage includes new synaptic connections between neurons, permanent changes in pre- and postsynaptic membranes, and a permanent increase or decrease in neurotransmitter synthesis. Furthermore, visual imaging studies suggest that there is greater branching of dendrites in regions of the brain thought to be involved with memory storage. Other studies suggest that protein synthesis somehow influences memory formation; drugs that prevent protein synthesis appear to block long-term memory formation.

Not all behaviors are learned, of course. The neural processes described above occur when animals or people learn new behaviors, or change their behaviors based on experience (that is, environmental feedback). As our learned behaviors change, our synapses change too. On the other hand, some behaviors are **innate**. These are all the actions we know how to do instinctively (or our body just does without us consciously thinking about it), not because someone taught us to do them (for example, breathing or pulling away from a hot stove). Further, innate behaviors are always the same among members of the species, even for the ones performing them for the first time.

Observational Learning

More advanced organisms, particularly humans, do not learn only through direct experience. **Observational learning,** also known as **social learning** or **vicarious learning**, is learning through watching and imitating others.

Modeling

Modeling is one of the most basic mechanisms behind observational learning. In modeling, an observer sees the behavior being performed by another person. Later, with the model in mind, the observer **imitates** the behavior she or he observed. You likely participated in this behavior as a child (or even now). Think back to when you were little and you played with your friends; perhaps you played house or pretended to be a superhero. Typically, you would play your role ("mom" or "Superman") according to the model you have seen: your mother, or Superman (on TV). As an adult, your appearance may be based on models in society; you dress, talk, and walk like your friends. Modeling is not limited to humans either; think about how lions learn to hunt in the wild. A lioness will take her cubs with her to hunt and her cubs watch her during the process and hunt based on what they observe.

Typically, the likelihood of imitating a modeled behavior is based on how successful someone finds that behavior to be, or the type of reinforcement that the model received for his behavior. However, individuals may choose to imitate behaviors even if they do not observe the consequences of the model's behavior. For instance, **Albert Bandura** (considered a pioneer in the field of observational learning) conducted a series of experiments using a Bobo doll (a large inflatable toy with a heavy base that will spring back up after being punched). Bandura showed children videos of adults either behaving aggressively toward the Bobo doll (punching, kicking, and shouting at the doll) or ignoring the doll altogether. Even when children did not see the consequences of the adult's behavior, they tended to imitate the behavior they saw. Later studies conducted by others support that humans are prone to imitation and modeling, and we are particularly likely to imitate those whom we perceive as similar to ourselves, as successful, or as admirable in some way. Therefore, modeling, and social learning in general, is a very powerful influence on individuals' behaviors.

Biological Processes that Affect Observational Learning

Mirror neurons have been identified in various parts of the human brain, including the premotor cortex, supplementary motor area, primary somatosensory cortex, and the inferior parietal cortex. In monkeys, mirror neurons fire when the monkey performs a task, as well as when the monkey observes another monkey performing the task. Humans also possess mirror neurons, and while there is still some debate about the exact function of these neurons, there are several hypotheses. Some believe that mirror neurons are activated by connecting the sight and action of a movement (that is, they are programmed to mirror). Some postulate that mirror neurons help us understand the actions of others and help us learn through imitation. It has also been proposed that mirror neurons in humans are responsible for **vicarious emotions**, such as empathy, and that a problem in the mirror neuron system might underlie disorders such as autism. However, this has yet to be proven, and there is clearly still much research needed to determine the exact function or functions of mirror neurons. Despite that, many believe that they are somehow involved in observational learning in animals, including humans.

Applications of Observational Learning to Explain Individual Behavior

As social organisms, human beings connect through observational learning. We learn from and behave like one another, but this mimicking is not perfect. There are individual differences between people and animals. Personality differences and psychological disorders can affect observational learning. For example, much of the research on observational learning has focused on violence and how observing violence increases violence in society, but not everyone who observes violence is violent. Cognition plays a role in how we use what we learn.

9.2 MEMORY

Encoding

Process of Encoding Information

As you may recall from information-processing models, information first enters a sensory register before encoding occurs. **Encoding** is the process of transferring sensory information into our memory system.

Working memory—where information is maintained temporarily as part of a particular mental activity (learning, solving a problem)—is thought to include a phonological loop, visuospatial sketchpad, central executive, and episodic buffer (Chapter 11). Working memory is quite limited, and this model helps to explain the **serial position effect**. This effect occurs when someone attempts to memorize a series, such as a list of words. In an immediate recall condition (shortly after the information is first presented), the individual is more likely to recall the first and last items on the list. These phenomena are called the

primacy effect and the **recency effect**. It is hypothesized that first items are more easily recalled because they have had the most time to be encoded and transferred to long-term memory. Last items may be more easily recalled because they may still be in the phonological loop, and thus may be readily available. When the individual is asked to recall the list at a later point, the individual tends to remember only the first items well. This may be because that was the only information that was transferred to long-term memory, whereas recent information from the phonological loop would quickly decay and be lost.

Processes That Aid in Encoding Memories

A **mnemonic** is any technique for improving retention and retrieval of information from memory. One simple process that aids memory is use of the phonological loop through **rehearsal**. If someone were to give you a phone number and you didn't have any way to record the information, you might repeat the digits over and over in your head until you were able to write them down. In some cases, such as the recital of the Pledge of Allegiance, repeated rehearsal can lead to encoding into long-term memory.

Chunking is a strategy in which information to be remembered is organized into discrete groups of data. For example, with phone numbers, one might memorize the area code, the first three digits, and the last four digits as discrete chunks. Thus, the number of "things" being remembered is decreased—in the case of a phone number, there are now three "things" to memorize instead of 10 individual digits. This is an important strategy because the limit of working memory is generally understood to be about seven digits. Even the process of remembering that a group of letters makes a particular word involves chunking.

When memorizing information, people make use of **hierarchies** for organization. For example, imagine that a child is learning about the different animals in the zoo. It would be useful to have a category of "birds" to include ostriches, penguins, etc. and a category of "big cats" to remember lions, tigers, and so on. As the child learns more, these hierarchies are reorganized to match incoming information. When words are organized into groups, recall significantly improves. For example, it would be easier to remember the list "chair, table, desk, lamp, recliner, sofa" if you realized that all of these words are pieces of furniture.

There is some evidence that the **depth of processing** is important for encoding memories. Information that is thought about at a deeper level is better remembered. For example, it is easier to remember the general plot of a book than the exact words, meaning that semantic information (meaning) is more easily remembered than grammatical information (form) when the goal is to learn a concept. On the other hand, rhyme can be useful in aiding phonological processing. Another useful mnemonic device is to use short words or phrases that represent longer strings of information. For example, ROYGBIV is an **acronym** that is helpful in memorizing the colors of the rainbow (red, orange, yellow, green, blue, indigo, violet).

The **dual-coding hypothesis** asserts that it is easier to remember words with associated images than either words or images alone. By encoding both a visual mental representation and an associated word, there are more connections made to the memory and an opportunity to process the information at a deeper level. For this reason, imagery is a useful mnemonic device. One aid for memory is to use the **method of loci**. This involves imagining moving through a familiar place, such as your home, and in each place, leaving a visual representation of a topic to be remembered. The images of the places are then called upon to bring into awareness the associated topics. Similarly, **the peg word method** involves assigning images to a sequence of numbers.

It is also easier to remember things that are personally relevant, known as the **self-reference effect**. We have excellent recall for information that we can personally relate to because it interacts with our own views or because it can be linked to existing memories. A useful tool for memory is to try to make new information personally relevant by relating it to existing knowledge.

Memory Storage

Types of Memory Storage

Different stores of memory include sensory memory, short-term memory, and long-term memory. **Sensory memory,** the initial recording of sensory information in the memory system, is a very brief snapshot that quickly decays. Three types of sensory memory are iconic memory, eidetic memory, and echoic memory. **Iconic memory** is brief photographic memory for visual information, which decays in a few tenths of a second. **Eidetic memory** is an ability found in some children to remember an image in vivid detail for several minutes after brief exposure. **Echoic memory** is memory for sound, which lasts for about 3–4 seconds. This is why sometimes in a conversation you might ask what someone said if you had trouble hearing him or her, only to hear and make sense of the words yourself a second later. Information from sensory memory decays rapidly if it is not passed through Broadbent's filter into short-term memory. **Short-term memory** is also limited in duration and in capacity. Recall capacity for an adult is typically around seven items, plus or minus two. This is why phone numbers with seven digits (excluding the area code) are conveniently remembered. As discussed earlier, although chunking increases the amount of information remembered by putting more information into each chunk, it is still subject to this limit of about seven chunks. Information in short-term memory is retained only for about 20 seconds, unless it is actively processed so that it can be transferred into long-term memory. **Long-term memory** is information that is retained sometimes indefinitely; it is believed to have an infinite capacity.

It is important to draw a distinction between short-term memory and working memory. Short-term memory, which is strongly associated with the hippocampus, is where new information sought to be remembered resides temporarily and is then encoded to long-term memory or forgotten. Thus, if you meet a new person, you will store the person's name in short-term memory and, perhaps through rehearsal, encode the name into long-term memory. Working memory, which is strongly associated with the prefrontal cortex, is a storage bin to hold memories (short-term or long-term) that are needed at a particular moment in order to process information or solve a problem. For example, if you need to mentally determine the area of a triangle, you will bring the formula and your knowledge of multiplication into your working memory while you process the result.

Implicit or **procedural memory** refers to conditioned associations and knowledge of how to do something, while **explicit** or **declarative memory** involves being able to "declare" or voice what is known. Explicit memory involves conscious recall of information, while implicit memory does not. For example, one could read a book on how to develop a great shot in basketball from cover to cover and be able to explain in great detail the necessary steps. However, this book knowledge would not likely translate into being able to execute the shot on the court without practice. Explaining the concept involves explicit or declarative memory, while not having practiced it indicates a lack of implicit or procedural memory. Semantic and episodic memory are two subdivisions of explicit memory. **Semantic memory** is memory for factual information, such as the capital of England. **Episodic memory** is autobiographical memory for information of personal importance, such as the situation surrounding a first kiss. Typically, semantic memory deteriorates before episodic memory does.

Figure 6 Types of long-term memory

The distinction between explicit and implicit memory is supported by neurological evidence. Brain structures involved in memory include the hippocampus, cerebellum, and amygdala. The hippocampus is necessary for the encoding of new explicit memories. The cerebellum is involved in learning skills and conditioned associations (implicit memory). The amygdala is involved in associating emotion with memories, particularly negative memories; for example, a fear response to a dentist's drill involves fear conditioning. The roles of the hippocampus, cerebellum, and amygdala are shown by studies on patients who have the capacity for either implicit or explicit memory (but not both). For example, amnesic patients with hippocampal damage may not have declarative memory for a skill they have recently learned (due to amnesia), and yet may be able to demonstrate the skill, indicating that implicit memory exists. Interestingly, the implicit memories that infants form are retained indefinitely, but the explicit memories that infants form are largely not retained beyond about age four—a phenomenon known as infantile amnesia. It is only later, after the hippocampus has fully developed, that explicit memories are retained long-term.

Retrieval

Recall, Recognition, and Relearning

Retrieval is the process of finding information stored in memory. When most people think of retrieval, they think of **recall**, the ability to retrieve information. **Free recall** involves retrieving the item "out of thin air," while **cued recall** involves retrieving the information when provided with a cue. For example, a test of free recall would be to ask a student to name all of the capital cities of the world. A test of cued recall would be to provide the student with a list of countries and then ask him or her to name all of the capital cities of the world. Another type of retrieval is **recognition**, which involves identifying specific information from a set of information that is presented. One recognition task would be a multiple-choice question. **Reproductive memory** is storage of the original stimulus input and subsequent recall (i.e., remembering something accurately without significantly altering it). Finally, **relearning** involves the process of learning material that was originally learned. Once we have learned and forgotten something, we are able to relearn it more quickly than when it was originally learned, which suggests that the information was in the memory system to be retrieved.

Retrieval Cues

Retrieval cues provide reminders of information. Within the network model of memory, we have already discussed how hints may activate a closely related node, making it easier to retrieve the node being searched for. Prior activation of these nodes and associations is called **priming**. Often, this process occurs without our awareness. For example, if you are shown several red items and then asked to name a fruit, you will be more likely to name a red fruit. The best retrieval cues are often contextual cues that had associations formed at the time that the memory was encoding, such as tastes, smells, and sights. Almost everyone has had the experience of not recognizing someone familiar because of seeing the person in another context. For example, running into your coffee shop barista at a concert might make it harder to recognize her or him. Or a man may associate happiness with beagles because he had one as a child. When looking in a shelter to adopt a dog decades later, he may find himself emotionally drawn to select a beagle. Although he may not consciously be thinking of his childhood dog, his memories predispose him to connect a beagle with feeling happy.

The Role of Emotion in Retrieving Memories

In addition to words, events, and sensory input serving as retrieval cues, emotion can also serve as a retrieval cue. What we learn in one state is most easily recalled when we are once again in that emotional state, a phenomenon known as **mood-dependent memory**. Thus, when someone is depressed, events in the past that were sad are more likely to emerge to the forefront of his or her mind. This plays a role in maintaining the cycle of depression. When we are happy, we tend to remember past times that were also happy. In addition, emotion can bias the recall of memories. If someone is angry at a friend, the person is more likely to feel that the friendship has always been rotten, whereas in a moment when the friendship feels joyful, the person is more likely to perceive the relationship as having always been a joyful one. Emotion has a powerful effect on the experience of memory, often leading to increased recall for emotionally intense experiences. **Flashbulb memories** are intense, vivid "snapshots" of an emotionally intense experience. These intense memories are often experienced by PTSD patients during recollection of the traumatic event.

Forgetting

Remembering information is achieved through the process of paying attention, encoding, retaining information (storage), and finally retrieval. Failure along any step of this process can cause forgetting. A failure to pay attention or encode means that the information never got into the memory system. A failure to store information is decay. A failure in retrieval could result from a lack of retrieval cues or interference.

Aging and Memory

Older adults vary in their memory abilities. Decline in memory is influenced by how active the person is: increased activity (both physical and mental) is a protective factor against neuronal atrophy. Memory loss may parallel the age-related loss of neurons. As we age, memory decline tends to follow some common trends, with certain types of memory being affected earlier. As you might expect, older adults have accumulated many experiences and so have a rich network of nodes and associations. Information that is meaningful and connects well to that existing web of information, and information that is skill-based, shows less decline with age. However, there is greater decline for information that is less meaningful and less richly connected.

Due to having a more extensive memory network, retrieval can also become trickier with time. Older adults show minimal decline in recognition, but greater decline in free recall. One type of recall is **prospective memory**, remembering to do things in the future. Prospective memory is stronger when there are cues in the environment. For example, an older adult may be asked to remember to take a particular medication three times a day. However, unless there is a reminder cue such as a readily visible pillbox or an alarm, it may be difficult to remember that there is a task that needs to be completed. Thus, the person fails to "remember to remember." Difficulty with prospective memory without cues also makes it difficult to complete time-based tasks, since one must remember to look at a clock or keep track of a schedule.

Memory Dysfunctions

Remember that memory has a neurological basis, with the hippocampus playing a role in the encoding of new explicit memories, the cerebellum playing a role in encoding implicit memories, and the amygdala helping to tie emotion to memories. Once information is in long-term memory, it is stored in various areas spread throughout the brain. Damage to parts of the brain by strokes, brain tumors, alcoholism, traumatic brain injuries, and other events can cause memory impairment. Patients with damage to the hippocampus could develop **anterograde amnesia**, an inability to encode new memories, or **retrograde amnesia**, an inability to recall information that was previously encoded (or both types of amnesia). In addition, neurological damage involving neurotransmitters can also cause memory dysfunction. One theory about the cause of Alzheimer's disease, for example, involves an inability to manufacture enough of the neurotransmitter acetylcholine, which results in, among other things, neuronal death in the hippocampus.

Decay

Memory decay results in a failure to retain stored information. Even if information is successfully encoded into memory, it can decay from our memory storage and be forgotten. However, decay does not happen in a linear fashion. Rather, the "forgetting curve" indicates that the longer the **retention interval**, or the time since the information was learned, the more information will be forgotten, with the most forgetting occurring rapidly in the first few days before leveling off. It is unclear why memories fade or erode with the passage of time. It is possible that the brain cells involved in the memory may die off, or perhaps that the associations among memories need to be refreshed in order not to weaken.

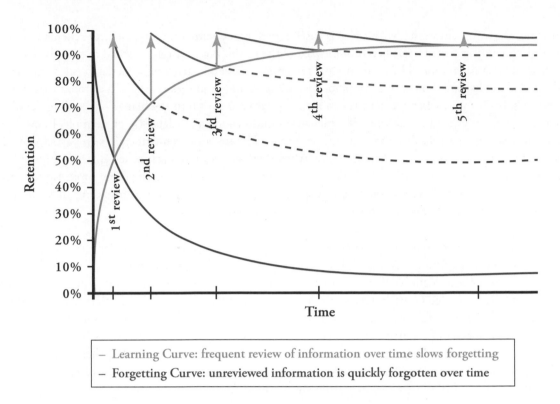

Figure 7 showing retention (y-axis) versus Time (x-axis) with labeled points for 1st review, 2nd review, 3rd review, 4th review, and 5th review.

- Learning Curve: frequent review of information over time slows forgetting
- Forgetting Curve: unreviewed information is quickly forgotten over time

Figure 7 Forgetting curve

Interference

Interference can result in a failure to retrieve information that is in storage. The passage of time may create more opportunity for newer learning to interfere with older learning, which is especially common if the learned information is similar. **Proactive interference** happens when information previously learned interferes with the ability to recall information learned later. For example, remembering where you had parked your car in a parking garage will be more difficult once you have parked in that parking garage for months in different locations. **Retroactive interference** happens when newly learned information interferes with the recall of information learned previously. For example, someone who has moved frequently may find that learning new addresses and directions interferes with his or her ability to remember old addresses and directions. Of course, old and new information do not always interfere. Sometimes, old information facilitates the learning of new information through **positive transfer**. For example, knowing how to play American football may make it easier for someone to learn how to play rugby.

Memory Construction and Source Monitoring

Our memories are far from being snapshots of actual experience. We already know that when memories are encoded, they pass through a "lens;" the mood and selective attention of the observer influence how they are encoded. Memory is once again altered when passing through the "lens" of retrieval. When we remember something, we do not pull from a mental photo album, but rather, we draw a picture, *constructing* the recalled memory from information that is stored. This process is not foolproof.

Sometimes the information that we retrieve is based more on a **schema** than on reality. A schema is a mental blueprint containing common aspects of some part of the world. For example, if asked to describe what your fourth-grade classroom looked like, you might "remember" a chalkboard, chalk, desks, posters encouraging reading, and books, based on your schema for such a classroom, even though the actual room may not have had posters. In this way, when we construct a memory, we tend to "fill in the blanks" by adding details that may not have been present at the time. We may also unknowingly alter details. For example, in eyewitness testimony, leading questions often cause witnesses to misestimate or misremember. When participants in an experiment were asked how fast cars were going when they *smashed* into each other, instead of just *hit* each other, they indicated higher speeds. Individuals in the first group also reported seeing broken glass and car parts, when there actually were none. After people are exposed to subtle misinformation, they are usually susceptible to the **misinformation effect**, a tendency to misremember.

Individuals may also misremember when asked to repeatedly imagine nonexistent actions and events. Simply repeatedly imagining that one did something can create **false memories** for an event. False memories are inaccurate recollections of an event and may be the result of the implanting of ideas. For example, if one repeatedly imagined being lost as a child in a shopping mall, this imagined occurrence would begin to feel familiar, and as it felt more familiar, it would take on the flavor of a real memory. In fact, it can be very difficult for people to distinguish between real memories and false memories by feeling, because both can be accompanied by emotional reactions and the sense of familiarity. The theory of **reconstructive memory** posits that rather than an episodic recall of events that took place, memory is a constructive process that involves building a memory from similar experiences, social expectations, perceptions, cues, and feelings, all of which are combined with recollection of the event itself to form a memory experience. For this reason, an individual's confidence in the validity of a memory has not been found to be a good indication of how valid it actually is.

When recalling information, people are also susceptible to forgetting one particular fact—the information's source. This is an error in **source monitoring**. For example, you may find yourself angry with an individual in your life for doing something hurtful, only to later realize that the action occurred in a dream. Or you may recognize someone, but have no idea where you have seen the person before.

Changes in Synaptic Connections Underlie Memory and Learning

Neuroscientists have had a difficult time in their search for a physical basis for memory. There has been no central location found for memories, and there seem to be no such thing as special memory neurons. The process of forming memories involves electrical impulses sent through brain circuits. Somehow, these impulses leave permanent neural traces that are physical representations of information. More and more evidence indicates that what is important for memory and for learning is the synapses—those sites where nerve cells communicate with one another through neurotransmitters.

9.3 HUMAN DEVELOPMENT

Developmental psychology is the study of how humans develop physically, cognitively, and socially, throughout their lifetime. As previously discussed, genetics and environment play an important role in human development.

Early Brain Development

During prenatal development, the brain actually produces more neurons than needed. At birth, humans have the highest number of neurons at any point in their life, and these are pruned throughout the ensuing lifetime. However, the immature brain does not have many **neural networks**, or codified routes for information processing (the types that are generated in response to learning and experience throughout a lifetime). During infancy and early childhood development, these neurons form neural networks, and networks are reinforced by learning and behavior. From ages 3 to 6, the most rapid growth occurs in the frontal lobes, corresponding to an increase in rational planning and attention. The association areas, linked with thinking, memory, and language, are the last cortical areas to develop. (For more information on cognitive development, see Jean Piaget in Chapter 11.)

Maturation is the sequence of biological growth processes in human development. Maturation, while largely genetic, is still influenced by environment. For example, while humans are programmed to learn how to speak, first using one-word utterances, then developing progressively more complex speech, severe deprivation can significantly delay this process, while an incredibly nurturing environment might speed it up. The developing brain allows for motor development; as the nervous system and muscles mature, more and more complex physical skills develop. The sequence of motor development is almost entirely universal. Babies learn to roll over, then sit, then crawl, then stand, then walk. The development of the cerebellum is a necessary precursor to walking, and most humans learn to walk around age one.

The average age of earliest conscious memory is roughly 3.5 years. Before this age, we are unable to remember much, if anything; this is referred to as **infantile amnesia**. Even though humans are unable to recall memories from this period, babies and young children are still capable of learning and memory. In one famous experiment, a researcher tied a string to an infant's foot and attached the other end of the string to a mobile. When the baby kicked its foot, the mobile moved. Babies demonstrated learning—they associated kicking with mobile movement—because they kicked more when attached to the mobile, both on the day of the experiment and the day after. Interestingly, if the babies were attached to a different mobile, they did not kick more; however, when attached to the same mobile a month later, they remembered the association and began kicking again.

Social Development and Attachment

Humans are social organisms. From approximately 8–12 months of age, young children display **stranger anxiety** (crying and clinging to caregiver). Around this time, infants have developed schemas for familiar faces, and when new faces do not fit an already developed schema, the infant becomes distressed. Infant-parent attachment bonds are an important survival impulse. Stranger anxiety seems to peek around 13 months for children and then gradually declines. For many years it was assumed that infants attached to their parents because they provided nourishment, but an accidental experiment actually countered this assumption.

In the 1950s, two psychologists (**Harry Harlow** and **Margaret Harlow**) bred monkeys for experiments. To control for environment and to reduce the incidence of disease, infant monkeys were separated from their mothers at birth (maternal deprivation) and provided with a baby blanket. When the blankets were removed for laundering the baby monkeys became very distressed because they had formed an intense attachment to the object. This physical attachment seemed to contradict the idea that attachment was formed based on nourishment, so the Harlows designed a series of experiments to further investigate. In one experiment, the Harlows fashioned two artificial mothers—one nourishing (a wire frame with a wooden head and a bottle) and the other cloth (wire frame with a wooden head and a cloth blanket wrapped around it). They found that the baby monkeys preferred the cloth mother, clinging to her and spending the majority of their time with her, and visiting the other mother only to feed. Harlow concluded that "contact comfort" was an essential element of infant/mother bonding, as well as to psychological development. Keep in mind, however, that even though these baby monkeys were provided with a surrogate wire mother, this mother was still largely inadequate. Therefore, when the monkeys from these experiments matured, they demonstrated social deficits when reintroduced to other monkeys. Harlow's monkeys demonstrated aggressive behavior as adults, were unable to socially integrate with other monkeys, and did not mate. If female monkeys were artificially inseminated, they would neglect, abuse, or even kill their offspring.[1]

Mary Ainsworth conducted a series of experiments called the "strange situation experiments," wherein mothers would leave their infants in an unfamiliar environment (usually a laboratory playroom) to see how the infants would react. These studies suggested that attachment styles vary among infants. **Securely attached** infants in the presence of their mothers (or primary caregivers) will play and explore; when the mother leaves the room, the infant is distressed, and when the mother returns, the infant will seek contact with her and is easily consoled. **Insecurely attached** infants in the presence of their mothers (or primary caregivers) are less likely to explore their surroundings and may even cling to their mothers; when the mother leaves, they will either cry loudly and remain upset or will demonstrate indifference to her departure and return. Observations indicate that securely attached infants have sensitive and responsive mothers (or primary caregivers) who are quick to attend to their child's needs in a consistent fashion. Insecurely attached infants have mothers (or primary caregivers) who are insensitive and unresponsive, attending to their child's needs inconsistently or sometimes even ignoring their children. In the Harlow monkey experiments described above, the cloth mother would be considered rather insensitive and unresponsive; when these monkeys were put into situations without their artificial mothers, they became terrified.

Psychologists believe that early interactions with parents and caregivers lay the foundation for future adult relationships. Securely attached infants grow up to demonstrate better social skills, a greater capacity for effective intimate relationships, and a superior ability to promote secure attachments in their children. Alternatively, children who are neglected or abused are *more likely* to neglect or abuse their own children. Note that more likely does not imply a destiny; most abused children do not grow up to abuse their own children. Humans display a large degree of resiliency, and most insecurely attached or abused children grow into normal adults.

Parenting styles vary but tend to fall largely into three categories: authoritarian, permissive, and authoritative:

- **Authoritarian** parenting involves attempting to control children with strict rules that are expected to be followed unconditionally. Authoritarian parents will often utilize punishment instead of discipline, and will not explain the reasoning behind their rules. Typically, authoritarian parents are very demanding, but not very responsive to their children, and do

---

[1] Note: this type of extreme deprivation experiment would no longer be considered ethical or humane today; research animals in captivity are treated much better.

not provide much warmth or nurturing. Children raised by authoritarian parents may display more aggressive behavior toward others, or may act shy and fearful around others, have lower self-esteem, and have difficulty in social situations.

- **Permissive** parents, on the other hand, allow their children to lead the show. With few rules and demands, these parents rarely discipline their children. Permissive parents are very responsive and loving toward their children, but are rather lenient; if rules exist, they are enforced inconsistently. Children raised by permissive parents tend to lack self-discipline, may be self-involved and demanding, and may demonstrate poor social skills.

- **Authoritative** parents listen to their children, encourage independence, place limits on behavior and consistently follow through with consequences when behavior is not met, express warmth and nurturing, and allow children to express their opinions and to discuss options. Authoritative parents have expectations for their children, and when children break the rules they are disciplined in a fair and consistent manner. Authoritative parenting is the "best" parenting style, as it tends to produce children that are happier, have good emotional control and regulation, develop good social skills, and are confident in their abilities.

Please remember that parenting style and children's dispositions are merely correlated; while it is possible that parenting style causes these outcomes in children, there are other possible explanations, as well [what are some potential alternative explanations for these results?[2]].

Adolescence

Despite the fact that infancy is crucial for development, development continues throughout our lifetime. **Adolescence**[3] is the transitional stage between childhood and adulthood; this period roughly begins at puberty and ends with achievement of independent adult status. Therefore, adolescence generally encompasses the teenage years. Adolescence involves many important physical, psychological, and social changes. The onset of puberty (typically around age 10 or 11 in girls, and age 11 or 12 in boys) involves surging estrogens and androgens (sex hormones) that cause a cascade of physical changes. In girls, increased estrogen causes the development of secondary sex characteristics (increased body and pubic hair, increased fat distribution, breast development) as well as the initiation of the menstrual cycle. In boys, increased testosterone (the primary androgen) also causes the development of secondary sex characteristics (increased body and pubic hair, increased muscle mass, voice deepening, enlargement of the penis and testes), and the onset of ejaculation. While the sequence of events in puberty is fairly predictable, the onset of these events is less so, which can be distressing. For example, early puberty for a girl means that she will begin developing breasts and menstruating before her peers do, which can be psychologically upsetting.

During adolescence, the brain undergoes three major changes: cell proliferation (in certain areas, particularly the prefrontal lobes and limbic system), synaptic pruning (of unused or unnecessary connections), and myelination (which strengthens connections among various regions). The prefrontal cortex—responsible for abstract thought, planning, anticipating consequences, and personality—continues to develop

---

[2] It is possible that certain children have a genetic disposition to be easygoing, confident, and socially adjusted, so the authoritative parent has an "easy time" raising this easy child, and their resultant behavior is attributed to the parent when, in actuality, there was something innate about the child that caused the parent to respond to him in that way.

[3] From the Latin word *adolescere*, which means "to grow up."

9.3

during this period.[4] The limbic system—involved in emotion—develops more rapidly than the prefrontal cortex during adolescence, which may explain behavior that appears to be emotionally, rather than rationally, driven. Though it may seem contradictory, adolescents are actually improving their self-control, judgment, and long-term planning abilities during this time.

Adulthood and Later Life

While the transition to "adulthood" is not marked by any definitive biological event (indeed, the term is essentially defined by society), attainment of adulthood is marked by a feeling of comfortable independence. Interestingly, while childhood and adolescence are marked by clear developmental milestones and attainment of physical abilities, adulthood is less clearly defined. For example, if you met a 4-year old and a 14-year old, you would probably be able to reasonably guess at some of the actions they were and were not capable of, and the differences between them would be drastic. If, on the other hand, you met a 40-year old and 50-year old, it may be much harder to pinpoint the difference, if there was much of one at all.

---

[4] In fact the frontal lobes are not completely developed until roughly age 26!

Chapter 9 Summary

- Nonassociative learning occurs when an organism is repeatedly exposed to a stimulus and includes habituation and sensitization.

- Associative learning occurs when an organism learns that an event, object, or action is connected with another; the two major types are classical conditioning and operant conditioning.

- Classical conditioning pairs a neutral stimulus with an unconditioned stimulus to generate a conditioned stimulus and conditioned response (for example, Pavlov's dogs). In acquisition the response is learned, in extinction the response is "lost," and in spontaneous recovery, an extinct response occurs again when the stimulus is presented after some length of time.

- Taste aversion is a very strong and long-lasting association between a specific taste or smell and illness; taste aversion challenges some of the tenets of classical conditioning because it is learned quickly (after one time) and is very slow to extinguish.

- Operant conditioning uses reinforcement and punishment to mold behavior and eventually cause associative learning; B. F. Skinner and his work with rats and pigeons in a "Skinner box" is a famous example of operant conditioning.

- Reinforcement increases the likelihood that a preceding behavior will be repeated; positive reinforcement is a desirable stimulus that occurs immediately following a behavior, whereas negative reinforcement is an undesirable stimulus that is removed immediately following a behavior.

- A fixed-ratio schedule provides the reinforcement after a set number of instances of the behavior while a variable-ratio schedule provides the reinforcement after an unpredictable number of occurrences.

- A fixed-interval schedule provides the reinforcement after a set amount of time, while a variable-interval schedule provides the reinforcement after an inconsistent amount of time.

- Punishment is a consequence that follows a behavior and decreases the likelihood that the behavior will be repeated; positive punishment presents an undesirable stimulus after an instance of the target behavior, while negative punishment removes a desirable stimulus after an instance of the target behavior.

- Insight learning occurs when previously learned behaviors are suddenly combined in unique ways.

- Latent learning occurs when previously unseen behavior can manifest quickly when required.

- Long-term potentiation occurs when, following brief periods of stimulation, a persistent increase in the synaptic strength between two neurons leads to stronger electrochemical responses to a given stimulus.

- Observational learning is a social process; in modeling, an observer sees behavior and later imitates it; Albert Bandura's Bobo doll experiment is a famous example of modeling.

- Mirror neurons have been identified in various parts of the human brain and are believed to fire when we observe another person performing a task.

- Short-term memory is limited in duration and in capacity; recall capacity for an adult is typically around seven items, plus or minus two.

- Long-term memory is information that is retained sometimes indefinitely; it is believed to have an infinite capacity. Long-term memory consists of implicit (procedural) memory and explicit (declarative) memory; explicit memory includes episodic and semantic memory.

- The spreading activation theory of memory posits that during recall, nodes (concepts) are activated, which are connected to other nodes, and so on.

- Anterograde amnesia is an inability to encode new memories, while retrograde amnesia is an inability to recall information that was previously encoded.

- Important information about attachment was discovered through studies conducted by Mary Ainsworth; the impact of deprivation was discovered through studies conducted by Harry and Margaret Harlow.

CHAPTER 9 FREESTANDING PRACTICE QUESTIONS

1. Retroactive interference occurs when:

A) old information interferes with learning new material.
B) new material interferes with recalling old material.
C) new information decays over time.
D) old information decays over time.

2. Which of the following types of memory does not affect behavior consciously and can be measured only indirectly?

A) Nondeclarative memory
B) Declarative memory
C) Episodic memory
D) Explicit memory

3. A five-year-old boy has formed a habit of writing on his parents' living room walls. Based on operant conditioning principles, which of the following types of punishment would be least effective in stopping this behavior?

A) Giving the child a time out immediately after he writes on the wall, every time the child writes on the wall.
B) Providing the child with a cookie at the end of each day that he abstains from writing on the walls.
C) Harshly scolding the child (an intense punishment) every time that the child writes on the wall.
D) Punishing the child occasionally, when the parents happen to notice writing on the wall.

4. Jay joins a social media website to lose weight, and he receives points based on the intensity of his daily exercise and praise from fellow website users for each workout he logs on the website. This increases his exercise frequency and intensity. Eventually he stops logging onto the website, but continues to exercise with increased frequency. This is an example of:

A) vicarious reinforcement.
B) operant conditioning.
C) innate behavior.
D) classical conditioning.

5. A student cramming for finals memorizes the steps in solving a physics problem early in the afternoon and then studies for his other subjects for several hours before his physics exam. When he arrives at the exam, he can no longer remember how to solve the physics equation. This is an example of:

A) retroactive interference.
B) proactive interference.
C) retrieval cues.
D) long-term potentiation.

6. A researcher studying several patients gives each of them the same maze to solve. Although each works independently on it for 30 minutes—with varying degrees of success—none of them recalls seeing the maze when presented with it the next day. Nonetheless, their overall speed and success in solving it has improved significantly. These patients are likely experiencing impairment in:

I. procedural memory.
II. episodic memory.
III. echoic memory.

A) I only
B) II only
C) I and II
D) II and III

7. Knowing how to ride a bike is a type of:

A) procedural, long-term, implicit memory.
B) explicit, short-term, procedural memory.
C) prospective, long-term, implicit memory.
D) procedural, mood-dependent, source memory.

8. An individual attempting to memorize a series of complex steps for the first time is most likely to have the most success if he uses:

A) priming that incorporates proactive interference.
B) chunking and serial position.
C) source-monitoring and rehearsal.
D) a mnemonic that incorporates spaced repetition of the steps.

CHAPTER 9 PRACTICE PASSAGE

Elizabeth Loftus is widely known as one of the leading experts in the field of false memories, especially regarding childhood sexual abuse. However, this particular topic is deeply controversial, with many experts divided over whether these memories are truly false, or if they are instead repressed to protect the individual from reliving further trauma. Loftus is most famous for her theory of the *misinformation effect*, which refers to the phenomenon in which exposure to incorrect information between the encoding of a memory and its later recall causes impairment to the memory. That is to say, if you witnessed a hit-and-run car accident, and heard a radio commercial for Ford before giving your testimony to the police, you might incorrectly recall that the offending vehicle was a Ford, even if it was not. Loftus' research has been used in many cases of eyewitness testimony in high-profile court cases to demonstrate the malleability of the human memory.

To test this theory, researchers in New York City set up a "crime" for participants to "witness" (unbeknownst to them). 175 local female college students were recruited to participate in a study about memory, and were directed to complete some computer tasks involving word and picture recall in a room overlooking an alley. While completing the computer tasks, participants witnessed a young woman being "mugged" by a young man in the alley outside the lab—both individuals were confederates of the researchers. After reporting the "crime" to the researchers, participants were escorted out of the lab and told that this crime would be reported to the local police, and that they might be called back in to give a testimony. For half of the participants, a research confederate acting as a custodial worker was present as they were being escorted out. For the other half, no decoys were present. Participants were randomly assigned to either the decoy or non-decoy groups. Participants who did not report the "crime" to the researchers were excluded from the study (25 women were excluded).

One week later, participants were called back to the lab to give their testimony to a police officer—another confederate. Participants were told that the police had several leads on who the mugger might be, and were asked to pick out the suspect from five different photo options. Included in the photo set were photos of the mugger, the custodial worker, and three neutral faces chosen to be similar to the two experimental faces. After recalling the event to the police officer and choosing a face, participants were debriefed (they were told that the mugging was fake) and awarded course credit for their participation. The results of this study are summarized in Table 1.

Table 1 Number of Positive Identifications in Photo Line-up

	Photo				
	"Mugger"	"Custodial Worker"	Neutral Photo #1	Neutral Photo #2	Neutral Photo #3
Decoy Group ($n = 75$)	18	37	7	5	8
Non-Decoy Group ($n = 75$)	23	13	12	14	13

1. What conclusions can be drawn from the data presented in Table 1?

A) The misinformation effect is present in the decoy group.
B) The non-decoy group had better memory than the decoy group.
C) There are no significant differences between the decoy and non-decoy groups.
D) No conclusions can be drawn from these data.

2. The inability to form new memories is called:

A) retrograde amnesia.
B) anterograde amnesia.
C) source amnesia
D) infantile amnesia.

3. Suppose that after selecting someone from the photo line-up, all of the subjects in the non-decoy group watched a ten-minute film presentation in which a "police officer" provided additional evidence about why the custodial worker was suspected to be the culprit responsible for the mugging. Half of the subjects had a "very handsome" police officer presenting the information, and the other half had an "unattractive" police officer presenting the same information. 85% of the subjects who watched the video with the handsome police officer either changed their answer to the custodial worker or confirmed that selection. 35% of the subjects who watched the video with the unattractive police officer changed their answer to the custodial worker. The elaboration likelihood model suggests that the discrepancy in the two groups is based on:

A) the peripheral route of information processing.
B) target characteristics.
C) message characteristics.
D) the central route of information processing.

4. What type of memory is used in a multiple-choice test, such as this one?

A) Recall
B) Recognition
C) Repressed
D) Déjà vu

5. What are the three main stages of memory, according to the information-processing perspective?

A) Encoding, storage, and retrieval
B) Recognition, detection, and regurgitation
C) Consolidation, reconsolidation, and recovery
D) Identification, encrypting, and reclamation

SOLUTIONS TO CHAPTER 9 FREESTANDING PRACTICE QUESTIONS

1. **B** Retroactive interference is a type of memory interference in which new information interferes with our ability to recall older material (choice B is correct). Proactive interference occurs when old information interferes with learning new material (choice A is wrong). Choices C and D refer to memory decay which occurs regardless of interference (choices C and D are wrong).

2. **A** Nondeclarative memory, or implicit memory, is a form of memory that is not conscious. It is the autopilot of memory (so it does not affect behavior consciously) and may be difficult to verbalize, making it measurable only indirectly (choice A is correct). Declarative memory, also referred to as explicit memory, involves long-term memories that can be consciously or intentionally called upon (choices B and D are wrong). Episodic memory is a type of declarative memory that is responsible for the recall of autobiographical events (choice C is wrong).

3. **D** Operant conditioning employs consequences to modify behavior. Reinforcement is more effective at modifying behavior than punishment is, but for both, the timing/schedule and intensity of the reinforcement or punishment is important. In general, delivering punishment consistently for every occurrence of the behavior produces more effective suppression of the behavior than does delivering punishment intermittently or inconsistently. Punishing the child only when the negative behavior happens to be noticed would not qualify as consistent and would thus not be very effective (choice D is correct). Immediacy, or delivering the punishment immediately after the act, will increase the effectiveness of the punishment, as will consistency (choice A would be more effective than D, and is therefore wrong). Positive reinforcement is generally more effective than punishment for increasing the frequency of a desired behavior (not writing on the walls) and diminishes the child's motivation to engage in the undesired response (choice B is more effective than D, and is therefore wrong). Finally, while severe punishment can have undesirable side effects, in general, the more intense the punishment, the more effective the punishment is in producing major, rapid, and long-lasting suppression (choice C is more effective than D, and is therefore wrong).

4. **B** Positive reinforcement (one type of operant conditioning) is accomplished when someone receives a reward after performing a task; after the person has performed the task and received the reward enough times, they will perform the task without the reward (choice B is correct). Vicarious reinforcement involves watching another person receive a reward for his or her behavior; there is no mention of Jay being motived by other people getting rewarded (choice A is wrong). An innate behavior is one that does not need to be conditioned, and therefore not what is being described in the question stem (choice C is wrong). Classical conditioning is accomplished by pairing two stimuli, one that is neutral with another that is unconditioned. Over time, the neutral stimulus becomes the conditioned stimulus. Since the question is not describing the pairing of two stimuli, nor is a stimulus presented before the behavior, classical conditioning does not explain the behavior described in the question stem (choice D is wrong).

5. **A** Retroactive interference occurs when new information interferes with the storage of information learned beforehand (choice A is correct). Proactive interference occurs when information that is learned first interferes with the ability to recall information learned subsequently; the opposite is described in this question (choice B is wrong). Retrieval cues are used to retrieve stored memories; there is no mention of retrieval cues in this question (choice C is wrong). Long-term potentiation is part of long-term memory storage; while a failure to remember information is partially a result of a failure to convert information

via long-term potentiation, it does not explain the interference of information learned after memorizing the steps to a physics problem (choice D is wrong).

6.   **B**   Item I is false: the subjects have no recall of the maze, meaning that their *declarative* memory (long-term, concerning specific facts, details, situations, and context) is not functioning properly; *procedural* memory, which concerns development of specific skills for how to do something, is biologically distinct from declarative memory, and must be functioning if they display improvement on the maze (choices A and C can be eliminated). Note that both remaining answer choices include Item II, so Item II must be true: episodic memory (part of declarative memory) includes memory of events that have been experienced personally. Amnesic patients with hippocampal damage may not have declarative memory for a skill they have recently learned (due to amnesia), and yet may be able to demonstrate the skill, indicating that implicit (procedural) memory exists, much like the patients described in the question stem. Item III is false: echoic memory, part of the short-term sensory memory system, is brief memory for sound. The question stem does not provide any information about the patients' ability to process or remember sound information (choice D can be eliminated, and choice B is correct).

7.   **A**   Procedural memory is related to actions, implicit memory is unconscious memory without conscious recall, and long-term memory is memory stored indefinitely. Each of these attributes applies to riding a bike (choice A is correct). Explicit memory is memory that involves conscious recall, which does not apply to riding a bike. Riding a bike is also part of long-term, not short-term or working memory (choice B is wrong). Prospective memory refers to remembering to perform planned actions (choice C is wrong). Mood-dependent memory refers to memories that are more easily accessed during the experience of similar moods and emotions. Source memory does not refer to a type of memory, but is a trap answer taken from "source monitoring error" (choice D is wrong).

8.   **D**   A mnemonic is a memory retention tool, and spaced repetition is known to reduce forgetting and allow for long-term retention (choice D is correct). Priming would be a memory aid, but would not help to memorize the steps independently of the presence of the aid. Proactive interference refers to forgetting and would reduce memory retention (choice A is wrong). Chunking would be a helpful tool, but serial position refers to the location of a word in a list and does not to refer to a memorization technique (choice B is wrong). Source-monitoring refers to knowing the source from which a memory came from and is not likely to help memorization of a series of complex steps. That is, knowing where one originally learned the steps does not address the problem of trying to memorize them (choice C is wrong).

SOLUTIONS TO CHAPTER 9 PRACTICE PASSAGE

1. **A** Based on the data presented in Table 1, one can reasonably conclude that the misinformation effect is present in the decoy group. The overwhelming majority of participants in that group positively identified the custodial worker as the mugger, most likely because his face was presented to them before the memory of the mugging could be fully encoded (choice A is correct). Although the non-decoy group chose the mugger at a higher rate than did the decoy group, this is not enough information to reasonably conclude that the non-decoy group has better memory (choice B is wrong). Forty-nine percent (37) of the subjects in the decoy group identified the custodial worker as the mugger, whereas only 17% (13) of the non-decoy subjects did so (choice C is wrong). Based on these findings, some conclusions can indeed be drawn from these data (choice D is wrong).

2. **B** Anterograde amnesia is defined as the inability to form new memories (choice B is correct). Retrograde amnesia is defined as the inability to retrieve information from one's past (choice A is wrong). Source amnesia is defined as the attribution of an event one has experienced, heard about, or imagined to the wrong source (choice C is wrong). Infantile amnesia is used to explain why individuals are typically unable to remember anything from before the age of 3; the human brain pathways are not yet fully developed enough to form memories at this age (choice D is wrong).

3. **A** The elaboration likelihood model theorizes that attitudes are formed by dual processes, via the central processing route or by the peripheral processing route. Since the subjects with the handsome police officer were far more likely to be persuaded that the photo of the custodial worker was the mugger, this suggests that both groups were focusing on characteristics of the person delivering the message (attractiveness). In the peripheral processing route, people are more likely to be persuaded by attractive messengers (choice A is correct). The central processing route involves focusing on the information of the message; in this scenario, the message was the same for both groups, so the central processing route does not explain the difference in outcome (choice D is wrong). Target characteristics describe the characteristics of the person receiving the message (motivation, interest); there is no information provided in the stem that would indicate that any characteristics of the two groups were responsible for the different outcome (choice B is wrong). Similarly, the message characteristics include specific features of the message itself (like length, logic, and evidence). Since the message was the same for the two groups, message characteristics do not explain the difference in outcomes (choice C is wrong).

4. **B** Multiple-choice tests rely most heavily on recognition memory; that is, test-takers do not have to generate the correct response, but rather have to recognize the correct response from several options (choice B is correct). On the flip side, a test that involved short-answer or essay questions would rely on recall memory, which requires individuals to retrieve previously learned information and repeat it in some context (choice A is wrong). Repressed memories are a phenomenon that is hotly debated in the legal and psychological fields, and would likely not come into play during a multiple-choice test (choice C is wrong). Déjà vu is the phenomenon in which cues from the current situation subconsciously trigger retrieval of an earlier experience, creating that "I've been here before" feeling. This phenomenon is not typically associated with testing (choice D is wrong).

5. **A** The three main stages of memory are encoding (receiving, processing, and combining information), storage (the creation of a permanent record of the encoded information), and retrieval (the recovery of the stored information in response to a particular cue or activity; choice A is correct). The other terms, while sometimes associated with the study of memory, are not part of the formal stages of memory (choices B, C, and D are wrong).

Chapter 10
Behavioral
Neuroscience

We now mostly take for granted that the brain is the primary seat of behavior, where our thoughts, feelings, reflections, and perceptions take place. However, it took many years for scientists and philosophers to arrive at this conclusion. Gradually, through work with patients who had suffered traumatic brain injury and strokes, it became clear to neurologists and psychologists that our brains contain regions that are largely responsible for specific functions. This lead to an effort to "map the brain" by compiling clinical data from lesions, using molecular techniques to study neural activity, and using brain imaging to determine functionality. These various methods show that the brain is more integrated and complex than anyone could previously have imagined, and different regions and networks play crucial roles in learning, memory, emotion, stress, and indeed, all behavior.

10.1 MEASUREMENT TOOLS FOR STUDYING THE BRAIN

Behavioral neuroscience is the area of psychology that looks for the neurophysiological correlates of behavior. This search can be broken down to two questions: "What parts of the brain are active during specific behaviors?" and "How do neurotransmitters and other chemicals affect behavior?" These two questions will remain central as we explore the way that the brain gives life to experiences we are all familiar with like fear, stress, happiness, confusion—in fact, there is probably no area of psychology that today does not fall within the purview of neuroscience and exploration of brain-behavior correlates. First, it is important to understand what tools researchers have at their disposal for exploring the brain. There are three general categories: molecular methods, brain lesions, and neuroimaging. Molecular methods are beyond the scope of the MCAT Psychology/Sociology section and some of these methods will be covered in Biology and Organic Chemistry. Let's take a closer look at the other two methods: the clinical study of brain lesions and neuroimaging.

Brain Lesions

A landmark case in the history of neuroscience was the case of Phineas Gage. In the 1800s, Phineas Gage, a 25-year-old railroad worker, suffered an accident in which a railroad tie blasted through his head, entering under his cheekbone and exiting through the top of his skull. Gage survived, but after the accident, he was described by friends and associates as "no longer himself," prone to impulsivity, unable to stick to plans, and seemingly unable to demonstrate empathy. People who knew him said he was like a completely different person. The accident had severely damaged his **prefrontal cortex,** an area of the brain that is now known to be involved in reflection, planning, emotional regulation, and **theory of mind**—the ability to understand the perspectives of others.

Phineas Gage Injury

The case of Phineas Gage was groundbreaking as it was a first step toward the discovery of the role of the prefrontal cortex in personality. Psychologists had also stumbled on an important methodology for mapping the brain: by observing the clinical changes in behavior that occurred after a lesion or accident, they could infer the role that the damaged area played in behavior and personality. The case study method (described in Chapter 3) has been critical to the study of behavioral neuroscience and discovering brain-behavior correlates. Throughout the 20th century, psychologists continued to study and document traumatic brain injuries such as Phineas Gage's as well as the effects of acute strokes. The rationale was simple: if damage to an area of the brain resulted in a change in behavior, then that area must be directly involved in, or part of a network of regions that is involved in, the functioning of that behavior.

Of course, this method had limitations because scientists could not conduct double-blind, randomized experimental studies (sign us up for the control group, please!) and researchers had to wait for a stroke or accident to occur, which could then only be studied one incident at a time. Later in the 20th century and continuing into the present, technological innovations have allowed neuroscientists to use various imaging techniques to study the brain in a more controlled fashion, and design studies—many of them experimental—to address specific hypotheses, rather than waiting for the data to come to them.

Neuroimaging Techniques

Neuroimaging techniques are either structural or functional. **Structural imaging** techniques provide a picture of the brain; they show anatomical regions and where they are located with respect to one another. They do not, however, offer any insight into which regions are active at any given time. For this, neuroscientists use **functional imaging** techniques, which demonstrate which parts of the brain are active, and to what extent, as experimental participants manifest a behavior. Let's look first at the two important types of structural techniques; Computerized Tomography (CT) and Magnetic Resonance Imaging (MRI).

Computerized Tomography (CT) scans, also known as CAT (computerized axial tomography) scans, use a computer to combine many cross-sectional (tomographic) images generated from the differential absorption of X-rays of an anatomical part, in this case the human brain, or a subsection of it. These differential absorptions are used to create a three-dimensional structural "snapshot" that appears as a series of cross-sectional images.

Magnetic Resonance Imaging (MRI) uses strong magnets which cause protons to align, spin, and generate a detectable radio-frequency signal that is measured by antennas close to the anatomy being examined. Regular MRI (in contrast to "functional" MRI, see below) provides only structural data, high quality "snapshots" that provide three-dimensional views of the target tissue. Structural MRI cannot be used to analyze the function of the brain across time.

When comparing CT scans and MRIs, advantages of CT scans include a very rapid acquisition of images of a large portion of the body, generally lower cost, more open and less noisy machinery, no requirement that subjects remain completely motionless, and no prohibition on implanted medical devices. For brain imaging, CT scans are preferred when speed is important, such as during a suspected stroke. Advantages of MRIs include higher resolution and therefore a more detailed image. MRI provides much more detail about soft tissues. Also, MRIs do not use X-rays, and do not include significant exposure to ionizing radiation, which make MRIs safer in most instances.

Figure 1   CT scan vs. MRI

The other important types of imaging techniques are functional: they provide insight into which brain regions are active during any given time. We'll look at four types of functional imaging: EEG, MEG, fMRI, and PET.

Electroencephalography (EEG) is a relatively noninvasive method of gathering functional information about brain activity. Electrodes are placed on the scalp to measure voltage fluctuations in the ionic currents of brain neurons. The resulting traces are known as electroencephalograms (EEGs), and each trace represents the net electrical signal of a large number of neurons. EEGs provide functional data about the brain's electrical neural oscillations (often referred to as "brain waves") that have extremely precise temporal resolution.

To prepare a subject for an EEG, a number of electrodes are placed on the subject's face and scalp, which allows the electrical potential of each electrode to be measured. Depending on a person's state of consciousness (awake, REM sleep, N1 sleep, N2 sleep, N3 sleep, etc.), the frequency, amplitude, and waveforms of the measured EEG traces differ. EEGs are useful in the diagnosis of seizures, sleep disorders, and other conditions that involve activity imbalances in certain parts of the brain.

Advantages of EEG compared to fMRI and PET (below) include less hardware bulk, lower hardware costs, relative tolerance of movement, much higher temporal resolution, non-aggravation of claustrophobia, and silence. However, disadvantages of EEG include far lower spatial resolution, poor measurement of neural activity that occurs below the cortex, poor signal-to-noise ratio, and significant additional preparation time.

EEG

Figure 2 EEG and results

Magnetoencephalography (MEG) is a functional neuroimaging technique for mapping brain activity that records the magnetic fields produced by the brain's electrical currents. MEG uses very sensitive magnetometers, typically using an array of SQUIDs (superconducting quantum interference devices).

MEG has more or less the same advantages and disadvantages as EEG compared to fMRI and PET. Compared to EEG, MEG has better spatial resolution of the brain activity it can detect, while EEG can detect activity in more areas of the brain. In addition, MEG requires expensive bulky machinery as well as a magnetically shielded room.

Functional magnetic resonance imaging (fMRI) uses a computer to combine a series of magnetic resonance images (see MRI, above) taken less than a second apart to provide a functional picture of how brain activity changes over time. fMRI can display changes in oxygen levels (which indicate blood flow) in various regions of the brain in real time and can be used to produce activation maps that indicate the areas of the brain involved in particular mental processes.

fMRI technology has several advantages over other methods of measuring brain structure (regular MRI) by providing evidence of real-time activity in the brain. fMRI is also considered safer than PET (below) because PET requires subjects to be injected with radioactive substances. The locational precision of fMRI data is more precise than PET and far more precise than EEG. fMRI is also generally more cost effective than PET. The major disadvantage of fMRI (as with MRI, above) is that the subject has to remain completely still in a noisy, cramped space while the imaging is performed. For example, it is not possible to query a subject to answer simple questions during the fMRI of the brain.

Positron emission tomography (PET) is a nuclear medicine imaging technique that produces a three-dimensional image of functional metabolic processes across time. PET scans require the subject to be injected with a positron-emitting radionuclide tracer, which is introduced into the body on a biologically active molecule, such as glucose. Three-dimensional images of the tracer concentration within the body are then constructed by computer analysis that allows the movement of, and changes in, the tracer concentration to be displayed in real time.

In modern PET-CT scanners, three-dimensional PET imaging is often augmented with a CT X-ray scan performed on the patient during the same session, in the same machine. This combination (as well as the less common PET/MRI combination) can provide a detailed structural image of the brain together with functional data. PET is a valuable technique for some diseases and disorders because it is possible to image specific radio-chemicals used for particular bodily functions. For example, if a patient is injected with a radioactive glucose analog, a PET scan can be used to image and then analyze the uptake of this specific glucose analog in the brain.

fMRI   PET scan

Figure 3   fMRI vs. PET

These are the primary methods of observing the brain itself. However, researchers are often also interested in understanding how the rest of the body is responding by measuring physiological markers that are associated with personality or behavior. For example, if a researcher were investigating the stress response, they would likely take data on electrical skin conductance, cortisol levels, heart rate, blood pressure, pupil dilation, etc. These indicators are also frequently used in behavioral neuroscience studies, especially research into stress and stress management, which we cover below.

10.2 BRAIN STRUCTURE AND NEUROTRANSMITTERS

Now that we have looked at some of the techniques neuroscientists use to study functionality in the brain, let's take a deeper look at what their work has revealed about the brain and behavior. We hope to understand not only what the anatomical parts of the brain are, but how those parts interact with one another to give rise to behavior. Then, we'll look more closely at the neurotransmitters in the brain and their functions as understood by neuroscientists.

Anatomical Organization of the Nervous System

The main anatomical division of the nervous system is between the **central nervous system (CNS)** and the **peripheral nervous system (PNS)**. The central nervous system is the brain and spinal cord. The peripheral nervous system includes all other axons, dendrites, and cell bodies. The great majority of neuronal cell bodies are found within the central nervous system. Sometimes they are bunched together to form structures called **nuclei** (not to be confused with the nucleic-acid-containing nuclei of cells). Somas located outside the central nervous system are found in bunches known as **ganglia**. In this section, we'll look at the anatomy of the central nervous system. The peripheral nervous system is covered in Chapter 12.

CNS Anatomical Organization

The CNS includes the **spinal cord** and the brain. The brain has three subdivisions: the **hindbrain,** the **midbrain**, and the **forebrain**. These four regions of the CNS (which will be discussed individually below) perform increasingly complex functions, with the forebrain considered the seat of complex behavior and planning. The entire CNS (brain and spinal cord) floats in **cerebrospinal fluid (CSF),** a clear liquid that serves various functions such as shock absorption and exchange of nutrients and waste with the CNS.

Figure 4 Medial cross-section of the brain

1) The spinal cord is connected to the brain and is protected by the CSF and the vertebral column. It is a pathway for information to and from the brain. Most sensory data is relayed to the brain for integration, but the spinal cord is also a site for information integration and processing. The spinal cord is responsible for simple spinal reflexes (like the muscle stretch reflex) and is also involved in primitive processes such as walking, urination, and sex organ function.

2) The hindbrain includes the medulla, the pons, and the cerebellum.
   - The **medulla** (or medulla oblongata) is located below the pons and is the area of the brain that connects to the spinal cord. It functions in relaying information between other areas of the brain, and regulates vital autonomic functions such as blood pressure and digestive functions (including vomiting). Also, the respiratory rhythmicity centers are found here.
   - The **pons** is located below the midbrain and above the medulla oblongata. It is the connection point between the brain stem and the cerebellum (see below). The pons controls some autonomic functions and coordinates movement; it plays a role in balance and antigravity posture.
   - The **cerebellum** (or "little brain") is located behind the pons and below the cerebral hemispheres. It is an integrating center where complex movements are coordinated. An instruction for movement from the forebrain must be sent to the cerebellum, where the billions of decisions necessary for smooth execution of the movement are made. Damage to the cerebellum results in poor hand-eye coordination and balance. Both the cerebellum and the pons receive information from the vestibular apparatus in the inner ear, which monitors acceleration and position relative to gravity.

3) The midbrain is a relay for visual and auditory information and contains much of the **reticular activating system** (RAS), which is responsible for arousal or wakefulness. Another term you should be familiar with is **brainstem**. Together, the medulla, pons, and midbrain constitute the brainstem, which contains important processing centers and relays information to and from the cerebellum and cerebrum.

4) The forebrain includes the **diencephalon** and the **telencephalon**.
   a) The diencephalon includes the thalamus and hypothalamus:
      - The thalamus is located near the middle of the brain below the cerebral hemispheres and above the midbrain. It contains relay and processing centers for sensory information.
      - The hypothalamus interacts directly with many parts of the brain. It contains centers for controlling emotions and autonomic functions, and has a major role in hormone production and release. It is the primary link between the nervous and the endocrine systems, and, by controlling the pituitary gland, it is the fundamental control center for the endocrine system (discussed later in this chapter).

   b) All parts of the CNS up to and including the diencephalon form a single symmetrical stalk, but the telencephalon consists of two separate cerebral hemispheres. Generally speaking, the areas of the left and right hemispheres have similar functions, with some exceptions. However, the left hemisphere primarily controls the motor functions of the right side of the body, and the right hemisphere controls those of the left side. Also, in most people, the left side of the brain is said to be dominant; it is generally responsible for speech. The right hemisphere is more involved in visual-spatial reasoning and music.

- The **cerebral hemispheres** are connected by a thick bundle of axons called the **corpus callosum**. A person with a cut corpus callosum has two independent cerebral cortices and to a certain extent two independent minds!
- The **cerebrum** is the largest region of the human brain and consists of the large, paired cerebral hemispheres. The hemispheres of the cerebrum consist of the **cerebral cortex** (an outer layer of gray matter) plus an inner core of white matter connecting the cortex to the diencephalon. The gray matter is composed of trillions of somas; the **white matter** is composed of myelinated axons (see Chapter 12 for information on somas, axons, and myelination). The cerebral hemispheres are responsible for conscious thought processes and intellectual functions. They also play a role in processing somatic sensory and motor information. The cerebral cortex is divided into four lobes, each of which is subdivided according to specific functions:

    i) The **frontal lobes** initiate all voluntary movement and are involved in complex reasoning skills and problem-solving.

    ii) The **parietal lobes** are involved in general sensations (such as touch, temperature, pressure, vibration, etc.) and in gustation (taste). The parietal lobes receive input from mechanoreceptors and proprioceptors.

    iii) The **temporal lobes** process auditory and olfactory sensation and are involved in short-term memory, language comprehension, and emotion.

    iv) The **occipital lobes** process visual sensation.

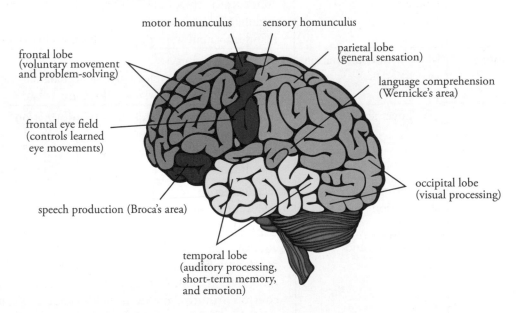

Figure 5 Principal areas of the cerebral cortex

Two other regions of the brain deserve mention:

- The **basal nuclei** (also called the "cerebral nuclei," and also sometimes referred to as the basal ganglia) are composed of gray matter and are located deep within the cerebral hemispheres. They include several functional subdivisions, but broadly function in voluntary motor control and procedural learning related to habits. The basal nuclei and cerebellum work together to process and coordinate movement initiated by the primary motor cortex; the basal nuclei are inhibitory (preventing excess movement), while the cerebellum is excitatory.

- The **limbic system** is located between the cerebrum and the diencephalon. It includes several substructures (such as the amygdala, the cingulate gyrus, and the hippocampus) and works closely with parts of the cerebrum, diencephalon, and midbrain. The limbic system is important for emotion and memory.

The information above describes the general functions of each region of the brain. Table 1, below, summarizes the brain functions and provides a little more specific detail for each region.

Table 1 Parts of the Brain

Structure	General Function	Specific Functions
Spinal cord	Simple reflexes	• controls simple stretch and tendon reflexes • controls primitive processes such as walking, urination, and sex organ function
Medulla	Involuntary functions	• controls autonomic processes such as blood pressure, blood flow, heart rate, respiratory rate, swallowing, vomiting • controls reflex reactions such as coughing or sneezing • relays sensory information to the cerebellum and the thalamus
Pons	Relay station and balance	• controls antigravity posture and balance • connects the spinal cord and medulla with upper regions of the brain • relays information to the cerebellum and thalamus
Cerebellum	Movement coordination	• integrating center • coordination of complex movement, balance and posture, muscle tone, spatial equilibrium
Midbrain	Eye movement	• integration of visual and auditory information • visual and auditory reflexes • wakefulness and consciousness • coordinates information on posture and muscle tone
Thalamus	Integrating center and relay station	• relay center for somatic (conscious) sensation • relays information between the spinal cord and the cerebral cortex
Hypothalamus	Homeostasis and behavior	• controls homeostatic functions (such as temperature regulation, fluid balance, appetite) through both neural and hormonal regulation • controls primitive emotions such as anger, rage, and sex drive • controls the pituitary gland
Basal nuclei	Movement	• regulate body movement and muscle tone • coordination of learned movement patterns • general pattern of rhythm movements (such as controlling the cycle of arm and leg movements when walking) • subconscious adjustments of conscious movements
Limbic system	Emotion, memory, and learning	• controls emotional states • links conscious and unconscious portions of the brain • helps with memory storage and retrieval

Structure	General Function	Specific Functions
Cerebral cortex	Perception, skeletal muscle movement, memory, attention, thought, language, and consciousness	• divided into four lobes (frontal, parietal, temporal, and occipital) with specialized subfunctions • conscious thought processes and planning, awareness, and sensation • perception and processing of the special senses (vision, hearing, smell, taste, touch) • intellectual function (intelligence, learning, reading, communication) • abstract thought and reasoning • memory storage and retrieval • initiation and coordination of voluntary movement • complex motor patterns • language (speech production and understanding) • personality
Corpus callosum	Connection	• connects the left and right cerebral hemispheres

The motor and sensory regions of the cortex are organized such that a very specific, small area of cortex controls a specific body part. A larger area is devoted to body parts which require more motor control or more sensation, such as facial muscles and fingers (Figure 6). For example, more cortex is devoted to the lips than to the entire leg. The body parts represented on the cortex can be sketched according to the body part controlled by each part of the cortex. When sketched out, this drawing looks like a distorted person, known as a **homunculus** (little man).

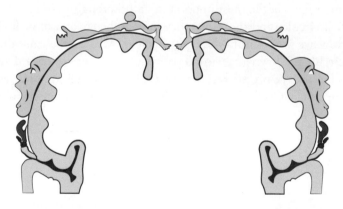

Figure 6 The sensory homunculus

Neurotransmitters

Neurotransmitters are chemicals released by neurons into synapses that affect the next neuron (or organ). They can generally can generally be divided into excitatory neurotransmitters, which increase the likelihood of the postsynaptic neuron firing, and inhibitory neurotransmitters, which decrease the likelihood of firing (for more detail on synaptic transmission, see Chapter 12). Although, be careful! The actual function of each neurotransmitter varies widely based on the part of the nervous system or part of the brain where it is active, and how it interacts with other neurotransmitters.

Table 2 Summary of Neurotransmitters

Neurotransmitter	Primary Functions
Dopamine	• Reward, mood, pleasure, smooth motor movements, focus and attention • Shortages can lead to depression, lethargy, and difficulty coordinating motion
Serotonin	• Mood, digestion, sleep, memory, sexual desire • Shortages can lead to aggression, compulsive behavior, overeating, and depression
Melatonin	• Circadian rhythm, sleepiness, sleep initiation (melatonin is technically a "neurotransmitter-like substance") • Shortages can lead to insomnia
Gamma Aminobutyric Acid (GABA)	• Primary inhibitory neurotransmitter in the brain • Shortages can lead to stress and anxiety, depression, ADHD, panic disorders, and a host of other disorders
Acetylcholine	• Excitation at neuromuscular junction, parasympathetic nervous system activity • Shortages can lead to dysfunction of the GI tract and paralysis
Epinephrine (adrenaline) and norepinephrine (noradrenaline)	• Two similar molecules both involved in fight-or-flight response, sympathetic nervous system activation (both are hormones and neurotransmitters) • Shortages can lead to fatigue, lack of focus, apathy
Glutamate	• Primary excitatory neurotransmitter the brain; learning, memory, long-term potentiation • Shortages can lead to fatigue, low concentration and energy

Dopamine and serotonin are two of the most important, and thoroughly studied, neurotransmitters in the brain. A summary of their circuits, and the effects they have on behavior, can be found in Figure 7 on the next page. Serotonin pathways project from the raphe nucleus, whereas there are three dopaminergic pathways: the **mesolimbic circuit** is known as a natural pathway for feelings of reward and pleasure (covered in more detail in addiction below), the **nigrostriatal circuit** is heavily involved in movement and coordination, and the **mesocortical circuit** is involved in higher cortical functions, thought, planning, and emotional regulation.

Figure 7   Dopamine and serotonin pathways in the brain

In addition to neurotransmitters, there are various hormones that impact behavior and produce psychological effects. Note that the primary difference between the two is that neurotransmitters are considered the signaling chemicals of the *nervous* system, and hormones are considered the signaling chemicals of the *endocrine* system, although there can be considerable overlap.

Table 3   Summary of Hormones

Hormone	Primary Functions
Cortisol	Stress, sympathetic nervous system response
Oxytocin	Trust, formation of social bonds, sexual reproduction, mother-infant bonding
Endorphins	Pleasure, arousal, pain suppression
Leptin	Regulation of energy, inhibition of hunger

Other differences between neurotransmitters and hormones can be seen in the table below:

Table 4   Neurotransmitters vs. Hormones

	Neurotransmitters	Hormones
Area of Operation	Synaptic cleft between neurons	Bloodstream
Produced by	Neurons	Endocrine glands
Activation Period	Extremely fast (a few milliseconds)	Can be longer (a few seconds to a few days)
Target Cells	Neighboring neurons or cells	Can be more distant cells throughout the body

10.3 NEUROSCIENCE OF EMOTION, MEMORY, STRESS, AND LANGUAGE

The Role of Biological Processes in Perceiving Emotion

Someone who openly expresses emotions is sometimes referred to as "wearing his heart on his sleeve." But while romantics tend to believe that emotion is purely a matter of the heart, it turns out that the brain is very much involved in emotional states. The generation and experience of emotions involve many brain regions. Mapping emotions to brain regions is difficult because thinking of different emotions as based in different parts of the brain has proven to be too simplistic. There is no "surprise center" in the brain. Rather, widespread areas of the brain appear to be associated with specific emotions. And instead of emotional "centers," there appear to be emotional "circuits" that involve many brain structures.

The Role of the Limbic System in Emotion

The limbic system is a collection of brain structures that lies on both sides of the thalamus; together, these structures appear to be primarily responsible for emotional experiences. The main structure involved in emotion in the limbic system is the **amygdala**, an almond-shaped structure deep within the brain. The amygdala serves as the conductor of the orchestra of our emotional experiences. It can communicate with the **hypothalamus**, a brain structure that controls the physiological aspects of emotion, such as sweating and a racing heart. It also communicates with the **prefrontal cortex**, located at the front of the brain, which controls approach and avoidance behaviors—the behavioral aspects of emotion (the prefrontal cortex is not, however, part of the limbic system). The amygdala plays a key role in the identification and expression of fear and aggression.

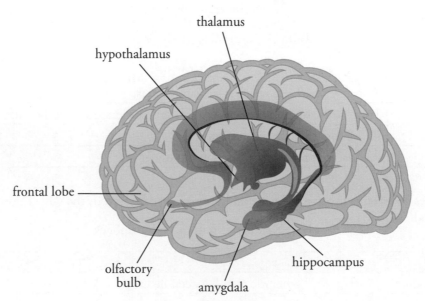

Figure 8 The limbic system

Emotion and the Autonomic Nervous System (ANS)

The **autonomic nervous system** is responsible for controlling the activities of most of the organs and glands, and controls arousal. It answers primarily to the hypothalamus. The sympathetic nervous system (SNS) provides the body with brief, intense, vigorous responses. It is often referred to as the "fight or flight" system because it prepares an individual for action. It increases heart rate, blood pressure, and blood sugar levels in preparation for action. It also directs the adrenal glands to release the stress hormones epinephrine and norepinephrine. The parasympathetic nervous system (PNS) provides signals to the internal organs during a calm resting state when no crisis is present. When activated, it leads to changes that allow for recovery and the conservation of energy, including an increase in digestion and the repair of body tissues.

Physiological Markers of Emotion (Signatures of Emotion)

Many physiological states associated with emotion have been discussed. These include heart rate, blood pressure, respiratory rate, sweating, and the release of stress hormones. An increase in these physiological functions is associated with the sympathetic (fight-or-flight) response. In order to measure autonomic function, clinicians can measure heart rate, finger temperature, skin conductance (sweating), and muscle activity. Keep in mind that different patterns tend to exist during different emotional states, but states such as fear and sexual arousal may display very similar patterns.

Emotions, Temperament, and Decision-Making

As mentioned earlier, the prefrontal cortex is critical for emotional experience, and is also important in temperament and decision-making. Increased activity in the prefrontal cortex is associated with a reduction in emotional feelings, especially fear and anxiety. It is the soft voice that calms down the amygdala when it is overly aroused. Methods of emotion regulation and stress relief often activate the prefrontal cortex. The prefrontal cortex also plays a role in **executive functions**—higher order thinking processes such as planning, organizing, inhibiting behavior, and decision-making. Damage to this area may lead to inappropriateness, impulsivity, and trouble with initiation. This area is not fully developed in humans until they reach their mid-twenties, explaining the sometimes erratic and emotionally-charged behavior of teenagers.

Another behavior that is connected to self-control and impulse regulation is addiction. **Addiction** has a strong biological basis. Many addictive drugs, as well as other pleasurable behaviors and primary reinforcers such as food or sex, share the characteristic of stimulating the release of dopamine in the nucleus accumbens. As such, the **nucleus accumbens** is often described as the primary center for reward in the brain, and dopamine is often thought of as the primary neurotransmitter in reward, although many other brain areas and chemicals also play a lesser role.

Other important cortical structures that have also been implicated in the experience of reward include the amygdala, a part of the limbic system that is involved in many different types of emotion, the insula, or insular cortex, which is closely connected to the striatum, and the lateral hypothalamus, which releases hormones such as endorphins that induce the physiological changes we often associate with pleasure and reward.

Emotion and Memory

Emotional experiences can be stored as memories that can be recalled by similar circumstances. The limbic system also includes the **hippocampus**, a brain structure that plays a key role in forming memories. When memories are formed, often the emotions that are associated with these memories are also encoded. Emotion can therefore aid and enhance memory and thus provides adaptive benefits. Take a second to

10.3

close your eyes and imagine someone whom you love very much. Notice the emotional state that arises with your memory of that person. Recalling an event can bring about the emotions associated with it. Note that this isn't always a pleasant experience. It has an important role in the suffering of patients who have experienced traumatic events. Similar circumstances to a traumatic event can lead to recall of the memory of the experience, referred to as "flashback." Sometimes this recall isn't even conscious; for example, for someone who was involved in a traumatic car accident, driving past the intersection where the incident occurred might cause increased muscle tension, heart rate, and respiratory rate.

However, memory also involves changes directly to the neural structures in the brain. Let's transition from our discussion of emotion to look more closely at memory and how it is stored within the brain by neurons and neural networks.

The Neuroscience of Memory

When something is learned, the synapses between neurons are strengthened and the process of **long-term potentiation** begins. Following brief periods of stimulation, neurons reorient themselves to increase the likelihood of firing within the connection, leading to an increase in the synaptic strength between two neurons and stronger electrochemical responses to a given stimulus. When long-term potentiation occurs, the neurons involved in the circuit develop an increased sensitivity, which results in increased potential for neural firing after a connection has been stimulated. This increased potential can last for hours or even weeks. Synaptic strength is thought to be the process by which memories are consolidated for long-term memory (so learning can occur). At a given synapse, long-term potentiation involves both presynaptic and postsynaptic neurons. For example, dopamine is one of the neurotransmitters involved in pleasurable or rewarding actions. In operant conditioning, reinforcement activates the limbic circuits that involve memory, learning, and emotions. Since reinforcement of a desired behavior is pleasurable, the circuits are strengthened as dopamine floods the system, making it more likely the behavior will be repeated.

After long-term potentiation has occurred, passing an electrical current through the brain doesn't disrupt the memory associations between the neurons involved, although other memories will be wiped out. For example, when a person receives a blow to the head resulting in a concussion, he or she loses memory for events shortly preceding the concussion. This is due to the fact that long-term potentiation has not had a chance to occur (and leave traces of memory connections), while old memories, which were already potentiated, remain.

Long-term memory storage involves more permanent changes to the brain, including structural and functional connections between neurons. For example, long-term memory storage includes new synaptic connections between neurons, permanent changes in pre- and postsynaptic membranes, and a permanent increase or decrease in neurotransmitter synthesis. Furthermore, visual imaging studies suggest that there is greater branching of dendrites in regions of the brain thought to be involved with memory storage. Other studies suggest that protein synthesis somehow influences memory formation; drugs that prevent protein synthesis appear to block long-term memory formation.

If our long-term memories contained isolated pockets of information without any organization, they might be more difficult to access. A person might have numerous memories for directions, people's faces, the definitions of tens of thousands of words, and other such content; with that much information, it could be nearly impossible to find anything. Just as hierarchies are a useful tool for processing information during the encoding process, it is believed that information is stored in long-term memory as an organized network. In this network exists individual ideas called **nodes**, which can be thought of like cities on a map. Connecting these nodes are **associations**, which are like roads connecting the cities. Not all roads are created equal; some are superhighways and some are dirt roads. For example, for a person living in a city, there may be a stronger association between the nodes "bird" and "pigeon" than between "bird" and "penguin." According to this model, the strength of an association in the network is related to how frequently and how deeply the connection is made. Processing material in different ways leads to the establishment of multiple connections. In this model, searching through memory is the process of starting at one node and traveling the connected roads until one arrives at the idea one is looking for. Retrieval of information improves if there are more and stronger connections to an idea. Because all memories are, in essence, neural connections, the road analogy provides a useful visual aid in understanding access to memories; strong neural connections are like better roads.

Like any neural connection, a node does not become activated until it receives input signals from its neighbors that are strong enough to reach a **response threshold**. The effect of input signals is cumulative: the response threshold is reached by the **summation** of input signals from multiple nodes. Stronger memories involve more neural connections in the form of more numerous dendrites, the stimulation of which can summate more quickly and powerfully to threshold. Once the response threshold is reached, the node "fires" and sends a stimulus to all of its neighbors, contributing to their activation. In this way, the activation of a few nodes can lead to a pattern of activation within the network that spreads onward. This process is known as **spreading activation**. It suggests that when trying to retrieve information, we start the search from one node. Then, we do not "choose" where to go next, but rather that activated node spreads its activation to other nodes around it to an extent related to the strength of association between that node and the others. This pattern continues, with well-established links carrying activation more efficiently than more obscure ones. The network approach helps explain why hints may be helpful. They serve to activate nodes that are closely connected to the node being sought after, which may therefore contribute to that node's activation. It also explains the relevance of contextual cues. If you are reading this book while jumping up and down on a trampoline, you are more likely to later recall this information if you are once again on the trampoline. This is because you would have developed some associations between the learned information and the cues in the environment when learning the information.

Not all behaviors are learned, of course. The neural processes described above occur when animals or people learn new behaviors, or change their behaviors based on experience (that is, environmental feedback). As our learned behaviors change, our synapses change too. On the other hand, some behaviors are **innate**. These are the things we know how to do instinctively (or our body just does without us consciously thinking about it), not because someone taught us to do them (for example, breathing or pulling away from a hot stove). Further, innate behaviors are always the same between members of the species, even for the ones performing them for the first time.

Neuroscientists have had a difficult time in their search for a physical basis for memory. There has been no central location found for memories, and there seem to be no such thing as special memory neurons. The process of forming memories involves electrical impulses sent through brain circuits. Somehow, these impulses leave permanent neural traces that are physical representations of information. More and more evidence indicates that what is important for memory and for learning is the synapses—those sites where nerve cells communicate with each other through neurotransmitters.

Neural Plasticity

It was once believed that after the brain develops in childhood, it remains fixed. However, scientists are finding that the brain is not a static organ. **Neural plasticity** refers to the malleability of the brain's pathways and synapses based on behavior, the environment, and neural processes. In fact, the brain undergoes changes throughout life. As you will see, changes in memory and learning are reflected physiologically by changes in the associations between neurons. Connections in the brain are constantly being removed and recreated. In fact, if someone sustains a brain injury, neurons will reorganize in an attempt to compensate for or work around the impaired connections. As an example, shortly after someone becomes blind, neurons that were devoted to vision take on different roles, potentially improving other sensory perception. Furthermore, while it was previously thought that neurons of the central nervous system were irreplaceable, **neurogenesis**, the birth of new neurons, has been found to occur to a small extent in the hippocampus and cerebellum. NMDA receptors (targets of the neurotransmitter glutamate) within the hippocampus are thought to play an important role in long-term potentiation and neural plasticity by inducing new connections, cell growth, and consolidation of new memories.

Memory and Learning

"What fires together, wires together." In other words, nearby neurons that fire impulses simultaneously form associations with one another. These associations can create neural nets, or patterns of activation, that represent information that is learned or stored in memory. Therefore, if any part of the neural net is activated, a memory may be recalled. This provides a neurological basis for the usefulness of retrieval cues discussed earlier. The process of learning and memory throughout the lifetime does not involve the enlarging of the brain or the gaining of neurons, but rather involves increased interconnectivity of the brain by increasing the synapses between existing neurons. As neurons fire together, more associations are formed. The strength of these associations is further based on the frequency with which simultaneous firing occurs, and other aspects such as the presence of emotion (which strengthens associations).

Neuroscience of Stress

In addition to the sympathetic fight-or-flight response, the hypothalamus, located just above the brain stem, releases corticotropin-releasing hormone (CRH), a messenger that stimulates the pituitary gland to release adrenocorticotropic hormone (ACTH). ACTH then signals the adrenal glands to release cortisol into the bloodstream. **Cortisol** is a glucocorticoid, a hormone that shifts the body from using sugar (glucose) as an energy source toward using fat as an energy source. This "glucose-sparing" effect keeps blood sugar levels high during stress situations (important because the only energy source the brain can use is glucose), thus ensuring that the brain will have enough fuel to stay active. This chain of events is a slower process than the near-instantaneous fight or flight response, and it is primarily triggered during long-term stress.

While short-term cortisol release can be helpful, prolonged release due to chronic stressors is harmful. Most notably, prolonged cortisol release inhibits the activity of white blood cells and other functions of the immune system. Thus, stress itself does not make us sick but rather increases the vulnerability for illness. It has been shown that stress can exacerbate the course of diseases including AIDS, cancer, and heart disease.

10.4 NEUROBIOLOGY OF NERVOUS SYSTEM DISORDERS

Schizophrenia

Recall that schizophrenia is a disorder characterized by positive symptoms, such as delusions and hallucinations, as well as negative ones, such as flat affect, disorganized speech, and avolition. Although schizophrenia presents as a thought disorder, it is important to remember that psychological characteristics have a physical or neurological basis; the division between these two is largely a conceptual one (based on an outdated **mind-body dualism** framework).

Additionally, *hypo*activation of the frontal lobes may be responsible for the negative signs of schizophrenia, creating a kind of pseudo-depression, flat affect, and impaired speech. Decreased working memory is also thought to be associated with decreased volume of the hippocampus. Individuals with schizophrenia have also been found to have smaller brains due to atrophy: schizophrenic individuals display increased ventricles (cavities in the brain), and enlarged sulci and fissures (less folding).

Further, the biochemical factor most associated with schizophrenia is excess levels of dopamine in the brain. The first drugs used for psychopathology, antipsychotics, were used to treat the positive symptoms of schizophrenia, such as hallucinations and delusions, by blocking the dopamine receptors, thus inhibiting the production of dopamine in the brain.

In addition to abnormal brain chemistry, abnormalities in brain structure may also play a role in schizophrenia. Enlarged brain ventricles are seen in some schizophrenics, indicating a deficit in the volume of brain tissue. There is also evidence of abnormally low activity in the frontal lobe, the area of the brain responsible for planning, reasoning, and decision-making. Some studies also suggest that abnormalities in the temporal lobes, hippocampus, and amygdala are connected to schizophrenia's positive symptoms. But despite the evidence of brain abnormalities, it is highly unlikely that schizophrenia is the result of any one problem in any one region of the brain.

Depression

Depression also appears to have a strong genetic basis—there is increased risk of developing depression when a first-degree family member has it. Depression has been linked to diminished functioning in pathways in the brain that involve the neurotransmitters dopamine, serotonin, and norepinephrine. Antidepressants thus target and try to stimulate these pathways. Depression can often accompany other neurological diseases, such as Parkinson's and traumatic brain injury, due to damage to similar or overlapping areas of the brain.

Stem Cell-based Therapy to Regenerate Neurons in the CNS

Cell death is a characteristic of most CNS disorders and neurodegenerative diseases. It has been theorized that neural stem cells, which have the capacity to differentiate into any of the cell types in the nervous system, hold the key to curing damage to the central nervous system caused by trauma or illness. Experiments have demonstrated that neural stem cells can migrate and replace dying neurons in the CNS. These studies hold promise for an eventual cure for diseases such as Parkinson's disease, Alzheimer's disease, multiple sclerosis, and Huntington's disease.

Chapter 10 Summary

- Neuroscientists use many different methods to understand how the brain is related to behavior and which brain regions are responsible for which functions.

- Structural imaging techniques give cross-sectional images of anatomical regions, whereas functional imaging provides insight into which brain regions are active during certain behaviors.

- Drug use causes increased dopamine activity in the nucleus accumbens, which can lead to drug addiction.

- The nervous system is divided into two parts: the central nervous system and the peripheral nervous system.

- The central nervous system is composed of the brain and spinal cord.

- Different brain regions, such as the thalamus, hippocampus, and amygdala, are responsible for specific functions.

- The central nervous system contains neurotransmitter systems that are important for modulating behavior.

- Important neurotransmitters are dopamine, serotonin, acetylcholine and others.

- The limbic system, made up of the amygdala, hippocampus, hypothalamus, thalamus, olfactory bulb, and frontal lobe, is known to play a critical role in emotion.

- The prefrontal cortex plays a critical role in executive functions such as long-term planning and emotional regulation.

- The hippocampus is critical in forming new memories.

- Physiological changes in neuron structure and neural network activation are associated with the formation of new memories.

- Spreading activation theory suggests that connections are made in memory with similar or related concepts.

- Stress has many important neurochemical implications, such as sympathetic nervous system activation and the release of cortisol, resulting in a fight-or-flight response.

- Nervous system disorders such as Alzheimer's, Parkinson's, depression, and schizophrenia are also correlated with neurophysiological changes.

CHAPTER 10 FREESTANDING PRACTICE QUESTIONS

1. Which imaging technique is best suited for measuring changes in brain activity that require the highest possible spatial resolution?

   A) Computerized tomography (CT)
   B. Positron emission tomography (PET)
   C) Electroencephalography (EEG)
   D) Functional magnetic resonance imaging (fMRI)

2. In an experiment, primates are injected with a newly synthesized chemical compound. Which of the following observed effects would provide the best evidence that this drug is a stimulant that is pharmacologically active in these primates?

   A) Increased alpha waves in the primates' brain
   B) Significant constriction of the primates' pupils
   C) Increased glucose metabolism in the primates' brains
   D) Increased absorption of norepinephrine agents inside neurons in the primates' brains

3. Which of the following structures of the human brain is LEAST likely to show increased activity when an extremely thirsty experimental participant drinks a glass of water?

   A) Reticular activating system
   B) Amygdala
   C) Hypothalamus
   D) Nucleus accumbens

4. A lesion in which of these areas is most likely to adversely affect an individual's vision?

   A) Occipital lobe
   B) Frontal lobe
   C) Hypothalamus
   D) Pons

5. Of the following, which neurotransmitter and hormone pair is most reliably associated with aggression?

   A) Serotonin and testosterone
   B) Glutamate and dopamine
   C) Melatonin and norepinephrine
   D) GABA and endorphins

6. Group A consists of socially anxious individuals sitting down to meet their peers on the first day of a new job. Group B consists of non-anxious individuals listening to white noise. In which of the following areas of the brain would we expect to see the largest difference in activity between these two groups?

   A) Cerebellum
   B) Thalamus
   C) Amygdala
   D) Basal ganglia

7. Each of the following has been demonstrated in the brains of schizophrenics EXCEPT:

   A) enlarged ventricles.
   B) smaller hippocampus.
   C) abnormal levels of acetylcholine.
   D) abnormal levels of dopamine.

8. Which part of the brain initiates signals to the endocrine system?

   A) Hippocampus
   B) Thalamus
   C) Prefrontal cortex
   D) Hypothalamus

CHAPTER 10 PRACTICE PASSAGE

Recent research has explored the neurophysiological correlates of various therapies to assess their efficacy. Reduced cortical mass in areas associated with negative emotions are interpreted as indications of effective therapeutic intervention. Also, researchers looked at the mass of various regions associated with emotional regulation, such that increased mass in these regions also suggested that the therapies had helped patients improve their ability to modulate emotional experience.

Study 1: Cognitive Behavioral Therapy

A team of researchers conducted an fMRI study that looked at activation levels in a cohort of 20 patients who were given a 10-week treatment protocol, meeting with a psychologist for 45 minutes in each session. During sessions, participants explored maladaptive thought patterns, and created a plan for more effective coping mechanisms that was encouraged by positive secondary reinforcement by the therapist at the next session. To track thoughts while subjects were alone during the week, participants were told to keep a journal. Pretest and posttest measures of cortical activity were measured and compared.

Study 2: Psychoanalytic Psychotherapy

Increase in cortical mass in areas associated with self-awareness and the top-down regulation of emotion was measured through the use of positron emission tomography (PET). At the end of the 3-month program, researchers saw changes in the mass of regions of the prefrontal cortex, amygdala, and hippocampal projections to the sensory cortices. Researchers conducted the study on 10 male and female participants who had grown up in single-parent homes, based on the premise that the absence of a parent made them good candidates for psychoanalytic therapy. Researchers hypothesized that awareness and analysis of repressed thoughts, and not emotional regulation, would mediate effectiveness of therapy and improved clinical outcomes.

Study 3: Behavioral Therapy

A reinforcement schedule was paired with aversion therapy, which was used to rewire the reward circuit in individuals with various types of addiction. 18 male and female undergraduate students who had been diagnosed with alcohol and drug addiction were given treatment. The treatment involved exposure to alcohol or the drug and nasal inhalation of an aversive agent meant to induce mild nausea. Application of the aversive treatment was potentially dangerous, so it was done in a supervised clinical environment twice a week according to a schedule. Researchers also checked in once a week at random

times to see if patients had successfully avoided drug or alcohol use, and gave points that could be used towards various prizes if they had. Afterwards, dopaminergic circuits and density of regions associated with impulse control were assessed.

1. Based on the information in the passage, and assuming validity of the research hypotheses, reductions in mass to which of the following regions would be evidence of the efficacy of a therapeutic intervention?

   A) Superior posterior frontal lobe
   B) Lateral hypothalamus
   C) Superior anterior parietal lobe
   D) Prefrontal cortex

2. Which of the following would be the most adequate substitute as a neuroimaging technique in the study on cognitive behavioral therapy?

   A) Magnetic resonance imaging (MRI)
   B) Positron emission tomography (PET)
   C) Electroencephalography (EEG)
   D) Magnetoencephalography (MEG)

3. Which of the following correctly describes the reinforcement schedule used in Study 3?

   A) Fixed interval
   B) Variable ratio
   C) Fixed ratio
   D) Variable interval

4. Data analysis revealed that of the three therapies, the psychoanalytic method was the least associated with growth of the prefrontal cortex. Which of the following is a potential problem with the conclusion that psychoanalysis was the least effective of the three therapies?

   A) The length of time of treatment
   B) Growth in the prefrontal cortex is evidence of reduced efficacy
   C) The neurophysiological exams used
   D) Study 2 did not include information on the reward circuit

5. If the hypothesis in Study 2 turned out to be correct, which of the following would most likely be the reason that the psychoanalytic psychotherapy had been effective?

A) Increased neural integration in the amygdala
B) Increased integration between the prefrontal cortex and limbic circuits
C) Increased rates of firing between hippocampal and primary sensory cortices
D) Increased volume of the prefrontal cortex

6. Suppose the subjects in Study 3 were presented with the addictive substances for which they received treatment. If the treatment was effective, one would expect measurements to show LESS cortical mass in each of the following, EXCEPT:

A) dopaminergic neurons in the basal ganglia.
B) dopaminergic neurons in the nucleus accumbens.
C) dopaminergic neurons in the ventral tegmental area.
D) serotonergic neurons in the amygdala.

SOLUTIONS TO CHAPTER 10 FREESTANDING PRACTICE QUESTIONS

1. **D** Imaging techniques that measure changes in brain activity require functional techniques, and CT scan is a structural technique (choice A is wrong). Although EEG has higher temporal resolution than the other imaging techniques, EEG has a very low spatial resolution compared to other functional techniques (choice C is wrong). Between fMRI and PET, fMRI is known to have the highest spatial resolution (choice D is correct). Although PET offers the advantage of measuring neuronal activity directly, the question stem is only concerned with spatial resolution (choice B is wrong).

2. **C** Pharmacological activity is best measured by the effect on neurotransmitters, which bind to receptors on the outside. Stimulants are known to increase blood metabolism; therefore, increased glucose metabolism would likely be measured (choice C is correct). Alpha waves are associated with a more relaxed state, which is unlikely to be induced by a stimulant (choice A is wrong). Also, stimulants are associated with pupil dilation, a sympathetic nervous system response, not pupil constriction, which is a parasympathetic response associated with depressants (choice B is wrong). Since pharmacological agents bind to receptors on the outside, internalization of the neurotransmitter is highly unlikely to occur. Rather, ions will be absorbed into the postsynaptic cell, not the neurotransmitter itself (choice D is wrong).

3. **A** Water is a primary reinforcer, and will therefore lead to activation of the reward circuit, especially in a participant who is extremely thirsty. Using the except/not/least technique, go through each answer choice one at a time. The reticular activating system is responsible for conscious awareness, not reward. Therefore, this structure is least likely to show increased activity and is the correct answer (choice A is correct). The amygdala, hypothalamus, and nucleus accumbens are all part of the brain's reward circuit (choices B, C, and D are wrong).

4. **A** The occipital lobe contains the primary visual cortex, and is the primary region for higher-order visual processing in the brain (choice A is correct). The frontal lobe is implicated in higher-level cortical functioning such as planning, attention, and emotional regulation. A lesion here would not be likely to affect vision (choice B is wrong). The hypothalamus' primary function is control of the endocrine system and hormone release, not visual processing or relay (choice C is wrong). The pons is associated with neurotransmitter synthesis and connectivity between the midbrain and hindbrain (choice D is wrong).

5. **A** Serotonin is a mood stabilizer, and depleted levels are known to be involved in aggressive behaviors. Testosterone is a hormone associated with aggressive behavior and fight-or-flight response (choice A is correct). Glutamate is an abundant neurotransmitter implicated in many behaviors, and some research shows associations with aggressive behavior, however, a relationship between dopamine and aggression has not been firmly established. In addition, glutamate and dopamine are neurotransmitters, so the answer choice does not include a hormone as indicated by the question stem (choice B is wrong). Norepinephrine is also known to be associated with sympathetic nervous system responses, such as fight or flight, however, melatonin release is associated with sleepiness and drowsiness, and decreases in melatonin would primarily result in sleeplessness and insomnia, not necessarily aggression (choice C is wrong). Increases in both GABA (usually inhibitory) and endorphins (pleasure and satisfaction) would have anti-aggressive effects, and low levels of neither is thought to be associated with aggression but primarily anxiety (GABA) and depression (endorphins) (choice D is wrong).

6. **C** The amygdala is associated primarily with negative emotions such as anxiety, so there would be a large difference in amygdala activity between anxious and relaxed groups of participants (choice C is correct). The cerebellum is primarily associated with movement (choice A is wrong), the thalamus is the brain's sensory relay station (choice B is wrong), and the basal ganglia are also associated with movement (choice D is wrong).

7. **C** Notice that this is an except/not/least question. Schizophrenia has not been associated with abnormal levels of acetylcholine (choice C is correct). It has, however, been associated with enlarged ventricles, a smaller hippocampus, and abnormal levels of dopamine (choices A, B, and D are wrong).

8. **D** The hypothalamus is the brain region most associated with control of the endocrine system (choice D is correct). The hippocampus is primarily associated with memory (choice A is wrong). The thalamus is primarily associated with sensory relay (choice B is wrong). The prefrontal cortex is primarily associated with executive control and emotional regulation (choice C is wrong).

SOLUTIONS TO CHAPTER 10 PRACTICE PASSAGE

1. **B** The passage states that reduction in mass in areas associated with negative emotionality would suggest that the therapy was effective. The lateral hypothalamus is part of the stress-release mechanism, leading to release of cortisol and other stress hormones, and is therefore known to be involved in negative primitive emotions such as anger and rage. Reduced mass in this area would make stressful or angry responses less likely (choice B is correct). The superior posterior frontal lobe is the location of the motor cortex and motor homunculus, responsible for motor control in the contralateral hemisphere (choice A is wrong). The superior anterior parietal lobe is the location of the sensory cortex and sensory homunculus, responsible for feeling and tactile awareness in the contralateral hemisphere (choice C is wrong). Increased activity in the prefrontal cortex is associated with improved emotional control and positive emotionality. Therefore, reduction in mass in this area would suggest that a given therapeutic intervention was not effective (choice D is wrong).

2. **B** The study on cognitive behavioral therapy used fMRI, and the description suggests that a functional technique with high resolution is needed to evaluate the hypotheses of the study. Of the answer choices, only PET is a functional imaging technique with high resolution (choice B is correct). MRI is a structural, not a functional technique, so it does not make a good substitute for fMRI as it would not produce functional data (choice A is wrong). EEG is a functional technique, but with low spatial resolution that would not let researchers draw conclusions about specific brain regions or areas deep in the cortex such as the limbic system (choice C is wrong). MEG is also a functional technique, but shares most of the benefits and limitations of EEG (choice D is wrong).

3. **D** For the reinforcement schedule of Study 3, the passage states that participants were contacted randomly and reinforced with tokens for successfully abstaining from drug or alcohol use. Because intervals of time are used, and not number of occurrences, this is an interval schedule (choices B and C are wrong). Because researchers contacted participants at random, and not fixed intervals, the reinforcement schedule is variable interval (choice D is correct, and choice A is wrong).

4. **A** Psychoanalytic psychotherapy is typically a long therapeutic intervention, requiring many months to many years to start to show results. Patients and therapists become part of a transference relationship in which patients will eventually transfer emotions associated with parents onto the therapist, and the therapist then works to bring these repressed feelings and behaviors further and further into conscious awareness. With such a lengthy process, three months may not have been enough time for patients to start to see results, so this would undermine the conclusion that psychoanalysis was not effective (choice A is correct). Growth in the prefrontal cortex is associated with increased emotional regulation, and therefore increased therapeutic effectiveness (choice B is wrong). The neurophysiological exams used are fMRI and PET, both functional exams with high spatial resolution. Although using the same type of exam would be preferable for points of comparison, both provide similar data about brain activity and would allow for valid comparisons and valid conclusions (choice C is wrong). The passage suggests that areas associated with negative emotionality and emotional regulation would be used to draw conclusions about therapeutic efficacy, and the reward circuit is associated with positive emotionality. Including it in Study 2, therefore, would not have provided much insight into the efficacy of therapy according to the research hypotheses (choice D is wrong).

5. **C** The study hypothesis states that awareness and analysis of repressed memories would be the determining factor of whether the therapy was effective. This suggests that integration of memory regions is the cause of improved outcomes. The hippocampus is involved in memory formation and transference into long-term memory, as well as memory recall processes in which long-term memory and short-term memory interact. Long-term memories are also believed to be stored in the area in which they are formed, so that the visual part of a long-term memory is stored in the occipital lobe, the auditory aspect is stored in the temporal lobe, etc. This indicates that integration between the hippocampus and these regions would lead to increased awareness of repressed memories, which the study hypothesizes improves therapeutic outcomes (choice C is correct). The amygdala is primarily associated with negative emotions, so increased integration there would suggest therapy was not effective (choice A is wrong). Increased integration between the prefrontal cortex and limbic circuits suggests improved emotional regulation, which the study hypothesizes is not the primary reason for improved outcomes (choice B is wrong). Increased volume of the prefrontal cortex would also suggest improved emotional regulation (choice D is wrong).

6. **A** This question constitutes an except/not/least question, so each answer choice should be evaluated one by one. If patients received treatment for addiction, you would expect less activation in the reward circuit in response to the addictive substance. Dopaminergic neurons in the basal ganglia are known to be primarily associated with movement, not reward. Therefore, it is not expected that there would be less cortical mass in this area. Therefore, choice A is a false statement and, in this case, the correct answer (choice A is correct). Dopaminergic neurons in the nucleus accumbens and ventral tegmental area are known to be associated with reward (choices B and C are wrong). The amygdala is also a part of the reward circuit, so although serotonin is not considered the primary neurotransmitter associated with reward and addiction, a decrease in cortical mass here would suggest that the substance was having less rewarding and addictive effects within the brain.

Chapter 11
Sensation, Perception, and Cognition

Organisms interact with their environments by taking in information (sensation) and deciding what information is important while filtering out the rest (attention), making complex decisions about that information (cognition), sometimes in a split-second, and reacting (behavior). Reacting includes a number of complex events, some conscious and some subconscious, some physical and some emotional. Humans are complex creatures, and emotion and stress play important roles in our interactions with the environment. Also, language is an important means for communicating with the environment for humans, and indeed, language is so important to what it means to be human, that it is difficult to imagine what "thinking" even means without language.

11.1 SENSATION

Types of Sensory Receptors

Sensory receptors are designed to detect one type of stimulus from either the interior of the body or the external environment. Each sensory receptor receives only one kind of information and transmits that information to sensory neurons, which can in turn convey it to the central nervous system. Sensory receptors that detect stimuli from the outside world are **exteroceptors** and receptors that respond to internal stimuli are **interoceptors**. A more important distinction between sensory receptors is based on the type of stimulus they detect. The types of sensory receptors are listed below.

1) **Mechanoreceptors** respond to mechanical disturbances. For example, **Pacinian corpuscles** are pressure sensors located deep in the skin. The Pacinian corpuscle is shaped like an onion. It is composed of concentric layers of specialized membranes. When the corpuscular membranes are distorted by firm pressure on the skin, the nerve ending becomes depolarized and the signal travels up the dendrite (note that these are graded potential changes—not action potentials). Another important mechanoreceptor is the **auditory hair cell**. This is a specialized cell found in the cochlea of the inner ear. It detects vibrations caused by sound waves. **Vestibular hair cells** are located within special organs called semicircular canals, also found in the inner ear. Their role is to detect acceleration and position relative to gravity. **Baroreceptors** are mechanoreceptors that respond to changes in pressure; these are commonly found in the walls of arteries.

2) **Chemoreceptors** respond to particular chemicals. For example, **olfactory receptors** detect airborne chemicals and allow us to smell things. Taste buds are **gustatory receptors**. Autonomic chemoreceptors in the walls of the carotid and aortic arteries respond to changes in arterial pH, PCO_2, and PO_2 levels.

3) **Nociceptors** are pain receptors. They are stimulated by tissue injury. Nociceptors are the simplest type of sensory receptor, generally consisting of a free nerve ending that detects chemical signs of tissue damage. (In that sense the nociceptor is a simple chemoreceptor.) Nociceptors may be somatic or autonomic. Autonomic pain receptors do not provide the conscious mind with clear pain information, but they frequently give a sensation of dull, aching pain. They may also create the illusion of pain on the skin when their nerves cross paths with somatic afferents from the skin. This phenomenon is known as **referred pain**.

4) **Thermoreceptors** are stimulated by changes in temperature. There are autonomic and somatic examples. Peripheral thermoreceptors fall into three categories: cold-sensitive, warm-sensitive, and thermal nociceptors, which detect painfully hot stimuli.

5) **Electromagnetic receptors** are stimulated by electromagnetic waves. In humans, the only examples are the rod and cone cells of the retina of the eye (also termed **photoreceptors**). In other animals, electroreceptors and magnetoreceptors are separate. For example, some fish can detect electric fields with electroreceptors, and magnetoreceptors allow animals to sense Earth's magnetic field, which can help them navigate during migration.

Encoding of Sensory Stimuli

All sensory receptors need to encode relevant information regarding the nature of the stimulus being detected. There are four properties that need to be communicated to the CNS:

1) Stimulus **modality** is the type of stimulus. As mentioned above, the CNS determines the stimulus modality based on which type of receptor is firing.

2) Stimulus **location** is communicated by the receptive field of the sensory receptor sending the signal. Localization of a stimulus can be improved by overlapping receptive fields of neighboring receptors. This works like a Venn diagram, and allows the brain to localize a stimulus activating neighboring receptors to the area in which their receptive fields overlap. Discrimination between two separate stimuli can be improved by lateral inhibition of neighboring receptors.

3) Stimulus **intensity** is coded by the frequency of action potentials. The dynamic range, or range of intensities that can be detected by sensory receptors, can be expanded by range fractionation—including multiple groups of receptors with limited ranges to detect a wider range overall. One example of this phenomenon is human cone cells responding to different but overlapping ranges of wavelengths to detect the full visual spectrum of light.

4) Stimulus **duration** may or may not be coded explicitly. *Tonic receptors* fire action potentials as long as the stimulus continues. However, these receptors are subject to adaptation, and the frequency of action potentials decreases as the stimulus continues at the same level (see below). *Phasic receptors* only fire action potentials when the stimulus begins and do not explicitly communicate the duration of the stimulus. These receptors are important for communicating changes in stimuli and essentially adapt immediately if a stimulus continues at the same level.

The ability to adapt to a stimulus is an important property of sensory receptors. This allows the brain to tune out unimportant information from the environment. **Adaptation** is a decrease in firing frequency when the intensity of a stimulus remains constant. For example, if you walk into a kitchen where someone is baking bread, the bread odor molecules stimulate your olfactory receptors to a great degree and you smell the bread baking. But if you remain in the kitchen for a few minutes, you stop smelling the bread; the continuous input to the olfactory receptors causes them to stop firing even though the odor molecules are still present. This is what allows us to "get used to" certain environments and situations, for example, cold pool water, loud background noise, etc. The receptors don't stop being able to respond; they can be retriggered if the stimulus intensity increases. For example, if you open up the oven door, you will smell the bread again. Likewise, if you are used to the background noise in a restaurant, but someone drops a plate, you'll hear it. In other words: the nervous system is programmed to respond to changing stimuli and not so much to constant stimuli, because for the most part, constant stimuli are not a threat, whereas changing stimuli might need to be addressed. (Note that nociceptors do not adapt under any circumstance. We can learn to ignore them, but pain is something that the nervous system wants us to do something about since it is an indication that something is wrong.)

Proprioceptors

This is a broad category including many different types of receptors. **Proprioception**[1] refers to awareness of self (that is, awareness of body position) and is closely related to your **kinesthetic sense** (your awareness of your body movement or "muscle memory," which is critical to learning and performing complex physical routines). An important example of a proprioceptor is the **muscle spindle**, a mechanoreceptor. This is a sensory organ specialized to detect muscle stretch. You are already familiar with it because it is the receptor that senses muscle stretch in the muscle stretch reflex. Other proprioceptors include **Golgi tendon organs**, which monitor tension in the tendons, and **joint capsule receptors**, which detect pressure, tension, and movement in the joints. By monitoring the activity of the musculoskeletal system, the proprioceptive component of the somatic sensory system allows us to know the positions of our body parts. This is most important during activity, when precise feedback is essential for coordinated motion. [What portion of the CNS would you expect to require input from proprioceptors?[2]]

Gustation and Olfaction

Taste and smell are senses that rely on chemoreceptors in the mouth and nasal passages. **Gustation** is taste, and **olfaction** is smell. Much of what is assumed to be taste is actually smell. (Try eating with a bad head cold.) In fact, taste receptors (known as **taste buds**) can only distinguish five flavors: sweet (glucose), salty (Na^+), bitter (basic), sour (acidic), and umami (amino acids and nucleotides). Each taste bud responds most strongly to one of these five stimuli. The taste bud is composed of a bunch of specialized epithelial cells, shaped roughly like an onion. In its center is a **taste pore**, with **taste hairs** that detect food chemicals. Information about taste is transmitted by cranial nerves to an area of the brain in the temporal lobe not far from where the brain receives olfactory information.

Olfaction is accomplished by olfactory receptors in the roof of the **nasopharynx** (nasal cavity). The receptors detect airborne chemicals that dissolve in the mucus covering the nasal membrane. Humans can distinguish thousands of different smells. Olfactory nerves project directly to the **olfactory bulbs** of the brain. The olfactory bulbs are located in the temporal lobe of the brain near the limbic system, an area important for memory and emotion (which may explain why certain smells can bring back vivid memories and feelings).

Interestingly, the perception of a smell as "good" or "bad" is entirely learned, based on experiences with those smells. There is no smell that is universally noxious to people (though the military has tried to find one in order to develop a "stink" bomb), because different smells can be associated with good or bad experiences based on culture and upbringing.

Pheromones are chemical signals that cause a social response in members of the same species. Though not well understood in humans, pheromones have been studied extensively in insects, particularly those species with complex social structures (such as bees and ants). Pheromones are an important means of communicating information; for example, alarm pheromones will alert the rest of the beehive of danger, food-trail pheromones allow ants to follow a trail to a promising food source, and sex pheromones play an important role in mating for most species. In humans, pheromones are much harder to study.

---

[1] *Proprio-* means *of or pertaining to the self*, as in "proprietary."

[2] The cerebellum, which is responsible for motor coordination.

Hearing and the Vestibular System

Structure of the Ear

The **auricle**, or **pinna**, and the external **auditory canal** comprise the **outer ear**. The **middle ear** is divided from the outer ear by the **tympanic membrane** or eardrum. The middle ear consists of the **ossicles**, three small bones called the **malleus** (hammer), the **incus** (anvil), and the **stapes** (stirrup). The stapes attaches to the **oval window**, a membrane that divides the middle and **inner ear**. Structures of the inner ear include the **cochlea**, the **semicircular canals**, the **utricle**, and the **saccule**. The semicircular canals together with the utricle and saccule are important to the sense of balance. The **round window** is a membrane-covered hole in the cochlea near the oval window. It releases excess pressure. The **Eustachian tube** (also known as the **auditory tube**) is a passageway from the back of the throat to the middle ear. It functions to equalize the pressure on both sides of the eardrum and is the cause of the "ear popping" one experiences at high altitudes or under water.

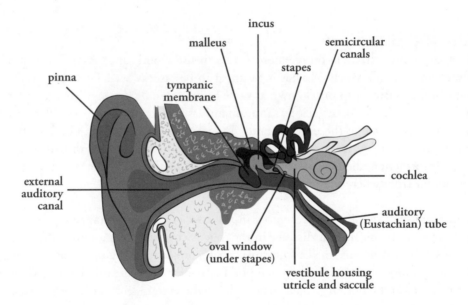

Figure 1 The ear

Mechanism of Hearing

Sound waves enter the external ear to pass into the auditory canal, causing the eardrum to vibrate. The malleus attached to the eardrum receives the vibrations, which are passed on to the incus and then to the stapes. The bones of the middle ear are arranged in such a way that they amplify sound vibrations passing through the middle ear. The stapes is the innermost of the three middle-ear bones, contacting the oval window. Vibration of the oval window creates pressure waves in the **perilymph** and **endolymph**, the fluids in the cochlea. Note that sound vibrations are first conveyed through air, next through bone, and then through liquid before being sensed. The pressure waves in the endolymph cause vibration of the **basilar membrane**, a thin membrane extending throughout the coiled length of the cochlea. The basilar membrane is covered with the auditory receptor cells known as **hair cells**. These cells have **cilia** (hairs) projecting from their apical (top) surfaces (opposite the basilar membrane). The hairs contact the **tectorial membrane** (tectorial means "roof"), and when the basilar membrane moves, the hairs are dragged across the tectorial membrane and they bend. This displacement opens ion channels in the hair cells, which results in neurotransmitter release. Dendrites from bipolar auditory afferent neurons are stimulated by hair cells, and tectorial membrane together are known as the **organ of Corti**. The outer ear and middle ear convey sound waves to the cochlea, and the organ of Corti in the cochlea is the primary site at which auditory stimuli are detected.

Summary: From Sound to Hearing sound waves → auricle → external auditory canal → tympanic membrane → malleus → incus → stapes → oval window → perilymph → endolymph → basilar membrane → auditory hair cells → tectorial membrane → neurotransmitters stimulate bipolar auditory neurons → brain → perception

Pitch (frequency) of sound is distinguished by which *regions* of the basilar membrane vibrate, stimulating different auditory neurons. The basilar membrane is thick and sturdy near the oval window and gradually becomes thin and floppy near the apex of the cochlea. Low frequency (long wavelength) sounds stimulate hair cells at the apex of the cochlear duct, farthest away from the oval window, while high-pitched sounds stimulate hair cells at the base of the cochlea, near the oval window. **Loudness** of sound is distinguished by the *amplitude* of vibration. Larger vibrations cause more frequent action potentials in auditory neurons.

Locating the source of sound is also an important adaptive function. Having two ears allows for stereophonic (or three-dimensional) hearing. The auditory system can determine the source of a sound based on the difference detected between the two ears. For example, if a horn blasts to your right, your right ear will receive the sound waves slightly sooner and slightly more intensely than your left ear. Sound stimuli are processed in the **auditory cortex**, located in the temporal lobe of the brain.

In humans, audition is highly adaptive. While we are able to hear a wide range of sounds, those sounds with frequencies within the range corresponding to the human voice are heard best, and we are able to differentiate variations among human voices. For example, when answering the phone, you will recognize your mom's voice within a fraction of a second.

- If a sensory neuron leading from the ear to the brain fires an action potential more rapidly, how will the brain perceive this change?
- In some cases of deafness, sound can still be detected by conduction of vibration through the skull to the cochlea. If the auditory nerve is severed, can sound still be detected by conductance through bone?
- If the bones of the middle ear are unable to move, would this impair the detection of sound by conductance through bone?

Equilibrium and Balance

The vestibular complex is made up of the **three semicircular canals**: the **utricle**, the **saccule**, and the **ampullae**. All are essentially tubes filled with endolymph; like the cochlea, they contain hair cells that detect motion. However, their function is not to detect sound, but rather rotational acceleration of the head. They are innervated by afferent neurons which send balance information to the pons, cerebellum, and other areas. The vestibular complex monitors both static equilibrium and linear acceleration, which contribute to your sense of balance.

Vision: Structure and Function

The eye is the structure designed to detect visual stimuli. The structures of the eye first form an image on the retina, which detects light and converts the stimuli into action potentials to send to the brain. Light enters the eye by passing through the **cornea**, the clear portion at the front of the eye. Light is bent or **refracted** as it passes through the cornea (which is highly curved and thus acts as a lens), since the refractive index of the cornea is higher than that of air. The cornea is continuous at its borders with the white of the eye, the **sclera**. Beneath the sclera is a layer called the **choroid**. It contains darkly-pigmented cells; this pigmentation absorbs excess light within the eye. Beneath the choroid is the **retina**, the surface upon which light is focused.

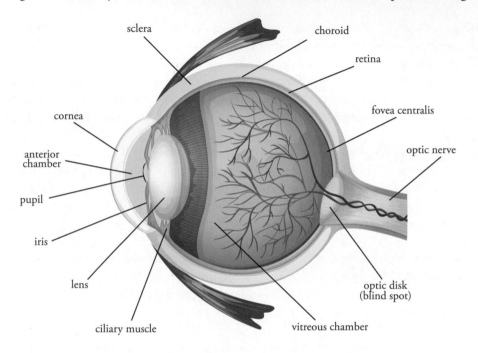

Figure 2   The eye

Just inside the cornea is the **anterior chamber** (front chamber), which contains a fluid termed **aqueous humor**. At the back of the anterior chamber is a membrane called the **iris** with an opening called the **pupil**. The iris is the colored part of the eye, and muscles in the iris regulate the diameter of the pupil. Just behind the iris is the **posterior chamber**, also containing aqueous humor. In the back part of the posterior chamber is the **lens**. Its role is to fine-tune the angle of incoming light, so that the beams are perfectly focused upon the retina. The curvature of the lens (and thus its refractive power) is varied by the **ciliary muscle**.

Light passes through the **vitreous chamber** en route from the lens to the retina. This chamber contains a thick, jelly-like fluid called **vitreous humor**. The retina is located at the back of the eye. It contains electromagnetic receptor cells (photoreceptors) known as **rods** and **cones** and which are responsible for detecting light. The rods and cones synapse with nerve cells called **bipolar cells**. In accordance with the name "bipolar," these cells have only one axon and one dendrite. The bipolar cells in turn synapse with **ganglion cells**, whose axons comprise the **optic nerve**, which travels from each eye toward the occipital lobe of the brain where complex analysis of a visual image occurs. In Figure 3, you may notice that light has to pass through two layers of neurons before it can reach the rods and cones. The neurons are fine enough to not significantly obstruct incoming rays.

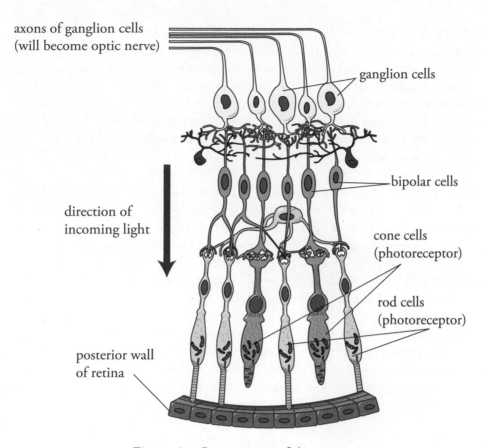

Figure 3 Organization of the retina

The point on the retina where many axons from ganglion cells converge to form the optic nerve is the **optic disk**. It is also known as the **blind spot** (Figure 4) because it contains no photoreceptors. Another special region of the retina is the **macula**. In the center of the macula is the **fovea centralis** (focal point), which contains only cones and is responsible for extreme visual acuity. When you stare directly at something, you focus its image on the fovea.

A ● ● B

Cover your left eye and focus your right eye on dot A while holding the page about 5 inches away from your face. Move the page forward and back. You will find that at a certain distance, dot B becomes invisible. You are placing dot A on the fovea by focusing on it, and at the correct distance, dot B becomes focused on the blind spot.

Figure 4 Demonstrating the blind spot

The Photoreceptors: Rods and Cones

Rods and cones, named because of their shapes, contain special pigment proteins that change their tertiary structure upon absorbing light. Each protein, called an opsin, is bound to one molecule and contains one molecule of **retinal**, which is derived from vitamin A. In the dark, when the rods and cones are resting, retinal has several *trans* double bonds and one cis double bond. In this conformation, retinal and its associated opsin keep a sodium channel open. The cell remains depolarized. Upon absorbing a photon of light, retinal is converted to the **all-trans form**. This triggers a series of reactions that ultimately closes the sodium channel, and the cell hyperpolarizes.

Rods and cones synapse on bipolar cells. Because of their depolarization in the dark, both types of photoreceptors release the neurotransmitter **glutamate** onto the bipolar cells, inhibiting them from firing. Upon the absorption of a photon of light and subsequent hyperpolarization, the photoreceptor stops releasing glutamate. Because glutamate has an inhibitory effect on the bipolar cells, when glutamate is no longer present, the bipolar cell can depolarize (removal of inhibition causes excitation in this system). This then causes depolarization of the ganglion cells and an action potential along the axon of the ganglion cell. All of the axons of the ganglion cells together make up the optic nerve to the brain.

Night vision is accomplished by the rods, which are more sensitive to dim light and motion, and are more concentrated in the periphery of the retina. Cones require abundant light and are responsible for color vision and high-acuity vision, and hence are more concentrated in the fovea. Color vision depends on the presence of three different types of cones. One is specialized to absorb blue light, one absorbs green, and one absorbs red. The brain perceives hues by integrating the relative input of these three basic stimuli.

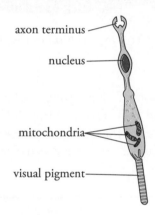

axon terminus

nucleus

mitochondria

visual pigment

Figure 5   Rod cell structure

Defects in Visual Acuity

Normal vision is termed **emmetropia**. Too much or too little curvature of the cornea or lens results in visual defects. Too much curvature causes light to be bent too much and to be focused in front of the retina. The result is **myopia**, or nearsightedness. Myopia can be corrected by a concave (diverging) lens, which will cause the light rays to diverge slightly before they reach the cornea. **Hyperopia**, farsightedness, results from the focusing of light behind the retina. Hyperopia can be corrected by a convex (converging) lens, which causes light rays to converge before reaching the cornea. **Presbyopia** is an inability to **accommodate** (focus). It results from loss of flexibility of the lens, which occurs with aging.

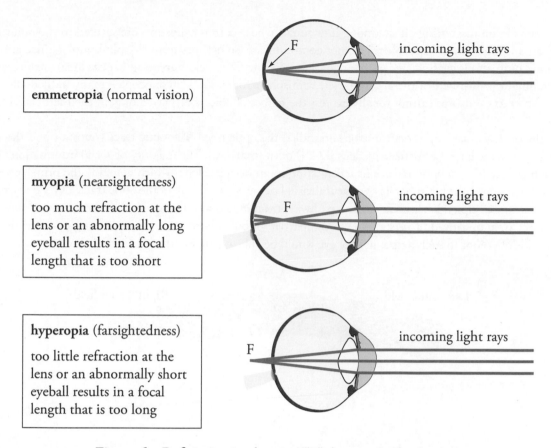

emmetropia (normal vision)

myopia (nearsightedness)

too much refraction at the lens or an abnormally long eyeball results in a focal length that is too short

hyperopia (farsightedness)

too little refraction at the lens or an abnormally short eyeball results in a focal length that is too long

Figure 6   Deficits in visual acuity ("F" denotes the focal point)

Primary Visual Pathways

The photoreceptors and other neuronal cells of the retina send varied types of information to the brain including the light intensity, colors, and spatial distribution of the information received. The neural signals initially processed by the retina travel via the axons of the ganglion cells and leave the posterior poles of the eyes as the optic nerves. The area where the axons exit the eye is called the optic disc. Since no receptors exist in this region, it is technically a blind spot. However, when both eyes are open, each eye's blind spot is filled in with neuronal information provided by the other eye.

At the point where the optic nerves unite, the optic chiasm is found. At the optic chiasm, fibers carrying information from the nasal half of each retina (the half of each retina nearer to the nose) cross over to the opposite side of the brain. Information from the nasal half of the retina of the left eye (the left eye's information about the left visual field) crosses over to the right side of the brain. Information from the nasal half of the retina of the right eye (the right eye's information about the right visual field) crosses over to the left side of the brain. Information from the temporal part of each eye (the half of each retina further from the nose) does not cross over at the optic chiasm. Thus, the left side of the brain receives all information about the right visual field of each eye, and the right side of the brain receives all information about the left visual field of each eye.

This results in an interesting effect among individuals whose corpus callosums are severed to the point that their left and right brain hemispheres cannot communicate (sometimes termed "split-brain"). Since areas of the brain most strongly associated with language processing (Wernicke's area and Broca's area) are located in the dominant hemisphere of the brain (the left hemisphere for about 97% of people), many individuals with severed corpus callosums cannot vocally express the names of objects displayed only in their left visual field.

After the optical chiasm, the optical axons are called the optic tract. The optic tract wraps around the midbrain to get to the lateral geniculate nucleus (LGN) of the thalamus. The majority of visual information flows through the LGN into optic radiations terminating in an occipital lobe, which contains the primary visual cortex. Each side of the brain has its own neural visual pathway consisting of the optic tract, LGN body, optic radiations, and occipital lobe. Each of these pathways contain neural information from both eyes. If the right optic tract were destroyed, a person would lose partial vision in both eyes, the right temporal and the left nasal fields of vision. In such a case, neither eye would be able to perceive the left field of vision.

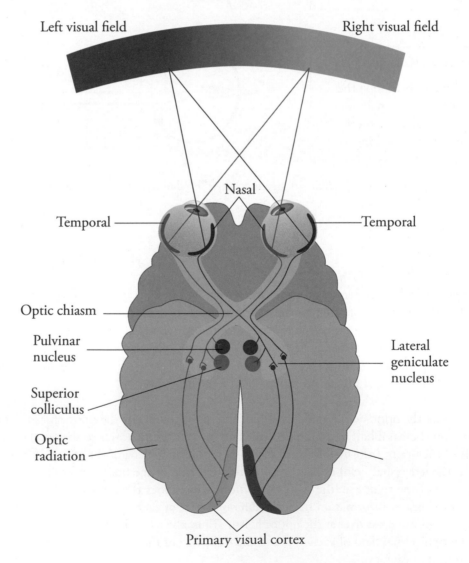

Figure 7   Visual pathways in the brain

Table 1   Summary of Sensory Modalities

Modality	Receptor	Receptor type	Organ	Stimulus
Vision	• rods and cones	• electromagnetic	• retina	• light
Hearing	• auditory hair cells	• mechanoreceptor	• organ of Corti	• vibration
Olfaction	• olfactory nerve endings	• chemoreceptor	• individual neurons	• airborne chemicals
Taste	• taste cells	• chemoreceptor	• taste bud	• food chemicals
Touch (a few examples)	• Pacinian corpuscules • free nerve endings • temperature receptors	• mechanoreceptor • nociceptor • thermoreceptor	• skin	• pressure • pain • temperature
Interoception (two examples)	• aortic arch baroreceptors • pH receptors	• baroreceptor • chemoreceptor	• aortic arch • aortic arch / medulla oblongata	• blood pressure • pH

11.2   PERCEPTION

Vision: Information Processing and Perception

For humans, vision is the primary sense; even if other information (such as sound or smell) counters visual information, we are more likely to "believe our eyes." The processing of visual information is extremely complex, and highly reliant on expectations and past experience. Neurons in the **visual cortex** fire in response to very specific information; feature-detecting neurons are specific neurons in the brain that fire in response to particular visual features, such as lines, edges, angles, and movement. This information is then passed along to other neurons that begin to assimilate these distinct features into more complex objects, and so on. Therefore, **feature-detection theory** explains why a certain area of the brain is activated when looking at a face, a different area is activated when looking at the letters on this page, etc. In order to process vast amounts of visual information quickly and effectively, our brain employs **parallel processing**, whereby many aspects of a visual stimulus (such as form, motion, color, and depth) are processed simultaneously instead of in a step-by-step or serial fashion. [Note: parallel processing is also employed for other stimuli as well.] The occipital lobe constructs a holistic image by integrating all of the separate elements of an object, in addition to accessing stored information. For example, the brain is simultaneously processing the individual features of an image, while also accessing stored information, to rapidly come to the conclusion that you are not only viewing a face, but you are specifically viewing your mom's face. All of this requires a tremendous amount of resources; in fact, the human brain dedicates approximately 30% of the cortex to processing visual information, while only 8% is devoted to processing touch information, and a mere 3% processes auditory information!

Depth perception is the ability to see objects in three dimensions despite the fact that images are imposed on the retina in only two dimensions. Depth perception allows us to judge distance, oftentimes with amazing accuracy. Experiments conducted on babies using something called a visual cliff demonstrate that depth perception appears to be largely innate. For these visual cliff experiments, babies were placed on a clear glass surface above a steep drop-off (Figure 8). The glass surface would allow the babies to safely crawl over the steep drop to their mothers, but most babies would not venture out over the visual cliff, indicating that their depth perception was developed enough to understand that the drop was dangerous.

Figure 8 Visual cliff experiments show depth perception in infants

Binocular cues and monocular cues are responsible for our ability to perceive depth and distance. **Binocular cues** are depth cues that depend on information received from both eyes and are most important for perceiving depth when objects are close to us in our visual field.

Retinal disparity is a binocular cue whereby the brain compares the images projected onto the two retinas in order to perceive distance. The greater the difference or disparity between the images on the two retinas, the shorter the distance to the observer. For example, suppose you are looking at a tree far in the distance, and hold your thumb about 18 inches in front of your face (feel free to try this!). When you focus on the tree far in the distance (or any object farther away than your thumb), your thumb appears to "double" (you see two sort of see-through versions of your thumb while you focus on the object farther from you). These two versions of your thumb are the two different images from the two retinas. If you move your thumb farther from your face (while still focusing past it), the two images of your thumb get closer together. If you move your thumb closer to your face, the two images get farther apart. Now focus on your thumb. Your brain is still receiving two disparate representations of your thumb, but now it converges these two representations into one, and also provides information about how far your thumb is from your face. This is how retinal disparity works. Farther images have less disparity (the images from the two retinas are more similar, indicating to your brain that the object is farther away), while closer images have more disparity, indicating to your brain that they are closer to your face.

Convergence is another binocular cue that describes the extent to which the eyes turn inward when looking at an object; the greater the angle of convergence or inward strain, the closer the object. In other words, if you hold your thumb right in front of your nose, your eyes have to turn inward a great deal to focus on your thumb (this is known as going "cross-eyed"), which signals to your brain that the object you are focusing on is quite close.

Figure 9   Retinal disparity helps us to determine distance

Monocular cues are depth cues that depend on information that is available to either eye alone and are important for judging distances of objects that are far from us, since the retinal disparity is only slight. Since we cannot rely on binocular cues for objects at farther distances, we rely on any combination of the following monocular cues:

- **Relative Size**: If objects are assumed to be the same size, the one that casts the smaller image on the retina appears more distant. For example, in Figure 10, our brains assume the elk in the foreground are roughly the same size as those in the background; therefore, since some of the elk are perceived by our retinas as smaller, those that are smaller are perceived as farther away than those elk that are perceived by our retinas as larger.
- **Interposition**: If one object blocks the view of another, we perceive it as closer. In Figure 10, the horns of the elk in the foreground partially obscure the elk in the immediate background (and the elk in the immediate background is partially obscuring elk in the more distant background and so on); therefore, the elk that are partially blocking the view of other elk are perceived by our brains as closer.
- **Relative Clarity**: We perceive hazy objects as being more distant than sharp, clear objects. In Figure 10, the elk in the far background are fuzzier and less sharp than the elk in the foreground; therefore, we perceive the sharper elk as closer and the fuzzier elk as farther away.

Figure 10

- **Texture Gradient**: Change from a coarse, distinct texture to a fine, indistinct texture indicates increasing distance. In Figure 11, the poppies in the foreground appear as distinct flowers, but those in the background begin to sort of blend in together until it looks like a continuous stretch of red. The distinct poppies are perceived as closer and the indistinct poppies that all blend into a stretch of red are perceived as farther away.
- **Relative Height**: We perceive objects that are higher in the visual field as farther away. In Figure 11, the red area of poppies higher in the visual field (and on the hill) are perceived as farther away than the poppies at the bottom of the visual field.

Figure 11

- **Relative Motion**: As we move, stable objects appear to move as well. Objects that are near to us appear to move faster than objects that are farther away. This is easily demonstrated whenever you are in a car or train—the farther away something is on the horizon, the slower it moves past you, while nearby objects fly past. This difference in motion cues our brains that the objects moving quickly by are close, while those moving by more slowly are farther away.
- **Linear Perspective**: Parallel lines appear to converge as distance increases. The greater the convergence, the greater the perceived distance. This is seen in Figure 12, where the parallel lines of the rail tracks appear to get closer together, which signals our brains that as the lines converge, the distance increases.

- **Light and Shadow**: Closer objects reflect more light than do distant objects. The dimmer of two identical objects will seem farther away. In Figure 12, the closer rail tracks are brighter than the more distant tracks, signaling our brains that the brighter tracks are closer, while the dimmer tracks are farther away.

Figure 12

Absolute Thresholds

We are very sensitive to certain types of stimuli. The minimum stimulus intensity required to activate a sensory receptor 50% of the time (and thus detect the sensation) is called the **absolute threshold**. In other words, for each special sense, the 50% recognition point defines the absolute threshold. (Note that this threshold can vary among individuals and different organisms—the absolute smell threshold for a human and a dog differs greatly.) Absolute thresholds also vary with age. For example, as we age, we gradually lose our ability to detect higher-pitched sounds. [What is the anatomical reason for this?[3]]

---

[3] Loud sounds can mechanically harm the hair cells, causing them to die. When this occurs, the hair cell can no longer send sound signals to the brain. In people, once a hair cell dies, it will never regrow. The hair cells that detect higher frequency sounds are the smallest and the most easily damaged; therefore, as people age and more hair cells are damaged and lost, hearing loss occurs. Since the smallest hair cells are the ones most likely lost, loss of sensitivity to high-pitched sounds is common in older people.

Difference Thresholds

Absolute thresholds are important for detecting the presence or absence of stimuli, but the ability to determine the change or difference in stimuli is also vital. The **difference threshold** (also called the *just noticeable difference*, or JND) is the minimum noticeable difference between any two sensory stimuli, 50% of the time. The magnitude of the initial stimulus influences the difference threshold; for example, if you lift a one-pound weight and a two-pound weight, the difference will be obvious, but if you lift a 100-pound weight and 101-pound weight, you probably won't be able to tell the difference. Indeed, **Weber's law** dictates that two stimuli must differ by a constant *proportion* in order for their difference to be perceptible. Interestingly, the exact proportion varies by stimulus; but for humans, two objects must differ in weight by 2% [in the weight example above, what is the minimum weight needed to detect a difference between it and the 100-pound weight?[4]], two lights must differ in intensity by 8%, and two tones must differ in frequency by 0.3%.

Signal Detection Theory

Detecting sensory stimuli not only depends on the information itself, but also on our psychological state, including alertness, expectation, motivation, and prior experience. **Signal detection theory** attempts to predict how and when someone will detect the presence of a given sensory stimulus (the "signal") amidst all of the other sensory stimuli in the background (considered the "noise"). There are four possible outcomes: a hit (the signal is present and was detected), a miss (the signal was present but not detected), a false alarm (the signal was not present but the person thought it was), and a correct rejection (the signal was not present and the person did not think it was). Signal detection can have important life-or-death consequences—imagine how crucial it is for doctors to be able to detect the signal (perhaps a tumor on a CT scan) from the noise.

Gestalt Psychology

Gestalt is the German word for "form" or "shape," and has come to mean, in English, an organized whole perceived as more than the sum of its individual parts. Therefore, in psychology, gestalt refers to the idea that the whole exceeds the sum of its parts; in other words, when humans perceive an object, rather than seeing lines, angles, colors, and shadows, they perceive the whole—a face or a table or a dog. Importantly, gestalt does not explain *how* the brain is able to perceive in such a way, merely that it does. There are many different gestalt principles to explain perceptual organization; below the most common are covered. (Note that gestalt principles can be applied to any sensory modality, but they are most often described using visual perception examples, as we have here).

Emergence. Look at the image in Figure 13. This is essentially a series of black irregular shapes on a white background. Those are the individual *parts* of the image. However, the whole that our brain perceives is a dog. You did not recognize the dog by first identifying its parts and constructing the whole ("there is the nose, there is the collar, there is a leg, this must be a dog!"), rather, the dog appears as a whole, all at once—it sort of pops out at you. This is an example of the gestalt principle of emergence. According to this gestalt principle, when attempting to identify an object, we first identify its outline, which then allows us to figure out what the object is. Only after the whole emerges do we start to identify the parts that make up the whole, such as the dog's face, legs, or the chain attached to his collar in Figure 13.

---

[4] 102 pounds, which is 2% heavier than 100 pounds.

Figure 13

Figure 14

Multistability. The image in Figure 14 is also a great example of the gestalt principle of multistability or multistable perception, which is the tendency for ambiguous images to pop back and forth unstably between alternative interpretations in our brains. Other examples include the images of two impossible objects in Figure 15. Again, gestalt does not explain *how* images appear multistable, only that they *do*.

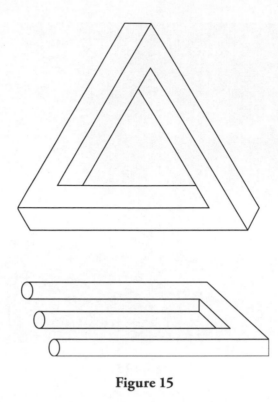

Figure 15

Gestalt Laws of Grouping. There are also several gestalt grouping laws meant to help explain how we tend to perceive things. While there are more than five laws, the five most common are discussed here. The **law of proximity** suggests that things that are near one another seem to be grouped together. Nearby objects tend to be perceived as a unit or group (see A in Figure 16: do you perceive 25 individual dots, or a square composed of dots? The law of proximity predicts that you perceive a square composed of dots). The law of similarity suggests that things that are similar tend to appear grouped together. In other words, we tend to perceive similar items as a unit or group (see B in Figure 16 below: what do you see? According to the law of similarity, you are likely to perceive the columns as important, and will perceive columns composed of circles and squares). The **law of continuity** (also known as the law of good continuation) suggests that we perceive smooth, continuous lines and forms, rather than disjointed ones. For example, in Figure 16, the law of continuity predicts that we will perceive the image in C as two overlapping circles, rather than two black semicircular lines and a red football shape in the middle. Even though the lines are different colors, we still tend to perceive the lines as continuous, forming two circles. The gestalt **law of closure** predicts that we will perceive things as complete logical entities, because our brains will fill in the gaps in the information. For example, what do you see in D in Figure 16? The law of closure predicts that you will perceive a triangle! The **gestalt law of common fate** predicts that objects moving in the same direction, or moving in synchrony, are perceived as a group or unit. This applies to things like a group of dancers moving in unison or a flock of birds all moving together (like E in Figure 16). The gestalt **law of connectedness** predicts that things that are joined or linked or grouped are perceived as connected. In Figure 16, F shows the same set of circles in the shape of a square as in A, but the box around some of those circles connects them in our brains. The law of connectedness predicts that we are likely to perceive those nine circles as connected and differentiated from the rest.

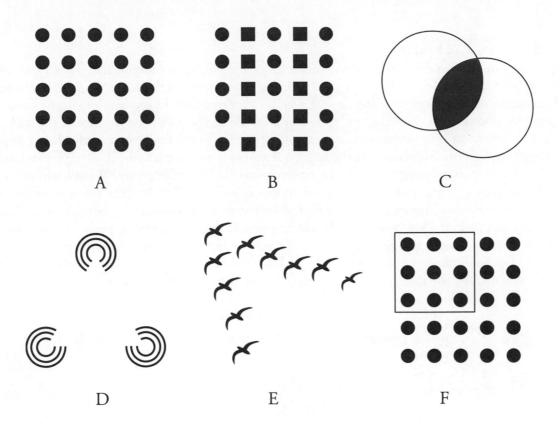

Figure 16

If a lot of these gestalt principles and laws seem similar to you, it is because there is a fair amount of over-lap (it doesn't help that they are described as either principles or laws by different sources, called by mul-tiple different names, and exemplified by many of the same images.). Therefore, familiarize yourself with the basic principles here and try not to get too wrapped up in differentiating between each individual law or principle—our visual perception is the result of many of these principles or laws working simultane-ously!

Perceptual Processing

Bottom-up processing begins with the sensory receptors and works up to the complex integration of information occurring in the brain. Bottom-up processing is also known as data-driven processing; information enters the eyes in one direction (this sensory input is the "bottom"), and is then turned into an identifiable image by the brain (this final image is the "top"). We tend to use more of a bottom-up approach when we have no or little prior experience with a stimulus. **Top-down processing** occurs when the brain applies experience and expectations to interpret sensory information. Instead of focusing on the sensory input (the "bottom"), we can use our prior experience and knowledge to impose our expectations on the stimulus, which tends to occur with stimuli with which we are more familiar. Note that the brain in fact uses a combination of the two: information is received in a bottom-up fashion from sensory receptors, while the brain is superimposing assumptions in a top-down manner.

11.3   ATTENTION

Imagine the attention to detail necessary to perform a complicated procedure such as a heart transplant. These details may include the tools being utilized, the various monitors, the incision site, the support staff, the status of the patient, etc. There might also be countless other things that the surgeon could pay attention to...the trim on the walls, the numbers on the clock, the glasses on the face of the nurse...in fact, if the surgeon *did* pay attention to these things, he or she would find it more difficult to complete the surgery successfully. How is it that the surgeon is able to avoid distractions, choosing instead to pay attention to only particular inputs out of the many available in the environment? What limits people in general from paying attention to all objects and entities at once? Further, imagine that the surgeon was chewing gum while performing the surgery (not recommended!). This would likely not have an impact on the surgeon's performance; however, if the surgeon were giving a speech while performing the surgery (definitely not recommended!), the surgeon's performance would likely be impaired. All of the above are examples of different aspects of attention. Let's look at two unique components of attention—selective attention and divided attention—and the models that have been used to explain each.

Figure 17   Broadbent Filter Model of Selective Attention

Selective Attention

Selective attention is the process by which one input is attended to and the rest are tuned out. This is necessary because we do not have the capacity to pay attention to everything in our environments. A resource model suggests that we only have a limited capacity to pay attention and so must devote our resources carefully.

One way that selective attention has been studied is using a dichotic listening setup. A person wears headphones and each ear hears a different dialogue. The individual is instructed to listen to information coming into one ear, called the **attended channel**, and to ignore input to the other ear, the **unattended channel**. When people do this, they are able to remember some of the message from the attended ear but lose almost everything from the unattended ear. The same observation has been made with visual stimuli; when people are told to focus on one visual aspect, they may miss other visual details.

Donald Broadbent thought of the brain as a processing system with a limited capacity and sought to map out the steps that went into creating memories from raw sensory data. He developed the **Broadbent Filter Model of Selective Attention** (Figure 17). In this model, inputs from the environment first enter a sensory buffer. One of these inputs is then selected and filtered based on physical characteristics of the input (e.g., sensory modality). This theoretical filter is designed to keep us from becoming overloaded and overwhelmed with information. Other sensory information stays in the sensory buffer briefly, but then quickly decays. At this point in the process, the information is still raw data that has just been filtered—it has not yet been transformed. It is in the next step, when the information enters short-term memory storage, where semantic (meaning-making) processes occur.

In the dichotic listening task described above, only information from the attended ear is allowed to pass through the filter. If an input in the sensory buffer does not go through the filter, the theory proposes that it remains briefly but then quickly decays and disappears.

To make matters more complicated, it seems that some unattended inputs are still detected. Imagine you are in a conversation with someone at a party in a room full of people. You are not aware of the content of any of the other conversations until suddenly you hear the name of your best friend mentioned in a conversation behind you. This phenomenon is known as the **cocktail party effect**. It happens when information of personal importance from previously unattended channels catches our attention. This observation cannot be well accounted for by the filter model of attention. Later adaptations of the original model have thus suggested that information from the unattended ear is not completely filtered out, but rather dampened, like turning the volume down on a television. Information from the unattended ear can still be processed at some level.

Anne Treisman's Attenuation Model tried to account for the cocktail party effect. Treisman believed that rather than a filter, the mind has an attenuator, which works like a volume knob—it "turns down" the unattended sensory input, rather than eliminating it.

Figure 18 Treisman Attenuation Model of Selective Attention

The cocktail party effect has also been explained through the concept of **selective priming**. This idea suggests that people can be selectively primed to observe something, either by encountering it frequently or by having an expectation. If one is primed to observe something, one is more likely to notice it when it occurs. Over the course of our lifetimes, we have frequently encountered our own names and the names of our friends and are thus primed to hear them. The more something is primed, the more it will be picked up despite distractions. Researchers have also studied priming by providing people with stimuli, sometimes subliminally, and testing whether these stimuli have an impact on later performance.

For example, if asked to read a list of words including the word "lettuce" before embarking on a word completion task, subjects are more likely to complete "LET____" with T-U-C-E to make the word "lettuce" than people who were not initially primed with the list of words. Even if people are not conscious of remembering the stimuli, it can still have an impact on later performance.

Visual attention has often been explained via a **spotlight model**. In this model, the spotlight is a beam that can shine anywhere within an individual's visual field. It is important to note that this beam describes the movement of attention, not the movement of the eyes. Shifts in attention actually precede the

11.3

corresponding eye movements. The shifting of attention requires us to unlock the beam from its current target, move the focus, and lock onto a new target.

Information from visual perception is processed in the brain by feature detectors that examine the different aspects of an object, such as color, shape, orientation, etc. One problem with visual processing is called the **binding problem**—the problem of how all these different aspects are assembled together and related to a single object, rather than something else in the visual field. Visual attention is the solution to this problem. If our visual attention is on a particular object such as a cup, then the feature detectors' input of shape, color, etc. will all be related to the object being attended to—the cup. It has been found that when people are distracted while viewing two items, they may have issues with binding; for example, the color of one item may be attributed to the other.

Divided Attention

Divided attention concerns when and if we are able to perform multiple tasks simultaneously. It turns out that this depends on the characteristics of the activities one is trying to multitask. The **resource model of attention** says that we have a limited pool of resources on which to draw when performing tasks, both modality-specific resources and general resources. In general, if the resources required to perform multiple tasks simultaneously exceed the available resources to do so, then the tasks cannot be accomplished at the same time. Three factors are associated with performance on multi-tasking: task similarity, task difficulty, and task practice.

Imagine listening to a talk radio program while trying to write a paper. It is likely that these two activities would be very difficult to pay attention to at the same time. They would interfere with each other because of their task similarity, in this case, the use of the same modality for processing. One activity requires verbal input, while the other requires verbal output. However, if instead you were listening to classical music, you might be able to write a paper at the same time because you would be doing two dissimilar tasks; one requires auditory input resources, while the other requires verbal output.

Task difficulty also plays a role. If a task is more difficult, it requires more resources in general and would be hard to do simultaneously with another task without passing resource capacity. Imagine driving a car while conversing with your passengers. When driving through familiar neighborhoods in a single lane (an easy task), you may have no trouble carrying on a conversation. However, if you are about to enter a complicated intersection involving a lane change and a quick turn, attention to the conversation may have to stop or you may become silent or miss what was said during that time. Alternatively, while deep in conversation, it is easy to miss a turn!

11.4   COGNITION

Information-Processing Models

With the advent of computers, psychologists were influenced to think about the human mind as if it were a computer processor. Contrary to behaviorism, which is concerned mostly with the link between stimulus and response, **information-processing models** focus on what happens between the ears. These models have a few basic assumptions. They assume that information is taken in from the environment and processed through a series of steps including **attention**, **perception**, and **storage into memory**. Along the way, information is systematically transformed. Thus, our minds are like mental computer programs or assembly lines that change, store, use, and retrieve information.

Two theories of attention and perception were described above (Broadbent filter model of selective attention and the Treisman attenuation model of selective attention). **Alan Baddeley's model** sought to better define short-term memory, which he renamed **working memory**. In his model, working memory consists of four components—a phonological loop, a visuospatial sketchpad, an episodic buffer, and a central executive. The **phonological loop** allows us to repeat verbal information to help us remember it. This may be what you use to remember a phone number that someone tells you when you have nothing with which to write it down. The **visuospatial sketchpad** serves a similar purpose for visuospatial information through the use of mental images. The **episodic buffer** is theorized to integrate information from the phonological loop and visuospatial sketchpad with a sense of time, and to interface with long-term memory stores. In other words, the episodic buffer is responsible for combining information from a variety of sources into coherent episodes (hence the name, episodic buffer). For example, if a man sees a station wagon much like the one his father used to drive, he is able to make this connection through the interaction between his memory of his father's car and his current visual experience in the episodic buffer. The **central executive** is the overseer of the entire process and orchestrates it by shifting and dividing attention.

Figure 19   Baddeley Model of Working Memory

Cognitive Development

Piaget's Stages of Cognitive Development

Jean Piaget was one of the first developmental psychologists who studied cognitive development in children; he argued against the prevailing belief that children were much like miniature adults in their thought processes and abilities. He thought that the process of cognitive development involved forming **schemas**, or mental frameworks that shape and are shaped by our experience. As we encounter new experiences, Piaget believed that we either **assimilate** those experiences by fitting them into our existing schemas or we **accommodate** by adjusting our schemas to take into account the new experiences. For example, if a young girl believes that there is a monster under the bed but her parent turns on the light to reveal that there is nothing there, the girl can take two paths. She can assimilate this experience by believing that the monster still exists but runs away from light, or accommodate her schema by agreeing that there must be no monster.

Piaget's theory included four developmental stages. They are as follows:

1) **Sensorimotor Stage:** from birth to roughly age 2. Babies and young infants experience the world through their senses and movement, such as looking, touching, mouthing, and grasping. During this time, they learn about **object permanence**—the understanding that things continue to exist when they are out of sight. They also demonstrate stranger anxiety: distress when confronted with an unfamiliar person.

2) **Preoperational Stage:** roughly from ages 2 to 7. During this time, children learn that things can be represented through symbols such as words and images. This accompanies their learning during pretend play and development of language, but they still lack logical reasoning. They also are egocentric, meaning they do not understand that others have different perspectives.

3) **Concrete Operational Stage:** roughly from ages 7 to 11. Children learn to think logically about concrete events. This helps them learn the principle of **conservation**: the idea that quantity remains the same despite changes in shape. For example, if water from a wide bowl is poured into a thin cylinder, it still has the same volume despite the difference in height. They also grasp mathematical concepts during this time.

4) **Formal Operational Stage:** roughly from age 12 through adulthood. People learn abstract reasoning (e.g., hypothesizing) and moral reasoning.

Cognitive Changes in Late Adulthood

During early and middle adulthood, most cognitive abilities remain stable or increase. Beyond the age of 60, the following cognitive declines have been noted:

1) The elderly show some memory declines in recall, while their recognition abilities remain relatively intact. **Recall** involves retrieving information from memory without any clues, while **recognition** involves retrieving information from memory with clues. Asking an eyewitness to describe the face of a suspect is a test of recall; asking an eyewitness to identify a suspect out of a lineup is a test of recognition.

2) Time-based tasks can also be challenging for older adults, such as a regimen involving medication taken three times a day.

3) Older adults also have slower information-processing abilities, as evidenced by slower reaction times and speech.

Role of Culture in Cognitive Development

The process of learning is in many ways the process of internalizing information provided by a given culture. Higher mental processes may have their roots in broader social processes. Thus, instead of the individual developing and learning how to utilize developed skills in a social context, consider the possibility that the individual learns social relationships and converts these into mental capabilities. The developing individual and the environment are in a reciprocal relationship in which the social context can shape thinking and behavior. For example: the expression of thoughts is limited by the thinker's language. Furthermore, internalized speech is only developed after a child speaks out loud and receives feedback from others in the environment. As you can imagine, different languages result in different ways of thinking. Multilingual people have even been shown to perform differently on personality tests depending on the language in which the test is given.

Influence of Heredity and Environment on Cognitive Development

Heredity and the environment interact during the course of an individual's life to create a developmental trajectory. One way of thinking about this is that genetics provides the biological predispositions, or raw material that an individual has. Sociocultural influences then help mold and channel this potential into the development of particular capabilities. The amount and quality of schooling and the richness of the child's environment can heavily influence performance on tests of cognitive functioning. Thus, neither "nature" (genetics) nor "nurture" (environment) may be sufficient to explain the developmental path of an individual—it may instead be explained by a complex interaction. For an example, consider the case of language. Noam Chomsky convincingly argued that children could not learn the wealth of vocabulary that they quickly acquire simply through environmental influence; genetics and heredity are also involved. At the same time, the quality of reading education in school influences a child's ability to acquire this skill.

Biological Factors that Affect Cognition

Many aspects of cognitive functioning can be traced back to structures in the brain. Sensory information provides the raw material for cognitive processes and is transmitted to the parietal, occipital, and temporal lobes of the brain (discussed in Chapter 10). In fact, the inability to recognize objects through sensory mechanisms (a vital aspect of perception and cognition) despite intact function of the underlying sense itself is called **agnosia**; it is often due to damage at the occipitoparietal border. The frontal lobes play a role in executive functions, including planning, organizing, inhibiting impulses, and thinking flexibly. The hippocampus has been shown to be involved in the formation of new memories. Furthermore, emotional arousal is necessary to provide the motivation and alertness necessary to complete tasks and is managed by the amygdala and the rest of the limbic system. The interconnectivity of these various regions underlies our cognitive skills.

Problem-Solving and Decision-Making

Types of Problem-Solving and Problem-Solving Approaches

What detours can I take to get out of this traffic jam? How do I change a flat tire? Should I hitchhike with this stranger? A strange morning commute may require us to use various strategies for solving problems. For some problems, we may use a strategy of **trial and error**. For others, we may rely on following an **algorithm**, a step-by-step procedure. For others, we may use mental shortcuts, called **heuristics**. At times, we may use a combination of these strategies. For example, when changing a tire, an algorithm may be followed until it is discovered that a needed wrench is missing. At this point, other tools may be pulled out and experimented with through trial and error until an appropriate one for the bolts is found. Sometimes we use problem-solving strategies consciously, while at other times this is an unconscious process. For example, we may not be actively thinking about a problem, but may be struck later in the shower with a sudden flash of inspiration called **insight**.

Barriers to Effective Problem-Solving

Think about a time when you struggled with solving a problem to no avail. There are two cognitive tendencies that can lead us astray when looking for solutions: confirmation bias and fixation.

Confirmation bias is a tendency to search only for information that confirms our preconceived thinking, rather than information that might not support it. This can prevent you from approaching a problem from multiple perspectives, because you are more likely to view it from one way—your way. As a result, this bias can lead to faulty decision-making; one-sided information may leave you without a complete picture of the situation. For example, suppose you are in charge of staffing the nurses at the hospital ER where you work, and you believe that during college football game nights there are more admissions than on other days. You will tend to take notice of admissions during college football game nights, but be inattentive to admissions during other nights of the month. A tendency to do this over time unjustifiably strengthens your belief, and it could lead to poor staffing decisions.

A second obstacle to problem-solving is **fixation**, an inability to see the problem from a fresh perspective. At times, fixation results from the existence of a **mental set**, a tendency to fixate on solutions that worked in the past though they may not apply to the current situation. For example, a parent trying to control their child's behavior may not realize that time-outs at age 15 are just not as effective as they were at age 5. Another type of fixation is **functional fixedness**, a tendency to perceive the functions of objects as fixed and unchanging. Thus, one may search high and low to find a box-cutter to open a package, when a readily available key would work just as well.

Heuristics, Biases, Intuition, and Emotion

It may not surprise you to know that humans are not always logical in their decision-making. Often we don't put a great deal of time and effort into a decision because the decision may be trivial, or because it must be made quickly, or because no clear logical path for problem-solving is available.

Mental shortcuts, or heuristics, can increase efficiency in decision-making and although they are helpful most of the time, they can also lead to errors in judgment. Who was a more prolific composer, Joseph Haydn or Ludwig van Beethoven? Most of us would assume Beethoven, because his name and possibly even examples of his work come more readily to mind. Haydn was actually Beethoven's teacher, and he composed nearly three times more music than did Beethoven! When you make a decision about something based on the examples that are most available in your mind, this is known as the **availability heuristic**. While the availability heuristic relies more on our memory of specific instances, the **representativeness heuristic** has more to do with our generalizations about people and events. For example, let's say you go to the post office three different times and each time a different employee is rude to you. You might conclude, "people who work at the post office are rude!" This would be an example of the representativeness heuristic—you have developed a generalization about postal workers. Another example: what does a taxicab look like? Most Americans would use the adjective "yellow" when describing a taxicab, because a yellow car fits our prototype of what a taxicab looks like. Again, this generalization is the result of the representativeness heuristic. The representativeness and availability heuristics may seem quite similar, but the representativeness heuristic is based more on generalizations (rather than specific examples), whereas the availability heuristic is based on how readily particular examples come to mind.

Another susceptibility is **belief bias**, which is the tendency to judge arguments based on what one believes about their conclusions rather than on whether they use sound logic. In other words, we tend to accept conclusions that fit with our beliefs and tend to reject conclusions that do not fit with our beliefs. For example, you probably believe that doctors are good people; therefore, if you read a story about a doctor who allegedly murdered his wife, no matter the strength of the evidence, you might be more inclined to believe that the death was an accident. On the other hand, you might easily believe that a drug-dealer killed his wife, despite the lack of any compelling evidence. Once these preexisting beliefs are formed, they become resistant to change through a phenomenon known as **belief perseverance**, a tendency to cling to beliefs despite the presence of contrary evidence.

Overconfidence and Belief Perseverance

The use of intuitive heuristics and a tendency to confirm preconceived beliefs combine to lead to **overconfidence**, an overestimation of the accuracy of knowledge and judgments. For example, after hearing that a classmate completed an assignment quickly, along with their belief that a particular class is easy, students can be overconfident in how much time it would take to complete assignments or write papers, estimating that they would take less time than they actually do. People can also be influenced by how information is **framed**. For example, one study found that consumers are more likely to buy meat advertised as 75% lean than that labeled 25% fat. Similarly, rather than informing customers that they will be charged a "fee" for using a credit card, a company may choose to offer those who use cash a "discount" to make the same situation more palatable.

11.5 CONSCIOUSNESS

Consciousness is something that science has not yet been able to pin down and with which religion has wrestled. It has been explained through concepts such as the soul by some and thought of as inseparable from the body by others. **Consciousness** is defined as the awareness that we have of ourselves, our internal states, and the environment. It is also important for reflection and exerts control by directing our attention. Thus, consciousness is always needed to complete novel and complex tasks, although we may complete practiced and simple tasks, such as driving a familiar path, with little conscious awareness. We may also be influenced by subconscious cues without them entering our consciousness. These subconscious cues can be a basis for first impressions of others and even for prejudice.

States of Consciousness

Alertness

Alertness and arousal involve the ability to remain attentive to what is going on. It is something that we often take for granted, however, many patients who arrive in an emergency room are not alert for various reasons. These can include head injuries and toxins. The ability to be alert is also impaired in a variety of disorders, including narcolepsy, attention deficit disorder, depression, and chronic fatigue syndrome. Even without these disorders, it is not possible to maintain a heightened state of alertness indefinitely, and alertness varies over a 24-hour cycle. Alertness and arousal are controlled by structures within the brainstem. These structures are known as the **reticular formation** (also known as the reticular activating system, or RAS).

Sleep

Stages of Sleep

Although the purpose of sleep and exact definition of sleep are unclear, the stages of sleep have been empirically determined. The best way to explain the stages of sleep is to put them in context of how they are measured and distinguished. **Polysomnography** (PSG) is a multimodal technique to measure physiological processes during sleep. PSG includes electroencephalogram (EEG—measures of electrical impulses in the brain), **electromyogram** (EMG—measures of skeletal muscle movements), **electrooculogram** (EOG— measures of eye movement), and other physiological indicators of sleep. Through experiments using PSG, research has shown there are several distinct stages of sleep.

When a person is awake, but sleepy and relaxed, the individual's EEG changes from when they are alert. In this relaxed state, the EEG shows **alpha waves**, which have low amplitudes and high frequencies (8–12 Hz; Figure 20). These waves are the first indicator that a person is ready to drift off to sleep: the body relaxes; the person feels drowsy and closes his or her eyes. Compare these waves to **beta waves**, the waves demonstrated during alert, focused, and active consciousness. These waves have even higher frequencies (between 12.5 Hz and 30 Hz) than alpha waves and also lower amplitudes.

When sleep begins, the first stage of non-REM (**rapid eye movement**) sleep is entered. This is called **Stage 1 sleep**. During this stage, the EEG is dominated by **theta waves**: waves of low to moderate intensity and intermediate frequency (3–7 Hz; Figure 20). Further, EOG measures slow-rolling eye movements and EMG measures moderate activity. The person becomes less responsive to stimuli and has fleeting thoughts.

Stage 2 sleep is denoted by a change to two distinct wave patterns on the EEG. Although a person still experiences theta waves, these waves are intermixed with these two patterns: K-complexes and sleep spindles. A **K-complex** typically has a duration of a half second and is large and slow. These each occur as a single wave amongst the theta waves. **Sleep spindles** are bursts of waves. They have a frequency of 12–14 Hz and are moderately intense. Like K-complexes, these spindles do not last long: only a half to one and a half seconds. During Stage 2, there is no eye movement and EMG measures moderate activity. This stage brings increased relaxation to in the body that is characteristic of sleep, such as decreased heart rate, respiration, and temperature.

During **Stage 3 and Stage 4 sleep**, a person transitions into slow wave sleep. Stage 3 and Stage 4 are characterized by **delta waves**, which are high amplitude, low frequency waves (0.5–3 Hz) and signify the deepest level of sleep. Initially, delta waves are mixed with higher-frequency waves, but as Stage 3 progresses to Stage 4, delta waves come to dominate. During slow wave sleep, a person continues to show no eye movement and moderate muscle movement. The heart rate and digestion slow, and growth hormones are secreted.

The final stage of sleep is **REM sleep**, which is characterized by bursts of quick eye movements. Also unique to REM sleep, the EEG measures waves that most resemble the beta waves seen in individuals when awake. However, the waves in REM sleep are sawtooth waves with low intensity and variable frequency. These waves are more jagged in appearance than beta waves, which are also low intensity, but high frequency (16–25 Hz). Unlike the conscious state, REM sleep is characterized by low (almost no) skeletal muscle movement: hence the name "**paradoxical sleep**." Although the person physiologically appears to be awake, their muscle movement does not corroborate, as the individual is nearly paralyzed except for sudden bursts or twitches. REM sleep is generally when dreams occur.

11.5

Figure 20   EEG wave forms during wakefulness and sleep

During normal sleep, an individual passes through the non-REM sleep stages, then enters into REM sleep, then passes back through the non-REM sleep stages. This may happen in sequence (Stages 1, 2, 3, 4, then REM), but it is also possible to jump between various stages while sleeping. Regardless, the average sleep cycle is about 90 minutes (for a typical adult), and includes periods of non-REM and REM sleep. We complete multiple sleep cycles per night. Periods of REM sleep are shortest early in the night, and get longer as the night progresses. Deep sleep (Stages 3 and 4) periods are longest early in the night and less frequent as the night progresses (Figure 21). The amount of sleep needed for optimal functioning changes throughout one's lifespan. Infants spend a much larger fraction of their sleep in REM than adults do (and need much more sleep—young babies spend about 16 out of every 24 hours sleeping!). Teens need, on average, about 9–10 hours a night of uninterrupted sleep. As we age, we require less and less sleep—it is not uncommon for individuals in their 60s and 70s to sleep about 6 hours a night. Without an adequate amount of sleep, the body is not able to complete all of the restorative phases needed for muscle repair, memory consolidation, and the release of various hormones, including those that regulate growth and appetite. When we do not get enough sleep, we wake up less prepared to concentrate, focus, and engage in decision-making.

Figure 21   Normal sleep stages throughout the night

Sleep and Circadian Rhythms

There are several possible explanations for why organisms sleep. Since humans (and most other non-nocturnal animals) are better suited to survival in the daytime when we can best use our vision to navigate and stay out of harm's way, sleep may have served as a survival mechanism to reduce nighttime activity (when our ancestors were more likely to become prey). A second theory is that sleep helps heal the body by restoring tissues, including those in the brain. While we are asleep, the brain is still active, and could be reorganizing connections and consolidating memories into long-term memory storage. A third idea is that sleep plays a role in growth. During sleep, the pituitary gland releases growth hormone, with lower levels of the hormone released as an individual ages. **Circadian rhythms** (sometimes referred to as the biological clock) are the biological waxing and waning of alertness over the 24-hour day. Most people feel their most alert during the mid-morning, experience an energy dip in early afternoon (when some people take siestas or grab a second cup of coffee!), and then feel alert again in the early evening; later in the evening, as alertness wanes, sleep becomes more and more enticing. Although this is a general description of the ebb and flow of alertness throughout the day, it varies by individual, and circadian rhythms also vary with age. Newborns can spend two-thirds of a day asleep. Older adults tend to peak in the morning and decline as the day progresses, while adolescents and young adults tend to be more energetic in the mid-to-late evening.

A key factor in how sleep is regulated involves exposure to light, which stimulates a nerve pathway from the retina to the suprachiasmatic nucleus (SCN) in the hypothalamus. The SCN signals other parts of the brain, which regulate body temperature and control the production and release of hormones. The SCN is essentially our internal clock; it helps regulate the pattern of neurophysiological activities that affect the entire body. When exposed to light at the beginning of the day, our body temperature begins to rise and hormones (like cortisol) are released; these signals indicate that it is time to wake up.

Melatonin is a hormone made by the **pineal gland** in the brain. Darkness causes the SCN to signal the pineal gland to start producing and releasing melatonin. As melatonin levels rise, you begin to feel tired. Melatonin levels stay elevated throughout the night; the light of a new day causes melatonin levels to fall. Bright light both regulates the function of the SCN and directly inhibits the release of melatonin. Artificial indoor lighting can also sometimes be bright enough to prevent the release of melatonin (which is why some studies suggest that turning off mobile devices an hour before bedtime can improve your sleep!).

Core body temperature fluctuates between about 96.8° and 100.4°F over a 24-hour period, and this is also regulated by the hypothalamus. For most of us with normal circadian rhythms, sleep tends to occur when the core temperature is dropping at the end of the day. The average adult experiences their lowest core body temperature about two hours before waking time in the morning.

Dreaming

As mentioned earlier, the REM stage of sleep is when dreams typically occur. This stage is absolutely necessary. Missing REM sleep for one night results in an increase in REM sleep later to make up for it, called **REM rebound**. Some of the dreams during the REM stage can be exciting, including lucid dreams (in which one might be aware that one is dreaming and have some conscious control of the dreams). Most dreams are about daily events, like missing an exam, playing a sport, or talking to a friend. But why is it that we dream? Freud believed that the plotlines of dreams, or **manifest content**, were symbolic versions of underlying **latent content**, unconscious drives and wishes that are difficult to express. Thus, he believed that dreams are a way of understanding our inner conflicts. Other theories for why dreams exist have emerged since Freud. Some studies have found that dreaming can improve learning and problem-solving. It was found that brain regions used by rats to navigate a maze while they were awake were also active while the rats slept, as if the rats were running the maze in their dreams. When they woke, the rats demonstrated improved performance compared to both their previous performances and the performances of other rats that did not get REM sleep. The same is true for human performance on tasks. You may find that a night of consolidating information you've learned while studying for the MCAT is beneficial to retaining that information. The **activation-synthesis theory** suggests that dreams are byproducts of brain activation during REM sleep. This theory allows for the possibility that dreams are far from purposeful. Finally, some proponents have suggested that the purpose of dreams is to provide a template of consciousness on which the mind can practice consciousness-development.

Sleep Disorders

While there may be some debate as to the purpose of sleep, it cannot be disputed that sleep is necessary when we consider how debilitating sleep disorders can be. Sleep disorders can be subdivided into dyssomnias and parasomnias.

Dyssomnias are abnormalities in the amount, quality, or timing of sleep, and include insomnia, narcolepsy, and sleep apnea. **Insomnia** is the most common sleep disorder and is characterized by difficulty falling or staying asleep. Insomnia is not the occasional inability to fall asleep due to anxiety or excitement, but rather a persistent problem that can stem from chronic stress. Common quick treatments are sedatives such as sleeping pills, but these have a risk of dependency and overdose, and become less effective with time. They also create abnormal sleep cycles that include less time in REM and slow-wave stages, which can lead to drowsy carry-over effects. Natural alternatives include relaxation before bedtime, avoiding stimulants and exercise in the evening, and sleeping on a regular schedule. Those with **narcolepsy** experience periodic, overwhelming sleepiness during waking periods that usually last less than 5 minutes. They can occur without warning at dangerous times, such as while driving or walking down stairs. Recent research suggests that the cause of narcolepsy is a dysfunction in the region of the hypothalamus that produces the neurotransmitter hypocretin (also called orexin). Narcolepsy has been treated with stimulants with modest success. **Sleep apnea** is a disorder that causes people to intermittently stop breathing during sleep, which results in waking after a minute or so without air. This process can repeat hundreds of times a night, and can deprive sufferers of deep sleep. Those with sleep apnea may not even be aware that they have it, although their partners may be, as it can be accompanied by heavy snoring. The incidence of sleep apnea is associated with obesity.

Parasomnias are abnormal behaviors that occur during sleep and include somnambulism and night terrors. **Somnambulism** (or sleepwalking) tends to occur during slow-wave sleep (Stage 3), usually during the first third of the night. There may be genetic predispositions for sleepwalking and sleeptalking. **Night terrors** also usually occur during Stage 3 (unlike nightmares, which occur during REM sleep toward morning). A person experiencing a night terror may sit up or walk around, babble, and appear terrified, although none of this is recalled the next morning. Both of these disorders are more likely to appear in children.

Hypnosis and Meditation

Hypnotism has been portrayed in so many different ways in movies and other media that it is important to separate fact from fiction. **Hypnotism** is an interpersonal interaction in which a hypnotist has a subject focus attention on what is being said, relax and feel tired, "let go," and accept suggestions easily through the use of vivid imagination. Nearly everyone is hypnotizable to some extent, although some have a stronger capacity. Hypnotized people do NOT acquire superhuman physical abilities—this is a myth. Hypnotism can promote recall of some long-term memories by putting someone in a relaxed state, but a patient is also susceptible to constructing **false memories**—that is, using imagination to create inaccurate memories. It cannot help a patient remember events from infancy. Finally, hypnotism cannot force people to commit extreme acts against their will or moral code, such as commit murder. Studies show that the presence of the authoritative hypnotist equally influences hypnotized and non-hypnotized people to commit acts that are of similar danger levels.

This does not imply that hypnotized people are "faking it." In fact, posthypnotic suggestions have been utilized to help alleviate headaches, asthma, and stress-related skin disorders. In addition, 50% of people can gain some pain relief from hypnosis. Hypnosis works not by preventing sensory input, but by blocking attention to those sensory inputs. People may experience physiological states such as pain or a pounding heart, but are not consciously aware of these sensations. Some studies indicate that hypnotism results in changes in brain activity, insinuating that it is an actual altered state of consciousness (although this idea is controversial). There are two theories for how it works. The **dissociation theory** suggests that hypnotism is an extreme form of divided consciousness. In hypnosis, just as in everyday life, many behaviors occur on autopilot. Have you ever driven somewhere and not recalled anything about the actual drive? Thus, hypnotism may be an extended form of this normal dissociation in which the individual is on autopilot and the hypnotist takes over the executive control, which directs action. The **social influence theory** suggests that people do, and report, what's expected of them. They are not consciously faking it, but are like actors who get caught up in their roles and thus behave in ways that fit them.

11.5

Meditation refers to a variety of techniques, many of which have been practiced for thousands of years, and which usually involve the training of attention. Meditators may focus intensely on one object of attention, such as their breathing, or they may broaden their attention and be aware of multiple stimuli, such as anything in their auditory field. Meditation has been utilized successfully to manage pain, stress, and anxiety disorders. **Mindfulness-based stress reduction** (MBSR) is a protocol commonly used in the medical setting to help alleviate stress. Meditators have increased alpha and theta waves while they are meditating (and to some extent an increase above baseline after they stop), with more experienced meditators showing greater improvements.

Consciousness-Altering Drugs

There are three main categories of psychoactive drugs: depressants, stimulants, and hallucinogenics. All of these drugs work by altering actions at the neuronal synapses, either enhancing, dampening, or mimicking the activity of the brain's natural neurotransmitters.

Depressants include alcohol, barbiturates (tranquilizers), and opiates. They work by depressing, or slowing down, neural activity. When drinking alcohol, people are more likely to be impulsive and may appear hyperactive, but this is due to the slowing of brain activity related to judgment and inhibition in the frontal lobe. In larger doses, alcohol can lead to deterioration in skilled motor performance, decreased reaction time, and slurring of speech [which brain area is impacted when this occurs?[5]]. Excessive drinking can lead to memory blackouts for recent memories (those that have not been consolidated into long-term memory). Alcohol also suppresses REM sleep, which may contribute to the loss of short-term memory and less restful sleep the night of drinking. Thus, a heavy drinker may not remember what happened the night before when they wake up the next morning. While impaired motor control after drinking has caused countless vehicular deaths, an "overdose" of alcohol can also cause death by depressing the respiratory control centers in the medulla to the point that breathing ceases. Alcohol works by stimulating GABA and dopamine systems. GABA is an inhibitory neurotransmitter and is associated with reduced anxiety, while dopamine leads to the feeling of minor euphoria. Prolonged and excessive alcohol use can actually shrink the brain.

---

[5]   The cerebellum, which is responsible for smoothing out motor commands from the primary motor cortex of the frontal lobe. The cerebellum controls precision, timing, coordination, and plays a role in muscle memory. The altered speech demonstrated with inebriation might lead you to believe that Broca's area is impaired; actually, slurred speech is the result of loss of motor control of the lips.

Both alcohol and **barbiturates** depress the sympathetic nervous system ("fight or flight") activity. Barbiturates are often prescribed as sleep aids. They are dangerous in combination with alcohol and prone to overdose—too much of a depressive effect can actually shut down life-sustaining organs. **Opiates**, which are derivatives of opium (including morphine and heroin), also depress neural functioning. They temporarily reduce pain by mimicking the brain's own pain relievers, neurotransmitters known as endorphins; pain is replaced with a blissful feeling. With prolonged use, the brain may stop producing endorphins, leading to a painful withdrawal from the drug.

Stimulants include caffeine, nicotine, cocaine, and amphetamines ("speed"). They typically work by either increasing the release of neurotransmitter, reducing the reuptake of neurotransmitter, or both. Their overall effect is to speed up body functions, resulting in increased energy, respiratory rate, heart rate, and pupil dilation. People use stimulants to stay awake, enhance physical performance, and boost mood. Cocaine works by causing a "rush," a release of the brain's supply of neurotransmitters including dopamine, serotonin, and norepinephrine. While this creates a brief period of intense pleasure, it is followed by a depressive crash. MDMA, also known as ecstasy, is a stimulant and a mild hallucinogen. It works by triggering the release of dopamine and serotonin, as well as by blocking the reabsorption of serotonin so that it stays in the synapse longer. It causes emotional elevation, but long-term effects include damage to serotonin-producing neurons. The resulting reduction in serotonin levels can cause a depressed mood.

Hallucinogens, also known as psychedelics, distort perceptions in the absence of any sensory input, creating hallucinations. These include LSD (lysergic acid diethylamide), mescaline, and, to a much lesser extent, marijuana. After taking LSD, a user may see vivid images and colors. The experience may peak with a feeling of being separated from one's body or experiencing imagined scenes as if they were reality. Emotions related to LSD can vary from euphoria to panic, depending on the person's mood and the context. Marijuana's active ingredient is THC, which affects functioning by stimulating cannabinoid receptors in the brain. It relaxes and disinhibits like alcohol, but it also acts as a hallucinogen by amplifying sensory perceptions including colors, sounds, tastes, and smells. Marijuana can also impair motor skills, reaction time, and judgment. Marijuana has been used medically to help with nausea and pain. Hallucinogens are thought to be the least addictive of the psychoactive drug classes.

Drug Addiction, Dependence, and Tolerance

The defining feature of drug addiction is a compulsion to use a drug repeatedly. Users can have psychological and/or physical dependence on drugs. A **psychological dependence** is often associated with the use of a drug in response to painful emotions related to depression, anxiety, or trauma. For example, an individual with social anxiety may feel compelled to drink alcohol excessively in order to lower anxiety at parties. Sometimes this dependence can be stopped by removing the individual from a painful situation. **Physical dependence** is evidenced by withdrawal. **Withdrawal** involves an uncomfortable and often physically painful experience without the use of a drug. This discomfort is alleviated when the user takes the drug, thus reinforcing further drug use. Alcohol withdrawal is especially dangerous—excessive users must be slowly detoxified, as stopping suddenly is life-threatening. Even caffeine addiction can cause withdrawal, with the user experiencing headache, fogginess, and irritability that end when more caffeine is taken.

Tolerance effects of drugs can vary. For example, alcohol abuse is associated with increased baseline blood pressure, potentially to dangerous levels. Alcohol is known to act as a stimulant for a brief period (up to two or three drinks) before depressant effects begin. Long-term abuse can lead an individual's intrinsic stress-reduction mechanisms to be debilitated. Caffeine, to take another example, is known to have acute effects, but does not change baseline measures such as blood pressure except at extreme doses above 600 mg.

Tolerance to caffeine will actually return an individual to baseline blood pressure after a period during which the individual demonstrates elevated levels. The effects of caffeine are therefore transient and reversible. Different drugs have different effects on baseline measures after tolerance.

11.6 LANGUAGE

One of the most characteristically *human* ways of interacting with the environment is to communicate using language. Indeed, our ability to learn and use language is often cited as the most defining human characteristic, that which distinguishes us from all the other animals. Even today, questions about what exactly language *is*, how it develops, and the role it plays in cognition remain important topics of debate and research.

Debates about these questions echo larger divisions in psychology. Behaviorists who argue that language is just another example of conditioned behavior are *empiricist* in their approach; they believe that the study of psychology should focus on directly observable environmental factors as opposed to abstract mental states. In contrast, nativists, who argue that language is a human ability prewired into the brain, are *rationalist* in their approach; they hold that certain ideas and capabilities cannot come from experience, and so must be innate. Still other researchers take a *materialist* approach to language and cognition, grounding their work in the belief that all discussion of "ideas," linguistic "expression," and the like is a set of convenient metaphors for real physical changes in the brain and actions of the body. Materialists believe that "only grey matter matters," and study thoughts and words by looking at what happens in the brain when people think, speak, write, and listen. In this section, we will define the ways these different schools of thought have explained how people learn language and how language relates to mental processes.

Theories of Language Development

Language acquisition is the term used by psychologists to refer to the way infants learn to understand and speak their native language (usually the language used by their parents). Language acquisition is the process of language learning in school or that of learning a foreign language. These other forms of language acquisition seem to work much differently.

B.F. Skinner's **behaviorist** model of language acquisition holds that infants are trained in language by operant conditioning (see Chapters 7 and 9 for more on behaviorism). Skinner argued that language use, though complex, is a form of behavior like any other, and so it is as subject to conditioning as a rat pulling a lever to receive a food pellet. Describing a beautiful sunset or persuading a friend to help you move obviously result in more complicated outcomes than receiving a food pellet after pulling a lever, but all three can be described as physical actions intended to produce effects (e.g., the production of sound using your vocal chords or the movement of your arm). How can learning to speak be analogous to learning other behaviors? Consider an infant babbling nonsense as its father repeats "bottle" while holding a bottle. By random chance, the baby will eventually make some noise like "bu-ba," at which point daddy will say "very good!" and smile delightedly before calling in mommy to praise their little genius. This positive reinforcement accomplishes two things: first, it conditions the infant to make the sound in association with the stimulus (the sight of the bottle), and second and more important, it encourages imitative behavior, so that the baby begins more regularly to copy the sounds made by the parent. This imitation is how the second, third, and five-hundredth words and phrases are learned progressively faster, as each subsequent "correct" utterance produces some reinforcing behavior like a hug or a piece of candy, whereas nonsense utterances achieve no reinforcement and are abandoned.

11.6

Linguist **Noam Chomsky** pointed out several major flaws with the application of behaviorism to language acquisition, and proposed an alternative to Skinner's model. Chomsky suggested that we all possess an innate feature unique to the human mind **(the language acquisition device)** that allows people to gain mastery of language from limited exposure during the sensitive developmental years in early childhood. This idea was later named "**universal grammar**" (UG). Chomsky's device was theoretical in that he provided no anatomical evidence for the exact location or structure of this device in the brain. However, research into the function of the device is empirical; linguists study UG by studying actual languages and actual cases of language acquisition. Their goal is to find the basic rules that apply to all or almost all languages and that are presumably innate in the brain, allowing the child to, for example, distinguish nouns, verbs, and adjectives without ever being taught these terms. It is important to note the distinction between language rules being prewired in the brain and language itself being hardwired: many songbirds, for example, are hatched knowing how to sing the territorial songs of their species, but no human is ever born knowing English or Mandarin. Rather, the theory states that humans have an innate ability to make grammatical distinctions and do so naturally when exposed to (not actively taught) language at a young age.

Influence of Language on Cognition

The relationship between language and cognition is still under debate. Some experts argue that language is first and foremost a social phenomenon, and that speech is not developmentally equivalent with thought. In other words, children first learn how to think and how to speak as separate enterprises, and only later is there overlap between the two. The first stage of acquiring language is immersion in "social speech," which is analogous to other social phenomena. This moves gradually into "egocentric speech" or "private speech," wherein children begin talking to themselves, experimenting with language as kind of thinking out loud. The final stage of language acquisition is "inner speech," the point at which a child's understanding of grammar and the relationship between words and objects is sufficiently advanced to allow him to think in words without mouthing them. This is a critical stage in the development of the relationship between language and thought. Prior to this point, speech and thought are separate activities, but at this point, some thought becomes "verbal," able to be expressed in words and clauses.

The **"linguistic relativity hypothesis"** asserts that not only do language and thought overlap, but cognition and perception are *determined* by the language one speaks. Unlike Chomsky's universal grammar, which emphasizes the commonality among all human languages, this hypothesis focuses on important distinctions among families of languages, such as Western European versus East Asian languages. Because of these distinctions, the argument goes, native speakers in these language groups conceptualize the world differently. The famous example is that Inuit peoples conceive of snow differently from English speakers, as evidenced by the fact that they have so many more words for snow. Subsequent research has called this "fact" into question, pointing out, for example, that Inuits do not have a very large number of words for snow compared to speakers of other languages and that skiers who speak different languages also have many different words in each to describe conditions of snow.

Different Brain Areas Control Language and Speech

Broca's area, located in the dominant hemisphere (usually left) of the frontal lobe of the brain, is involved in the complicated process of speech production. Broca's area was discovered when several people who had an injury to this area lost the ability to speak—a disorder now termed **Broca's aphasia**[6]. People with Broca's aphasia (also known as *expressive aphasia*) know what they want to say, but are unable to communicate it. They are typically able to comprehend words and simple sentences but are unable to generate fluent speech. Sometimes they can produce very simple, telegraphic speech ("Take. Car. Store."), or are limited to one or two words that they repeat over and over.

Wernicke's area, located in the posterior section of the temporal lobe in the dominant hemisphere of the brain (the left for most people), is involved in the comprehension of speech and written language. Wernicke's area was also discovered with the help of people with injuries to this area; in these individuals, speech production retains a natural sounding rhythm and syntax, but is completely meaningless. In other words, people with **Wernicke's aphasia** (also known as *receptive aphasia*) do not have a problem producing speech, but are incapable of producing intelligible, meaningful language. For example, someone with Wernicke's aphasia might say something like: "You know how go what moodle winkered and what you can't toodle doodle do so show him little litty round and cake you make more want to." A sentence such as this would be uttered with fluidity, with normal-sounding inflections. So, it would sound as though the person were merely speaking in an unknown language. As you might imagine, it is often difficult to decipher what the person is trying to communicate. People with Wernicke's aphasia usually have great difficulty understanding speech, and they are often unaware of their mistakes. Furthermore, these individuals usually have no body weakness or movement issues because their injury is not near the parts of the brain that control movement. Another type of aphasia, **conduction aphasia**, involves poor speech repetition despite intact comprehension and fluent speech.

Figure 22 Approximate locations of Broca's area and Wernicke's area in the brain

---

[6] From the Greek word aphatos meaning "speechlessness."

Chapter 11 Summary

- Humans have several types of receptors (mechanoreceptors, chemoreceptors, nociceptors, thermoceptors, electromagnetic receptors, and proprioceptors) that allow us to detect a variety of stimuli.

- Weber's law dictates that two stimuli must differ by a constant proportion in order for their difference to be perceptible.

- Gestalt psychology asserts that when humans perceive an object, rather than seeing lines, objects, colors, and shadows, they perceive the whole, not just the individual parts.

- The Broadbent filter model of selective attention proposes that all sensory input first enters a buffer, then is selectively filtered so that only some of the information is sent on for higher processing.

- Treisman's attenuation model proposed that rather than being filtered, sensory input is attenuated—turned up or turned down—before moving on to working memory.

- The resource model of attention asserts that there are limited resources for tasks in general.

- Baddeley's model of working memory considered working memory to have four components: a phonological loop, a visuospatial sketchpad, an episodic buffer, and a central executive (which oversees the process).

- Jean Piaget proposed a four-stage theory of cognitive development, which included: the sensorimotor stage, preoperational stage, concrete operations stage, and formal operations stage.

- Sleep progresses through four stages, each characterized by specific physiological differences.

- Broca's area is involved with speech production, while Wernicke's area is involved with speech comprehension.

CHAPTER 11 FREESTANDING PRACTICE QUESTIONS

1. Suppose that a researcher subliminally flashed words for negative and positive emotions (e.g., sad, happy) for a millisecond before showing subjects a neutral picture of people in a room. The words flashed so quickly that they were only perceived as a flash of light, but subjects were more likely to describe the scene in negative or positive terms (corresponding to the word that was flashed before the image), than subjects who did not see a subliminal word beforehand. What phenomenon does this describe?

A) Primacy effect
B) Priming
C) Divided attention
D) Episodic memory

2. If a two-year-old child repeatedly asks his mother for his favorite toy after it has been lost, what understanding has the child obtained, according to Piaget's theory of cognitive development?

A) Schemas
B) Conservation
C) Object permanence
D) Formal operations

3. The "candle problem" is a famous experiment whereby the subject is given a wax candle, a small cardboard box containing several thumbtacks, and a book of matches. The subject is asked to affix the candle to a corkboard so that wax will not drip onto the floor below. The only correct way to solve the task is to empty the box of thumbtacks, tack the box onto the corkboard, and light the candle and place it inside the box. Most subjects are unable to figure out the solution to this task, but if the thumbtacks are presented next to the box, not inside of it, they can solve the task easily. Why can't the subjects solve the task in the first scenario?

A) They are bound by a mental set that does not comprehend how to light a candle in this way.
B) They are unable to employ trial and error quickly enough to solve the task.
C) They are overconfident about their own strategies for solving the task.
D) They are unable to see alternative uses for the box containing the thumbtacks due to functional fixedness.

Figure 1 Average melatonin production (in ng/mL) over a 24-hour period by age group

4. A normal 15-year-old is participating in a sleep study and falls asleep at 10:30. This subject enters her first REM cycle at midnight. According to Figure 1 above, which of the following measures would most likely be recorded at midnight?

I. Melatonin levels of 90 ng/mL
II. Moderate to high EMG activity
III. EEG measures that include theta waves and K-complexes

A) I only
B) III only
C) I and III only
D) I, II, and III

5. Alcohol withdrawal syndrome occurs when an individual with a dependence on alcohol suddenly limits or stops alcohol consumption. Symptoms of withdrawal can be very dangerous, including seizures, uncontrollable shaking of the extremities, and other nervous system issues. What is the most plausible mechanism of action for these physical symptoms?

A) Chronic alcohol consumption causes down-regulation of GABA receptors, leading to a reduction in CNS inhibition, and excito-neurotoxicity.
B) Long-term alcohol abuse stimulates the autonomic nervous system, causing tremors.
C) Cessation of alcohol consumption leads to a reduction in dopamine production in the nucleus accumbens.
D) Alcohol is a hallucinogenic, and withdrawal acts by relaxing, disinhibiting, and amplifying sensory information.

6. A patient recently admitted to the ER is reported to have had a stroke. At present, he is having some trouble communicating with hospital staff. When he addresses the doctor, he seems to have great difficulty forming sentences. His speech is rather monotone and lacks many function words. This patient is most likely experiencing:

A) somnambulism.
B) Wernicke's aphasia.
C) Broca's aphasia.
D) receptive aphasia.

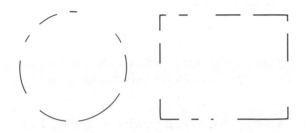

7. Instead of perceiving a series of lines in the figure above, humans perceive two shapes: a circle and a rectangle. What best accounts for this phenomenon?

A) The principles of Gestalt psychology
B) Bottom-up processing
C) Parallel processing
D) Weber's law

8. What structure in the middle ear generates vibrations that match the sound waves striking it?

A) Basilar membrane
B) Tympanic membrane
C) Cochlea
D) Malleus

9. In the human visual pathway, what cell type comprises the bundle of fibers called the optic nerve?

A) Photoreceptors
B) Bipolar cells
C) Ganglion cells
D) Fovea cells

10. After hearing a telephone number, one only has a few seconds to write it down before the information is lost. What aspect of Baddeley's information processing model accounts for this ability?

A) Phonological loop
B) Visuospatial sketchpad
C) Episodic buffer
D) Central executive

CHAPTER 11 PRACTICE PASSAGE

Guided meditation and deep-breathing exercises have long been used as effective techniques for stress reduction. The mechanism of action for this non-pharmacologic intervention is not entirely known, but scientists believe that the act of focusing ones thoughts and deep belly-breathing both serve to somehow inhibit the stress response activated by the hypothalamic-pituitary-adrenal axis. Practitioners of meditation are capable of reducing their heart and respiration rates seemingly on command.

Irritable Bowel Syndrome (IBS) is a disorder that causes a range of abdominal discomfort and bowel irregularities, but unlike bowel diseases with similar symptoms, there are no physical abnormalities; rather, the disorder appears to be the physical manifestation of psychological triggers. For example, IBS is often comorbid with anxiety disorders or episodes of extreme stress. Acute anxiety and stress are known triggers for IBS symptoms, which usually include severe abdominal cramping, bloating, gassiness, constipation and/or diarrhea (sometimes sufferers experience one or the other more frequently, and a minority of sufferers experience both in an alternating pattern). IBS symptoms usually begin during late teen or early adult years, and a majority of sufferers are women.

The current standard non-pharmacologic treatment for IBS is cognitive behavior therapy (CBT). CBT treats IBS sufferers by treating the emotional and psychological triggers that cause physical symptoms. A trained therapist uses a structured, goal-oriented plan to identify thought patterns and behaviors that trigger IBS symptoms, and provides patients with very specific tools for recognizing these, and also for implementing techniques to replace these negative thoughts and behaviors with more positive ones. In an attempt to determine if meditation is as beneficial as CBT for treating IBS, a recent six-month study was conducted on female IBS sufferers.

Eligible participants had active IBS symptoms for at least three months during the past year. Participants with and without a diagnosed anxiety disorder were recruited to participate in this study. Subjects were randomly assigned to one of three groups: a CBT group, a guided-meditation group, and a no-treatment group. Approximately 65% of the participants had an anxiety disorder, and these subjects were roughly equally represented in each of the three groups. The results of this study, measured by percent reduction of IBS symptoms after treatment, are summarized in Figure 1.

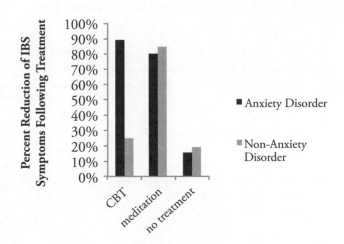

Figure 1   IBS symptom reduction for participants with and without anxiety disorders, by treatment condition

1. Based on the results of this study, what can be most reasonably concluded about the efficacy of CBT for IBS sufferers who do not have an anxiety disorder?

A) CBT is more effective than no treatment and more effective than meditation.
B) CBT and meditation combined provide the most effective treatment possible.
C) CBT is not as effective as meditation.
D) CBT is equally effective for IBS sufferers with and without anxiety disorders.

2. What is the role of the adrenal gland in the stress response?

A) The adrenal gland produces epinephrine and norepinephrine as part of the parasympathetic response to stressful triggers.
B) At the onset of a stressful event, the adrenal gland triggers a cascade of events in the hypothalamus and pituitary, resulting in activation of the sympathetic nervous system's "fight or flight" response.
C) The adrenal medulla produces cortisol, which helps regulate blood pressure and heart rate, in response to stress.
D) The adrenal medulla produces adrenaline in response to acute stressors and the adrenal cortex produces cortisol in response to longer-term, low-grade stressors.

3. The average individual diagnosed with IBS is a 40–50 year old female who is white, educated, married, and middle to upper-middle class. Based on this information, which of the following is most likely to be true about IBS?

A) IBS is underdiagnosed in less-affluent populations.
B) IBS rarely affects younger men and women.
C) There is a causal relationship between educational status and IBS.
D) Getting a divorce could be an effective treatment for married women who develop IBS.

4. Given the description of the study in this passage, which unknown factor might have the most influence on the validity of the results?

A) Sample size
B) Duration of IBS symptoms before entering the study
C) Participants' previous exposure to medication to treat IBS symptoms
D) Length of the treatment protocols

5. Suppose that a recent study, using advanced neuroimaging techniques, found increased activity in the anterior cingulate cortex during meditation. Given the types of physical responses to meditation described in the passage, what functions are likely associated with this area of the brain?

A) Sympathetic functions, including inhibition of the hypothalamus to prevent release of corticotropin releasing hormone (CRH)
B) Somatic functions, including control of the diaphragm
C) Autonomic functions, including heart rate and blood pressure
D) Rational cognitive functions, including decision-making

SOLUTIONS TO CHAPTER 11 FREESTANDING PRACTICE QUESTIONS

1. **B** The scenario in this question stem is describing priming, whereby subjects are provided with some sort of subliminal information (in this instance, the word for a negative or positive emotion) before another stimulus, and their response is impacted by the primed word (choice B is correct). The primacy effect refers to the phenomenon wherein people are more likely to recall the first information they hear or see, and less likely to recall later information (choice A is wrong). Divided attention refers to the ability to complete multiple tasks at once, and the ability to pay attention to one or both of those tasks; because the images were not flashed simultaneously, nor were the subjects even aware of the subliminal image, this scenario is not demonstrating divided attention (choice C is wrong). Episodic memory refers to the type of memory that would be encoded surrounding an event that is of personal significance; this scenario is not demonstrating episodic memory (choice D is wrong).

2. **C** A two-year-old is likely in the earliest stages of preoperational thought and has thus attained object permanence, the ability to understand that something still exists even if they cannot see it (choice C is correct). Schemas are mental frameworks for organizing concepts; while the child likely has a schema for "toy" that he fits his favorite toy into mentally, this does not describe why the child would ask for the toy after it is lost (choice A is wrong). Conservation (the ability to understand that quantity does not change despite a change in size or shape) is attained during the concrete operational stage (ages 7 to 11), and does not explain the described scenario (choice B is wrong). Formal operational thought occurs around age 12 (choice D is wrong).

3. **D** Functional fixedness is the inability to envision various possibilities for an object. In this scenario, when presented with a box of thumbtacks, the subjects do not see the box as a potential tool for solving the task, because they are fixed on the idea that the box is merely a tool for holding the thumbtacks (choice D is correct). A mental set is the tendency to focus on past solutions to a problem, even if they do not apply to the problem at hand; there is no evidence in the question stem that subjects are bound by a mental set (choice A is wrong). Similarly, there is no mention of a time constraint, and trial and error does not best describe what is happening in this scenario (choice B is wrong). There is no indication that overconfidence was a factor here either (choice C is wrong).

4. **A** Item I is true: according to Figure 1, 90 ng/mL of melatonin would be within the normal range for a 15-year-old at approximately midnight (choice B can be eliminated). Item II is false: during REM sleep, the brain stem inhibits movement, therefore EMG activity is very low or absent (choice D can be eliminated). Item III is false: theta waves and K-complexes are present during stage 2 sleep, but absent during REM sleep (choice C can be eliminated, and choice A is correct).

5. **A** Alcohol is a depressant (choice D is wrong) and inhibits neural activity. GABA receptors in the central nervous system respond to GABA, an inhibitory neurotransmitter. Alcohol acts on GABA receptors, inhibiting neuronal signaling. Chronic alcohol consumption causes a down-regulation of GABA receptors; therefore, once the artificial depressant (alcohol) is removed from the system, the CNS no longer has an inhibitory influence, and excito-neurotoxicity occurs, which can result in seizures and tremors (choice A is correct).

Alcohol is a depressant and does not stimulate the autonomic nervous system (choice B is wrong). While alcohol consumption does promote dopamine release in the nucleus accumbens (which stimulates the reward pathway in the brain and helps to explain why alcohol is addictive), and cessation of alcohol consumption would surely lead to a decrease in dopamine, this does not explain the physical symptoms of withdrawal described in the question stem (choice C is wrong).

6. **C** Broca's aphasia is characterized by difficulty producing speech; moreover, inflection and function words (such as pronouns or prepositions) may disappear (choice C is correct). Somnambulism is sleepwalking, which is not typically a result of stroke and does not explain the patient's impairments described in the question stem (choice A is wrong). In cases of Wernicke's aphasia, speech is preserved; however, some words are substituted for others or used incorrectly. Utterances may seem confusing or nonsensical (choice B is wrong). Receptive aphasia is another term for Wernicke's aphasia (choice D is wrong; note also that there cannot be two correct answers).

7. **A** Gestalt psychology proposes that humans tend to see objects in their entirety, and our visual processing systems and brain will superimpose larger organization or structure that makes holistic sense. The "shapes" are technically composed of a series of unconnected lines, but according to Gestalt psychologists, humans are more likely to use both top-down and bottom-up processing to perceive them as a complete circle or a complete rectangle (choice A is correct). Bottom-up processing begins with the sensory receptors and works up to the complex integration of information occurring in the brain; while bottom-up processing is a requirement of perceiving the lines in the figure, it does not explain why we see two shapes instead of a bunch of unconnected lines (choice B is wrong). Parallel processing refers to the fact that the brain is capable of processing multiple sensory inputs simultaneously and Weber's law explains how much two stimuli must differ in order for their difference to be perceptible; neither accounts for the phenomenon described in the question stem (choices C and D are wrong).

8. **B** The tympanic membrane (also known as the eardrum), located in the middle ear, generates vibrations that match the sound waves striking it (choice B is correct). Vibrations generated in the tympanic membrane pass through three small bones—the malleus (the hammer), the incus (anvil), and the stapes (stirrup); these bones magnify the incoming vibrations by focusing them onto a structure known as the oval window (choice D is wrong). Once the vibrations pass through the oval window, they enter the cochlea, a fluid-filled spiral structure in the inner ear (choice C is wrong). The base of the cochlea is lined with a long, fluid-filled duct known as the basilar membrane (choice A is wrong). Sound waves passing along the basilar membrane cause it to move up and down, stimulating hair cells in the organ of Corti. These hair cells, in turn, connect with the acoustic, or auditory nerve.

9. **C** The axons of ganglion cells in the retina make up the optic nerve, which carries visual information to the brain (choice C is correct). Photoreceptors are specialized cells in the retina that transduce light energy into nerve cell activity; they synapse with bipolar cells (which synapse with ganglion cells), but neither is part of the optic nerve (choices A and B are wrong). The fovea is the area of highest visual acuity and contains a high concentration of cones, which are a type of photoreceptor, and do not comprise the optic nerve (choice D is wrong).

10. **A** According to Alan Baddeley's information processing model, the phonological loop is the component of working memory that allows us to remember auditory information for a very brief amount of time before it is either processed or lost; therefore, this is the best explanation for why, after hearing a telephone number, we only have a few seconds to write it down before forgetting it (choice A is correct). The visuospatial sketchpad works similarly to the phonological loop, but is specific for visual, not auditory, information (choice B is wrong). The episodic buffer does not store auditory information for short periods of time (the phonological loop does), but rather allows information from the phonological loop and visuospatial sketchpad to interact, incorporates a temporal element to information, and communicates with long-term memory (choice C is wrong). The central executive is the overseer of the entire system, responsible for shifting and dividing attention; while the central executive is responsible for the ability to focus on the important information—the telephone number—it is not the part of the system that explains why this information decays so quickly if it isn't written down (choice D is wrong).

SOLUTIONS TO CHAPTER 11 PRACTICE PASSAGE

1. **C** According to Figure 1, CBT appears to be far less effective than meditation at reducing IBS symptoms for participants without an anxiety disorder (choice C is correct, and choice A is wrong). It is also far less effective for participants without an anxiety disorder than it is for participants with an anxiety disorder (choice D is wrong). CBT and meditation were not tested in combination (choice B can be eliminated).

2. **D** The adrenal glands are endocrine glands above the kidneys; in response to stress, they release hormones. The adrenal medulla (inner portion) produces epinephrine and norepinephrine (choice C is wrong) in response to direct input from the sympathetic nervous system (not the parasympathetic, choice A is wrong). This is the body's response to acute stress. The adrenal cortex (outer portion) produces corticosteroids, including cortisol; the amount of cortisol released increases as a result of long-term stress (choice D is correct). The hypothalamus and pituitary gland release hormones that trigger the release of hormones from the adrenal gland, not the other way around (choice B is wrong).

3. **A** Since the passage states at the end of the second paragraph that "IBS symptoms usually begin during late teen or early adult years," choice B is wrong, and we might conclude that these individuals are not being diagnosed because they are less affluent, and have perhaps less access to medical care (choice A is correct). In fact, many psychiatric illnesses and disorders are underdiagnosed in less affluent populations. Based solely on the information provided, you cannot conclude that there is a causal relationship between the listed factors and IBS (choice C is wrong), nor can you assume that any of these factors increase one's risk for developing IBS, such that eliminating one of the factors (marriage) will cause the IBS to go away (choice D is wrong). Correlation does not imply or prove causation.

4. **A** In statistics, validity refers to whether the results of a given study are able to answer the question being posed by that study. In the case of this study, the question is whether meditation is as effective as the current standard therapy (CBT) at reducing IBS symptoms for participants with and without an anxiety disorder. Based on the description provided in the passage, we do not know all of the specifics about this study, though we do know that the

study duration is six months (choice D is wrong). While we do not know the overall duration of IBS symptoms for participants, we do know that participants must have had active IBS for at least three months in the past year (choice B is wrong). Prior exposure to medication to treat IBS symptoms is of unknown importance, but the sample size of this study is definitely not known, and the results cannot prove that meditation is as effective as CBT without an appropriately large sample size (choice A is better than choice C).

5.   **C**   The first paragraph of the passage describes the physical responses to meditation as reduced heart rate and respiration rate. Thus, it is most likely that the anterior cingulate cortex plays a role in autonomic functions (in this case parasympathetic activity, so choice A is wrong, and choice C is correct), including the regulation of heart rate, resting respiratory rate, and blood pressure. While practitioners of meditation can reduce their respiratory rate, and while this might involve the somatic nervous system (the diaphragm is a skeletal muscle), this would not account for the reduction in heart rate (choice B is wrong). The anterior cingulate cortex is involved with rational cognitive functions, however this does not help to explain how activity in this area during meditation might inhibit the stress response (choice D is wrong).

Chapter 12
Biological Processes
in the Brain

All human behavior has a biological foundation; psychological, sociological, and biological drivers influence how we perceive and respond to our environment. The ability to receive and process sensory information is dependent on several specialized cells, receptors, and biochemical pathways. The mechanisms of sensation can be understood largely from a biological perspective. The way we perceive, interpret, and respond to sensory information, however, can be infinitely more complex. It is important to keep a psychological, social, and cultural perspective in mind when understanding perception and behavior. This chapter covers the biological foundations of behavior, including the nervous system and endocrine system, as well as some of the genetic and environmental factors that play a role in behavior.

12.1 NEURONAL STRUCTURE AND FUNCTION

Neurons are specialized cells that transmit and process information from one part of the body to another. This information takes the form of electrochemical impulses known as **action potentials**. The action potential is a localized area of depolarization of the plasma membrane that travels in a wave-like manner along an axon. When an action potential reaches the end of an axon at a synapse, the signal is transformed into a chemical signal with the release of neurotransmitter into the synaptic cleft, a process called **synaptic transmission** (Section 12.2). The information of many synapses feeding into a neuron is integrated to determine whether that neuron will in turn fire an action potential. In this way, the action of many individual neurons is integrated to work together in the nervous system as a whole.

Structure of the Neuron

The basic functional and structural unit of the nervous system is the **neuron** (Figure 1). The structure of these cells is highly specialized to transmit and process **action potentials**, the electrochemical signals of the nervous system (Figure 3). Neurons have a central cell body, the **soma**, which contains the nucleus and is where most of the biosynthetic activity of the cell takes place. Slender projections, termed **axons** and **dendrites**, extend from the cell body. Neurons have only one axon (as long as a meter in some cases), but most possess many dendrites. Neurons with one dendrite are **bipolar neuron**; those with many dendrites are **multipolar neuron**. Neurons generally carry action potentials in one direction, with dendrites receiving signals and axons carrying action potentials away from the cell body. Axons can branch multiple times and terminate in **synaptic knobs** that form connections with target cells. When action potentials travel down an axon and reach the synaptic knob, chemical messengers are released and travel across a very small gap called the **synaptic cleft** to the target cell. The nature of the action potential and the transmission of signals across the synaptic cleft are key aspects of nervous system function. [In Figure 1, in what direction does an action potential travel in the axon shown?[1] What's the difference between a neuron and a nerve?[2]]

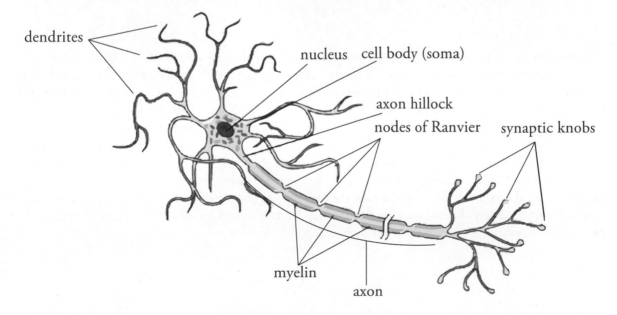

Figure 1 A multipolar neuron

---

[1] Action potentials travel from the cell body down the axon, or from left to right in Figure 1.

[2] A neuron is a single cell. A nerve is a large bundle of many different axons from different neurons.

The Action Potential

The Resting Membrane Potential

The **resting membrane potential** is an electric potential across the plasma membrane of approximately −70 millivolts (mV), with the interior of the cell negatively charged with respect to the exterior of the cell. Two primary membrane proteins are required to establish the resting membrane potential: the Na^+/K^+ ATPase and the potassium leak channels. The **Na^+/K^+ ATPase** pumps three sodium ions out of the cell and two potassium ions into the cell with the hydrolysis of one ATP molecule. The result is a sodium gradient with high sodium outside of the cell and a potassium gradient with high potassium inside the cell. **Leak channels** are channels that are open all the time and that simply allow ions to "leak" across the membrane according to their gradient. Potassium leak channels allow potassium, but no other ions, to flow down their gradient out of the cell. The combined loss of many positive ions through Na^+/K^+ ATPases and the potassium leak channels leaves the interior of the cell with a net negative charge, approximately 70 mV more negative than the exterior of the cell; this difference is the resting membrane potential. Note that there are very few sodium leak channels in the membrane (the ratio of K^+ leak channels to Na^+ leak channels is about 100:1), so the cell membrane is virtually impermeable to sodium.

The resting membrane potential establishes a negative charge along the interior of axons (along with the rest of the neuronal interior). Thus, the cells can be described as **polarized**: negative on the inside and positive on the outside. An action potential is a disturbance in this membrane potential, a wave of **depolarization** of the plasma membrane that travels along an axon. Depolarization is a change in the membrane potential from the resting membrane potential of approximately −70 mV to a less negative, or even positive, potential. After depolarization, **repolarization** returns the membrane potential to normal. The change in membrane potential during passage of an action potential is caused by movement of ions into and out of the neuron through ion channels. The action potential is therefore not strictly an electrical impulse, like electrons moving in a copper telephone wire, but an electro*chemical* impulse.

Depolarization

Key proteins in the propagation of action potentials are the **voltage-gated sodium channels** located in the plasma membrane of the axon. In response to a change in the membrane potential, these ion channels open to allow sodium ions to flow down their gradient into the cell and depolarize that section of membrane. These channels are opened by depolarization of the membrane from the resting potential of −70 mV to a **threshold potential** of approximately −50 mV. Once this threshold is reached, the channels are opened fully, but below the threshold, they are closed and do not allow the passage of any ions through the channel. When the channels open, sodium flows into the cell, down its concentration gradient, depolarizing that section of the membrane to about +35 mV before inactivating. Some of the sodium ions flow down the interior of the axon, slightly depolarizing the neighboring section of membrane. When the depolarization in the next section of membrane reaches threshold, those voltage-gated sodium channels open as well, passing the depolarization down the axon (Figure 2).

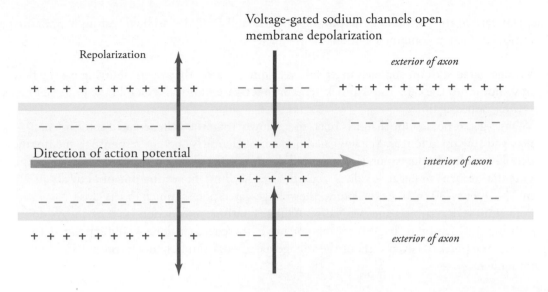

Figure 2 The action potential is a wave of membrane depolarization

Repolarization

With the opening of voltage-gated sodium channels, sodium flows into the cell and depolarizes the membrane to positive values. As the wave of depolarization passes through a region of membrane, the membrane does not remain depolarized (Figure 3).

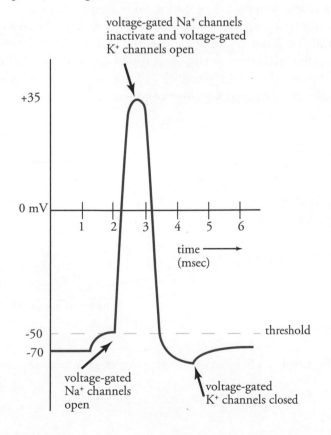

Figure 3 The action potential at a single location

After depolarization, the membrane is **repolarized**, re-establishing the original resting membrane potential. A number of factors combine to produce this effect:

1) Voltage-gated sodium channels inactivate very quickly after they open, shutting off the flow of sodium into the cell. The channels remain **inactivated** until the membrane potential nears resting values again.

2) Voltage-gated potassium channels open more slowly than the voltage-gated sodium channels and stay open longer. Voltage-gated potassium channels open in response to membrane depolarization. As potassium leaves the cell down its concentration gradient, the membrane potential returns to negative values, actually overshooting the resting potential by about 20 mV (to about −90 mV). At this point, the voltage-gated potassium channels close.

3) Potassium leak channels and the Na^+/K^+ ATPase continue to function (as they always do) to bring the membrane back to resting potential. These factors alone would repolarize the membrane potential even without the voltage-gated potassium channels, but it would take a lot longer.

Saltatory Conduction

The axons of many neurons are wrapped in an insulating sheath called **myelin** (Figure 4). The myelin sheath is not created by the neuron itself, but by cells called **Schwann cells**, a type of glial cell, that exist in conjunction with neurons, wrapping layers of specialized membrane around the axons. Note that Schwann cells are found in the peripheral nervous system (PNS). In the central nervous system (CNS), myelination of axons is accomplished via similar cells called oligodendrocytes. No ions can enter or exit a neuron where the axonal membrane is covered with myelin. There is no membrane depolarization and no voltage-gated sodium channels in regions of the axonal plasma membrane that are wrapped in myelin. There are periodic gaps in the myelin sheath, however, called **nodes of Ranvier** (Figures 1, 4, and 5). Voltage-gated sodium and potassium channels are concentrated in the nodes of Ranvier in myelinated axons. Rather than impeding action potentials, the myelin sheath dramatically speeds the movement of action potentials by forcing the action potential to jump from node to node. This rapid jumping conduction in myelinated axons is termed **saltatory conduction**.

myelin (Schwann cell)

axon

nodes of Ranvier

Figure 4   A Schwann cell wrapping an axon with myelin

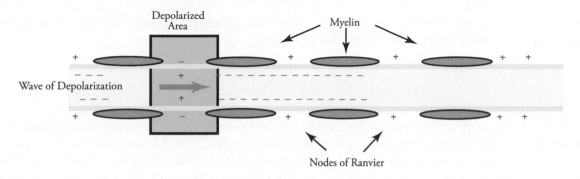

Figure 5   Propagation of the AP in a myelinated axon (cross section)

Glial Cells

As mentioned above, the myelin sheath is formed by a type of glial cell called a Schwann cell. However, Schwann cells are not the only type of glial cell. **Glial cells** are specialized, non-neuronal cells that typically provide structural and metabolic support to neurons (Table 1). Glia maintain a resting membrane potential but do not generate action potentials.

Table 1   Types of Glial Cells and Their Functions

Cell Type	Location	Primary Functions
Schwann cells	PNS	Form myelin—increase speed of conduction of APs along axon
Oligodendrocytes	CNS	Form myelin—increase speed of conduction of APs along axon
Astrocytes	CNS	Guide neuronal development Regulate synaptic communication via regulation of neurotransmitter levels
Microglia	CNS	Remove dead cells and debris
Ependymal cells	CNS	Produce and circulate cerebrospinal fluid

Equilibrium Potentials

During the action potential, the movement of Na^+ and K^+ ions across the membrane through the voltage-gated channels is *passive*; driven by gradients. The **equilibrium potential** is the membrane potential at which this driving force (the gradient) does not exist; in other words, there would be no net movement of ions across the membrane. Note that the equilibrium potential is specific for a particular ion. For example, the Na^+ equilibrium potential is *positive*, approximately +50 mV. Na^+ ions are driven inward by their concentration gradient. However, if the interior of the cell is too positive, the positively-charged ions are repelled; in other words, the *electrical* gradient would drive sodium *out*. These forces, the chemical gradient driving sodium in and the electrical gradient driving sodium out, balance each other at about +50 mV, so this is the equilibrium potential for Na^+.

K^+, however, has a *negative* equilibrium potential. K^+ ions are driven outward by their concentration gradient. However, if the interior of the cell is too negative, the positively-charged ions cannot escape the attraction; the electrical gradient drives potassium *in*. The chemical gradient driving potassium out and the electrical gradient driving potassium in balance each other at about −90 mV, so this is the equilibrium potential for K^+.

The equilibrium potential for any ion is based on the electrochemical gradient for that ion across the membrane, and can be predicted by the **Nernst equation**:

$$E_{ion} = \frac{RT}{zF} \ln \frac{[X]_{outside}}{[X]_{inside}}$$

where E_{ion} is the equilibrium potential for the ion, R is the universal gas constant, T is the temperature (in Kelvin), z is the valence of the ion, F is Faraday's constant, and $[X]$ is the concentration of the ion on each side of the plasma membrane. Note that the relative concentrations of the ion on each side of the membrane create the *chemical* gradient, while the valence (charge of the ion) helps determine the *electrical* gradient.

Note that the fact that the resting membrane potential is –70 mV reflects both the differences in the equilibrium potentials for Na$^+$ and K$^+$, and also the relative numbers of leak channels for these two ions. If the cell were completely permeable to K$^+$, the resting potential would be about –90 mV. The fact that the resting potential is *very close* to the K$^+$ equilibrium potential indicates that there are a large number of K$^+$ leak channels in the membrane; the cell at rest is almost completely permeable to potassium. However, the resting potential is slightly more positive than –90 mV, indicating that there are a few Na$^+$ leak channels allowing Na$^+$ in. There are not very many Na$^+$ leak channels, though, otherwise the resting potential would be much more positive—closer to the Na$^+$ equilibrium potential. (This is in fact what we see when the cell *does* become completely permeable to Na$^+$ at the beginning of the action potential; the membrane potential shoots upward to +35 mV.)

The Refractory Period

Action potentials can pass through a neuron extremely rapidly, thousands each second, but there is an upper limit to how soon a neuron can conduct an action potential after another has passed. The passage of one action potential makes the neuron nonresponsive to membrane depolarization and unable to transmit another action potential, or **refractory**, for a short period of time. There are two phases of the refractory period, caused by two different factors. During the **absolute refractory period**, a neuron will not fire another action potential no matter how strong a membrane depolarization is induced. During this time, the voltage-gated sodium channels have been *inactivated* (not the same as *closed*) after depolarization. They will not be able to be opened again until the membrane potential reaches the resting potential and the Na$^+$ channels have returned to their "closed" state. During the **relative refractory period**, a neuron can be induced to transmit an action potential, but the depolarization required is greater than normal because the membrane is **hyperpolarized**. When repolarization occurs, there is a brief period in which the membrane potential is more negative than the resting potential (Figure 3), caused by voltage-gated potassium channels that have not closed yet. Because it is further from threshold, a greater stimulus is required to open the voltage-gated sodium channels to start an action potential.

12.2 SYNAPTIC TRANSMISSION

A **synapse** is a junction between the axon terminus of a neuron and the dendrites, soma, or axon of a second neuron. It can also be a junction between the axon terminus of a neuron and an organ. There are two types of synapses: electrical and chemical. **Electrical synapses** occur when the cytoplasms of two cells are joined by gap junctions. If two cells are joined by an electrical synapse, an action potential will spread directly from one cell to the other. Electrical synapses are not common in the nervous system, although they are quite important in propagating action potentials in smooth muscle and cardiac muscle. In the nervous system, **chemical synapses** are found at the ends of axons where they meet their target cell; here, an action potential is converted into a chemical signal. The following steps are involved in the transmission of a signal across a chemical synapse in the nervous system (Figure 6), as well as at the junctions of neurons with other cell types, such as skeletal muscle cells:

1) An action potential reaches the end of an axon, the synaptic knob.
2) Depolarization of the presynaptic membrane opens voltage-gated calcium channels.
3) Calcium influx into the presynaptic cell causes exocytosis of neurotransmitter stored in secretory vesicles.
4) Neurotransmitter molecules diffuse across the narrow synaptic cleft (small space between cells).
5) Neurotransmitter binds to receptor proteins in the postsynaptic membrane. These receptors are ligand-gated ion channels.
6) The opening of these ion channels in the postsynaptic cell alters the membrane polarization.
7) If the membrane depolarization of the postsynaptic cell reaches the threshold of voltage-gated sodium channels, an action potential is initiated.
8) Neurotransmitter in the synaptic cleft is degraded and/or removed to terminate the signal.

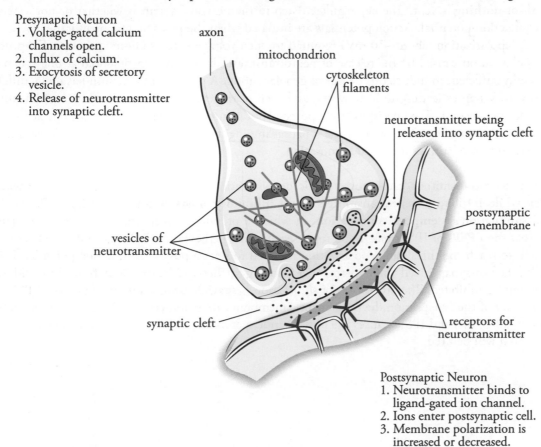

Presynaptic Neuron
1. Voltage-gated calcium channels open.
2. Influx of calcium.
3. Exocytosis of secretory vesicle.
4. Release of neurotransmitter into synaptic cleft.

axon

mitochondrion

cytoskeleton filaments

neurotransmitter being released into synaptic cleft

postsynaptic membrane

vesicles of neurotransmitter

synaptic cleft

receptors for neurotransmitter

Postsynaptic Neuron
1. Neurotransmitter binds to ligand-gated ion channel.
2. Ions enter postsynaptic cell.
3. Membrane polarization is increased or decreased.

Figure 6 A typical synapse

An example of a chemical synapse that is commonly used is the **neuromuscular junction** between neurons and skeletal muscle. The neurotransmitter that is released at the neuromuscular junction is **acetylcholine (ACh)**. When an action potential reaches such a synapse, acetylcholine is released into the synaptic cleft. The acetylcholine binds to the acetylcholine receptor on the surface of the postsynaptic cell membrane. When acetylcholine binds to its receptor, the receptor opens its associated sodium channel, allowing sodium to flow down a gradient into the cell, depolarizing the postsynaptic cell membrane. Meanwhile, acetylcholine in the synaptic cleft is degraded by the enzyme **acetylcholinesterase (AChE)**.

There are several different neurotransmitters and neurotransmitter receptors. Some of the other neurotransmitters are **gamma-aminobutyric acid (GABA)**, **serotonin**, **dopamine**, and **norepinephrine**. If a neurotransmitter, such as acetylcholine, opens a channel that depolarizes the postsynaptic membrane, the neurotransmitter is termed **excitatory**. Other neurotransmitters, however, have the opposite effect, making the postsynaptic membrane potential more negative than the resting potential, or hyperpolarized. Neurotransmitters that induce hyperpolarization of the postsynaptic membrane are termed **inhibitory.** (Note, however, that ultimately it is not the *neurotransmitter* that determines the effect on the postsynaptic cell, it is the *receptor* for that neurotransmitter and its associated ion channel. The same neurotransmitter can be excitatory in some cases and inhibitory in others.) Postsynaptic neurons may have many different receptors, allowing them to respond to many different neurotransmitters.

Summation

Once an action potential is initiated in a neuron, it will propagate to the end of the axon at a speed and magnitude of depolarization that do not vary from one action potential to another. The action potential is an "**all-or-nothing**" event. The key-regulated step in the nervous system is whether or not a neuron will fire an action potential. Action potentials are initiated when the postsynaptic membrane reaches the threshold depolarization (about −50 mV) required to open voltage-gated sodium channels. The postsynaptic depolarization caused by the release of neurotransmitter by one action potential at one synapse is not generally sufficient to induce this degree of depolarization. A postsynaptic neuron has many different neurons with synapses leading to it, however, and each of these synapses can release neurotransmitters many times per second. The "decision" by a postsynaptic neuron whether to fire an action potential is determined by adding the effect of all of the synapses impinging on a neuron, both excitatory and inhibitory. This addition of stimuli is termed **summation**.

Excitatory neurotransmitters cause postsynaptic depolarization, or **excitatory postsynaptic potentials (EPSPs)**, while inhibitory neurotransmitters cause **inhibitory postsynaptic potentials (IPSPs)**. One form of summation is **temporal summation**, in which a presynaptic neuron fires action potentials so rapidly that the EPSPs or IPSPs pile up on top of each other. If they are EPSPs, the additive effect might be enough to reach the threshold depolarization required to start a postsynaptic action potential. If they are IPSPs, the postsynaptic cell will hyperpolarize, moving further and further away from threshold, effectively becoming inhibited. The other form of summation is **spatial summation**, in which the EPSPs and IPSPs from all of the synapses on the postsynaptic membrane are summed at a given moment in time. If the total of all EPSPs and IPSPs causes the postsynaptic membrane to reach the threshold voltage, an action potential will be fired.

12.3 FUNCTIONAL ORGANIZATION OF THE HUMAN NERVOUS SYSTEM

The nervous system must receive information, decide what to do with it, and cause muscles or glands to act upon that decision. Receiving information is the **sensory** function of the nervous system (carried out by the peripheral nervous system, or **PNS**), processing the information is the **integrative** function (carried out by the central nervous system, or **CNS**), and acting on it is the **motor** function (also carried out by the PNS). **Motor neurons** carry information from the nervous system toward organs which can act upon that information, known as **effectors**. Notice that "motor" neurons do not lead only "to muscle." Motor neurons, which carry information away from the central nervous system and innervate effectors, are called **efferent** neurons (remember, efferents go to effectors). **Sensory neurons**, which carry information toward the central nervous system, are called **afferent** neurons.

Reflexes

The simplest example of nervous system activity is the **reflex**. This is a direct motor response to sensory input which occurs without conscious thought. In fact, it usually occurs without any involvement of the brain at all. In the simplest example, a sensory neuron transmits an action potential to a synapse with a motor neuron in the spinal cord, which causes an action to occur. For example, in the **muscle stretch reflex**, a sensory neuron detects stretching of a muscle (Figure 7). The sensory neuron has a long dendrite and a long axon, which transmits an impulse to a motor neuron cell body in the spinal cord. The motor neuron's long axon synapses with the muscle that was stretched and causes it to contract. That is why the quadriceps (thigh) muscle contracts when the patellar tendon is stretched by tapping it with a reflex hammer. A reflex such as this one, involving only two neurons and one synapse, is known as a **monosynaptic reflex arc.**

Something else also happens when a physician taps the patellar tendon. Not only does the quadriceps *contract*, but the hamstring also *relaxes*. If it did not, the leg would not be able to extend (straighten). The sensory neuron (that detects stretch) synapses with not only a motor neuron for the quadriceps, but also with an **inhibitory interneuron**. This is a short neuron which forms an inhibitory synapse with a motor neuron innervating the hamstring muscle. When the sensory neuron is stimulated by stretch, it stimulates both the quadriceps motor neuron and the inhibitory interneuron to the hamstring motor neuron. The interneuron inhibits the motor neuron for the hamstring. As a result, the quadriceps contracts and the hamstring relaxes (note that the hamstring part of the reflex—sensory neuron to interneuron to hamstring motor neuron—involves three neurons and two synapses, hence it is known as a **disynaptic reflex arc**). An interneuron is the simplest example of the integrative role of the nervous system. Concurrent relaxation of the hamstring and contraction of the quadriceps is an example of **reciprocal inhibition**.

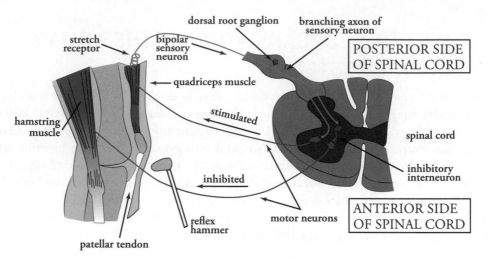

Figure 7 The muscle stretch reflex

Large-Scale Functional Organization

The peripheral nervous system can be subdivided into several functional divisions (Figure 8). The portion of this system concerned with conscious sensation and deliberate, voluntary movement of skeletal muscle is the **somatic** division. The portion concerned with digestion, metabolism, circulation, perspiration, and other involuntary processes is the **autonomic** division. The somatic and autonomic divisions both include afferent and efferent functions, although the sources of sensory input and the target of efferent nerves are different. The efferent portion of the autonomic division is further split into two subdivisions: **sympathetic** and **parasympathetic**. When the sympathetic system is activated, the body is prepared for "fight or flight." When the parasympathetic system is activated, the body is prepared to "rest and digest." Table 2 summarizes the main effects of the autonomic system. Notice that many sympathetic effects result from release of epinephrine into the bloodstream by the adrenal medulla. The parasympathetic system prepares you to rest and digest food.

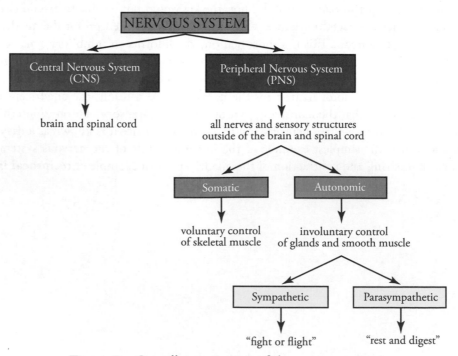

Figure 8 Overall organization of the nervous system

Table 2 Effects of the Autonomic Nervous System

Organ or System		Parasympathetic: rest and digest	Sympathetic: fight or flight
digestive system:	glands	stimulation	inhibition
	motility	stimulation (stimulates digestion)	inhibition (inhibits digestion)
	sphincters	relaxation	contraction
urinary system:	bladder	contraction (stimulates urination)	relaxation (inhibits urination)
	urethral sphincter	relaxation (stimulates urination)	contraction (inhibits urination)
bronchial smooth muscle		constriction (closes airways)	relaxation (opens airways)
cardiovascular system:			
heart rate and contractility		decreased	increased
blood flow to skeletal muscle		—	increased
skin		—	sweating and general vasoconstriction; emotional vasodilation (blushing)
eye:	pupil	constriction	dilation
	muscles controlling lens	near vision accommodation	accommodation for far vision
adrenal medulla		—	release of epinephrine
genitals		erection / lubrication	ejaculation / orgasm

PNS Anatomical Organization

All neurons entering and exiting the CNS are carried by 12 pairs of **cranial nerves** and 31 pairs of **spinal nerves**. Cranial nerves convey sensory and motor information to and from the brainstem. Spinal nerves convey sensory and motor information to and from the spinal cord. The different functional divisions of the nervous system have different anatomical organizations (Figure 9).

The **vagus nerve** is an important example of a cranial nerve, and one that you should be familiar with for the MCAT. The effects of this nerve upon the heart and GI tract are to decrease the heart rate and increase GI activity; as such, it is part of the *parasympathetic division* of the autonomic nervous system. It is a bundle of axons that end in ganglia on the surface of the heart, stomach, and other visceral organs. The many axons constituting the vagus nerve are preganglionic and come from cell bodies located in the CNS. On the surface of the heart and stomach they synapse with postganglionic neurons. The detailed terminology in this paragraph will make more sense to you as you read through the next couple of sections.

Somatic PNS Anatomy

The somatic system has a simple organization:

- *All* somatic motor neurons innervate skeletal muscle cells, use ACh as their neurotransmitter, and have their cell bodies in the brain stem or the ventral (front) portion of the spinal cord.

- *All* somatic sensory neurons have a long dendrite extending from a sensory receptor toward the soma, which is located just outside the CNS in a **dorsal root ganglion**. The dorsal root ganglion is a bunch of somatic (and autonomic) sensory neuron cell bodies located just dorsal to (to the back of) the spinal cord. There is a pair of dorsal root ganglia for every segment of the spinal cord, and thus the dorsal root ganglia form a chain along the dorsal (back) aspect of the vertebral column. The dorsal root ganglia are protected within the vertebral column but are outside the **meninges** (protective sheath of the brain and cord) and thus outside the CNS. An axon extends from the somatic sensory neuron's soma into the spinal cord. In all somatic sensory neurons, the first synapse is in the CNS; depending on the type of sensory information conveyed, the axon either synapses in the cord, or stretches all the way up to the brain stem before its first synapse!

Autonomic PNS Anatomy

Anatomical organization of autonomic efferents is a bit more complex. The efferents of the sympathetic and parasympathetic systems consist of two neurons: a preganglionic and a postganglionic neuron. The **preganglionic neuron** has its cell body in the brainstem or spinal cord. It sends an axon to an autonomic ganglion, located outside the spinal column. In the ganglion, this axon synapses with a **postganglionic neuron**. The postganglionic neuron sends an axon to an effector (smooth muscle or gland). *All* autonomic preganglionic neurons release acetylcholine as their neurotransmitter. *All* parasympathetic postganglionic neurons also release acetylcholine. Nearly all sympathetic postganglionic neurons release norepinephrine (NE, also known as noradrenaline) as their neurotransmitter.

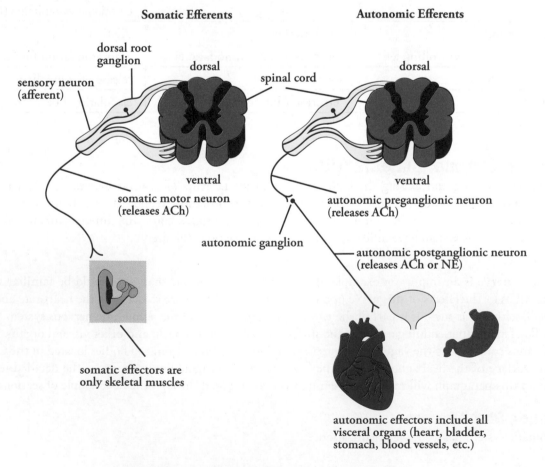

Figure 9   Anatomical organization of PNS efferents

All sympathetic preganglionic efferent neurons have their cell bodies in the thoracic (chest) or lumbar (lower back) regions of the spinal cord. Hence, the sympathetic system is also referred to as the *thoraco-lumbar system*. The parasympathetic system is known as the *craniosacral system*, because all of its preganglionic neurons have cell bodies in the brainstem (which is in the head or cranium) or in the lowest portion of the spinal cord, the sacral portion. In the sympathetic system, the preganglionic axon is relatively short, and there are only a few ganglia; these sympathetic ganglia are quite large. The sympathetic postganglionic cell sends a long axon to the effector. In contrast, the parasympathetic preganglionic neuron sends a long axon to a small ganglion which is close to the effector. For example, parasympathetic ganglia controlling the intestines are located on the outer wall of the gut. The parasympathetic postganglionic neuron has a very short axon, since the cell body is close to the target. These differences are visualized in Figure 10 and summarized in Table 3.

Figure 10 Pre- and post-ganglionic fibers of the autonomic nervous system

The autonomic afferent (sensory) neurons are similar to the somatic afferent neurons with one exception: they can synapse in the PNS (at the autonomic ganglia) with autonomic efferent neurons in what is known as a "short reflex." (Recall that the first synapse of somatic afferent neurons is in the CNS.)

Table 3 Sympathetic vs. Parasympathetic

	Sympathetic	**Parasympathetic**
General function	fight or flight, mobilize energy	rest and digest, store energy
Location of preganglionic soma	thoracolumbar = thoracic and lumbar spinal cord	craniosacral = brainstem ("cranial") and sacral spinal cord
Preganglionic axon neurotransmitter = acetylcholine (ACh)	short	long
Ganglia	close to cord, far from target	far from cord, close to target
Postganglionic axon (usual neurotransmitter)	long (norepinephrine [NE])	short (ACh)

The Adrenal Medulla

The **adrenal gland** is named for its location: "ad-" means "above" and "renal" refers to the kidney. There are two adrenal glands, one above each kidney. The adrenal has an inner portion known as the **medulla** and an outer portion known as the **cortex**. The cortex is an important endocrine gland, secreting **glucocorticoids** (the main one is cortisol), **mineralocorticoids** (the main one is aldosterone), and some sex hormones.

The **adrenal medulla,** however, is part of the sympathetic nervous system. It is embryologically derived from sympathetic postganglionic neurons and is directly innervated by sympathetic preganglionic neurons. Upon activation of the sympathetic system, the adrenal gland is stimulated to release **epinephrine**, also known as **adrenaline**. Epinephrine is a slightly modified version of *nor*epinephrine, the neurotransmitter released by sympathetic postganglionic neurons. Epinephrine is a hormone because it is released into the bloodstream by a ductless gland. But in many ways it behaves like a neurotransmitter. It elicits its effects very rapidly, and the effects are quite short-lived. Epinephrine release from the adrenal medulla is what causes the sudden flushing and sweating one experiences when severely startled. In general, epinephrine's effects are those listed in Table 4 for the sympathetic system. Stimulation of the heart is an especially important effect.

12.4   THE ENDOCRINE SYSTEM

The nervous system and endocrine system represent the two major control systems of the body. The nervous system is fast-acting with relatively short-term effects, whereas the endocrine system takes longer to communicate signals but has generally longer lasting effects. These two control systems are interconnected, as neurons can signal the release of hormones from endocrine glands. A primary connection between the nervous and endocrine systems is the **hypothalamic-pituitary axis**, which is described in more detail below.

Hormone Types: Transport and Mechanisms of Action

While the nervous system regulates cellular function from instant to instant, the endocrine system regulates physiology (especially metabolism) over a period of hours to days. The nervous system communicates via the extremely rapid action potential. The signal of the endocrine system is the **hormone**, defined as a molecule which is *secreted into the bloodstream* by an endocrine gland, and which has its effects upon *distant* target cells possessing the appropriate receptor. An **endocrine gland** is a *ductless* gland whose secretory products are picked up by capillaries supplying blood to the region. (In contrast, **exocrine glands** secrete their products into the external environment by way of ducts, which empty into the gastrointestinal lumen or the external world.) A **hormone receptor** is a polypeptide that possesses a ligand-specific binding site. Binding of ligand (hormone) to the site causes the receptor to modify target cell activity. *Tissue-specificity of hormone action is determined by whether the cells of a tissue have the appropriate receptor.*

Some signaling molecules modify the activity of the cell which secreted them; this is an **autocrine** activity (*auto-* means self). For example, a T cell secretes interleukin 2, which binds to receptors on the same T cell to stimulate increased activity.

Hormones can be grouped into one of two classes. *Hydrophilic* hormones, such as **peptides** and **amino-acid derivatives**, must bind to receptors on the cell surface, while *hydrophobic* hormones, such as the **steroid hormones**, bind to receptors in the cellular interior.

Peptide Hormones

Peptide hormones are synthesized in the rough ER and modified in the Golgi. Then they are stored in vesicles until needed, when they are released by exocytosis. In the bloodstream they dissolve in the plasma, since they are hydrophilic. Their hydrophilicity also means they cannot cross biological membranes and thus are required to communicate with the interior of the target cell by way of a second messenger cascade. To briefly review, the peptide hormone is a first messenger which must bind to a cell-surface receptor. The receptor is a polypeptide with a domain on the inner surface of the plasma membrane that contains the ability to catalytically activate a second messenger. The end result of second messenger activation is that the function of proteins in the cytoplasm is changed. A key feature of second messenger cascades is signal amplification, which allows a few activated receptors to change the activity of many enzymes in the cytoplasm.

Because peptide hormones modify the activity of existing enzymes in the cytoplasm, their effects are exerted rapidly, minutes to hours from the time of secretion. Also, the duration of their effects is brief.

There are two subgroups within the peptide hormone category: polypeptides and amino acid derivatives. An example of a polypeptide hormone is insulin, which has a complex tertiary structure involving disulfide bridges. It is secreted by the β cells of the pancreatic islets of Langerhans in response to elevated blood glucose and binds to a cell-surface receptor with a cytoplasmic domain possessing protein kinase activity. Amino acid derivatives, as their name implies, are derived from single amino acids and contain no peptide bonds. For example, tyrosine is the parent amino acid for the catecholamines (which include epinephrine) and the thyroid hormones. Despite the fact that these two classes are derived from the same precursor molecule, they have different properties. The catecholamines act like peptide hormones, while the thyroid hormones behave more like steroid hormones. Epinephrine is a small cyclic molecule secreted by the adrenal medulla upon activation of the sympathetic nervous system. It binds to cell-surface receptors to trigger a cascade of events that produces the second messenger cyclic adenosine monophosphate (cAMP) and activates protein kinases in the cytoplasm. Thyroid hormones incorporate iodine into their structure. They enter cells, bind to DNA, and activate transcription of genes involved in energy mobilization.

12.4

Steroid Hormones

Steroids are hydrophobic molecules synthesized from cholesterol in the smooth endoplasmic reticulum. Due to their hydrophobicity, steroids can freely diffuse through biological membranes. Thus, they are not stored but rather diffuse into the bloodstream as soon as they are made. If a steroid hormone is not needed, it will not be made. Steroids' hydrophobicity also means they cannot be dissolved in the plasma. Instead they journey through the bloodstream stuck to proteins in the plasma, such as albumin. The small, hydrophobic steroid hormone exerts its effects upon target cells by *diffusing through the plasma membrane to bind with a receptor in the cytoplasm*. Once it has bound its ligand, the steroid hormone-receptor complex is transported into the nucleus, where it acts as a sequence-specific regulator of transcription. Because steroid hormones must modify transcription to change the *amount* and/or *type* of proteins in the cell, their effects are exerted slowly, over a period of days, and persist for days to weeks.

Steroids regulating sexuality, reproduction, and development are secreted by the testes, ovaries, and placenta. Steroids regulating water balance and other processes are secreted by the adrenal cortex. All other endocrine glands secrete peptide hormones. (Note that although thyroid hormone is derived from an amino acid, its mechanism of action more closely resembles that of the steroid hormones.)

Table 4   Peptide vs. Steroid Hormones

	Peptides	**Steroids**
Structure	hydrophilic, large (polypeptides) or small (amino acid derivatives)	hydrophobic, small
Site of synthesis	rough ER	smooth ER
Regulation of release	stored in vesicles until a signal for secretion is received	synthesized only when needed and then used immediately, not stored
Transport in bloodstream	free	stuck to protein carrier
Specificity	only target cells have appropriate surface receptors (exception: thyroxine = cytoplasmic)	only target cells have appropriate cytoplasmic receptors
Mechanism of effect	bind to receptors that generate second messengers which result in modification of *enzyme activity*	bind to receptors that alter *gene expression* by regulating DNA transcription
Timing of effect	rapid, short-lived	slow, long-lasting

Organization and Regulation of the Human Endocrine System

The endocrine system has many different roles. Hormones are essential for gamete synthesis, ovulation, pregnancy, growth, sexual development, and overall level of metabolic activity. Despite this diversity of function, endocrine activity is harmoniously orchestrated. Maintenance of order in such a complex system might seem impossible to accomplish in a preplanned manner. Regulation of the endocrine system is not preplanned or rigidly structured, but is instead generally automatic. Hormone levels rise and fall as dictated by physiological needs. The endocrine system is ordered yet dynamic. This flexible, automatic orderliness is attributable to feedback regulation. The amount of a hormone secreted is controlled not by a preformulated plan but rather by changes in the variable the hormone is responsible for controlling.

Continuous circulation of blood exposes target cells to regulatory hormones and also exposes endocrine glands to serum concentrations of physiological variables that they regulate. Thus, *regulator* and that which is *regulated* are in continuous communication. Concentration of a species X in the aqueous portion of the bloodstream is denoted "serum [X]."

An example of feedback regulation is the interaction between the hormone calcitonin and serum $[Ca^{2+}]$. The function of calcitonin is to prevent serum $[Ca^{2+}]$ from peaking above normal levels, and the amount of calcitonin secreted is directly proportional to increases in serum $[Ca^{2+}]$ above normal. When serum $[Ca^{2+}]$ becomes elevated, calcitonin is secreted. Then when serum $[Ca^{2+}]$ levels fall, calcitonin secretion stops. The falling serum $[Ca^{2+}]$ level (*that which is regulated*) feeds back to the cells which secrete calcitonin (*regulators*). The serum $[Ca^{2+}]$ level is a **physiological endpoint** which must be maintained at constant levels. This demonstrates the role of the endocrine system in maintaining **homeostasis**, or physiological consistency.

An advantage of the endocrine system and its feedback regulation is that very complex arrays of variables can be controlled automatically. It's as if the variables controlled themselves. However, some integration (a central control mechanism) is necessary. Superimposed upon the hormonal regulation of physiological endpoints is another layer of regulation: hormones that regulate hormones. Such meta-regulators are known as **tropic hormones**.

For example, adrenocorticotropic hormone (ACTH) is secreted by the anterior pituitary. The role of ACTH is to stimulate increased activity of the portion of the adrenal gland called the **cortex**, which is responsible for secreting cortisol (among other steroid hormones). ACTH is a tropic hormone because it does not directly affect physiological endpoints, but merely regulates another regulator (cortisol). Cortisol regulates physiological endpoints, including cellular responses to stress and serum [glucose]. Feedback regulation applies to tropic hormones as well as to direct regulators of physiological endpoints; the level of ACTH is influenced by the level of cortisol. When cortisol is needed, ACTH is secreted, and when the serum [cortisol] increases sufficiently, ACTH secretion slows.

You may have noticed that in both of our examples the effect of feedback was *inhibitory*: the result of hormone secretion inhibits further secretion. Inhibitory feedback is called **negative feedback** or **feedback inhibition**. Most feedback in the endocrine system (and if you remember, most biochemical feedback in general) is negative. There are few examples of positive feedback which we will not discuss here.

There is yet another layer of control. Many of the functions of the endocrine system depend on instructions from the brain. The portion of the brain which controls much of the endocrine system is the **hypothalamus**, located at the center of the brain. The hypothalamus controls the endocrine system by releasing tropic hormones that regulate other tropic hormones, called **releasing and inhibiting factors** or **releasing and inhibiting hormones**.

For example (Figure 11), the hypothalamus secretes corticotropin-releasing hormone (CRH, also known as CRF, where "F" stands for factor). The role of CRH is to cause increased secretion of ACTH. Just as ACTH secretion is regulated by feedback inhibition from cortisol, CRH secretion, too, is inhibited by cortisol. You begin to see that regulatory pathways in the endocrine system can get pretty complex.

12.4

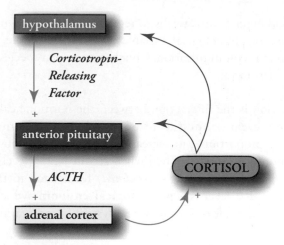

Figure 11   Feedback regulation of cortisol secretion

Understanding that the hypothalamus controls the anterior pituitary and that the anterior pituitary controls most of the endocrine system is important. Damage to the connection between the hypothalamus and the pituitary is fatal, unless daily hormone replacement therapy is given. This endocrine control center is given a special name: **hypothalamic-pituitary control axis** (Figure 12). The hypothalamus exerts its control of the pituitary by secreting its hormones into the bloodstream, just like any other endocrine gland; what's unique is that a special miniature circulatory system is provided for efficient transport of hypothalamic releasing and inhibiting factors to the anterior pituitary. This blood supply is known as the **hypothalamic-pituitary portal system**. You will also hear the term *hypothalamic-hypophysial portal system*. **Hypophysis** is another name for the pituitary gland.

A Note on Portal Systems: As a general rule, blood leaving the heart moves through only one capillary bed before returning to the heart, since the pressure drops substantially in capillaries. A portal system, however, consists of two capillary beds in sequence, allowing for direct communication between nearby structures. The two portal systems you need to understand are: the hypothalamic-pituitary portal system and the hepatic portal system (from the gastrointestinal tract to the liver).

One more bit of background information is necessary before we can delve into specific hormones. The pituitary gland has two halves: front (*anterior*) and back (*posterior*); see Figure 12. The **anterior pituitary** is also called the **adenohypophysis** and the **posterior pituitary** is also known as the **neurohypophysis**. It is important to understand the difference. The anterior pituitary is a normal endocrine gland, and it is controlled by hypothalamic releasing and inhibiting factors (essentially tropic hormones). The posterior pituitary is composed of axons which descend from the hypothalamus. These hypothalamic neurons that send axons down to the posterior pituitary are an example of **neuroendocrine cells**, neurons which secrete hormones into the bloodstream. The hormones of the posterior pituitary are ADH (antidiuretic hormone or vasopressin), which causes the kidney to retain water during times of thirst, and oxytocin, which causes milk let-down for nursing as well as uterine contractions during labor.

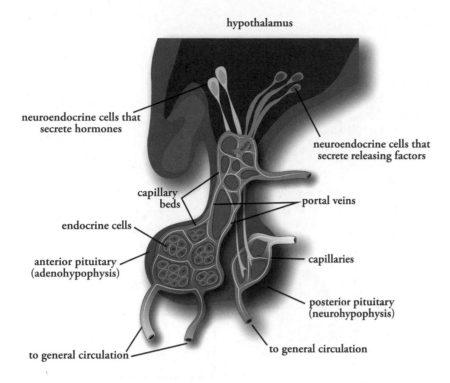

hypothalamus

neuroendocrine cells that
secrete hormones

neuroendocrine cells that
secrete releasing factors

capillary
beds

portal veins

endocrine cells

anterior pituitary
(adenohypophysis)

capillaries

posterior pituitary
(neurohypophysis)

to general circulation

to general circulation

Figure 12   The hypothalamic-pituitary control axis

Major Glands and Their Hormones

The major hormones and glands of the endocrine system are shown in Figure 13 and listed in Table 5. Many of these hormones will be discussed in detail in the MCAT Biology Review. The function of epinephrine has already been presented as part of the sympathetic nervous system response. In general, the hormones are involved in development of the body and in maintenance of constant conditions, homeostasis, in the adult.

Thyroid hormone and **cortisol** have broad effects on metabolism and energy usage. Thyroid hormone is produced from the amino acid tyrosine in the thyroid gland and comes in two forms, with three or four iodine atoms per molecule. The production of thyroid hormone is increased by thyroid stimulating hormone (TSH) from the anterior pituitary, which is regulated by the hypothalamus and the central nervous system in turn. The mechanism of action of thyroid hormone is to bind to a receptor in the cytoplasm of cells that then regulates transcription in the nucleus. The effect of this regulation is to increase the overall metabolic rate and body temperature, and, in children, to stimulate growth. Exposure to cold can increase the production of thyroid hormone. Cortisol is secreted by the adrenal cortex in response to ACTH from the pituitary. In general, the effects of cortisol tend to help the body deal with stress. Cortisol helps to mobilize glycogen and fat stores to provide energy during stress and also increases the consumption of proteins for energy. These effects are essential, since removal of the adrenal cortex can result in the death of animals exposed to even a small stress. Long-term high levels of cortisol tend to have negative effects, however, including suppression of the immune system.

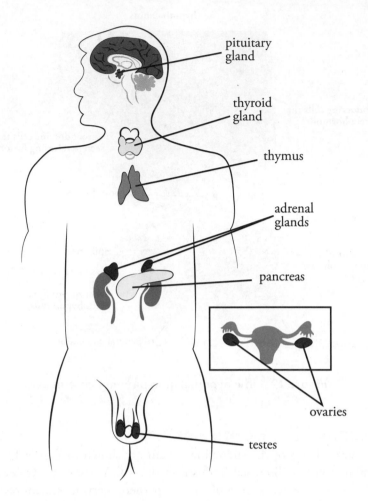

Figure 13   The major endocrine glands

Table 5 Summary of the Hormones of the Endocrine System

Gland	Hormone [class]	Target/effect
Hypothalamus	releasing and inhibiting factors (peptides)	anterior pituitary/modify activity
Anterior pituitary	growth hormone (GH) (peptide)	↑ bone & muscle growth, ↑ cell turnover rate
	prolactin (peptide)	mammary gland/milk production
tropic	thyroid stimulating hormone (TSH) (peptide)	thyroid/↑ synthesis & release of TH
	adrenocorticotropic hormone (ACTH) (peptide)	↑ growth & secretory activity of adrenal ctx
gonadotropic	luteinizing hormone (LH) (peptide)	ovary/ovulation, testes/testosterone synth.
	follicle stimulating hormone (FSH) (peptide)	ovary/follicle development, testes/spermatogenesis
Posterior pituitary	antidiuretic hormone (ADH, vasopressin) (peptide)	kidney/water retention
	oxytocin (peptide)	breast/milk let-down, uterus/contraction
Thyroid	thyroid hormone (TH, thyroxine) (modified amino acid)	child: necessary for physical & mental development; adult: ↑ metabolic rate & temp.
thyroid C cells	calcitonin (peptide)	bone, kidney; lowers serum $[Ca^{2+}]$
Parathyroids	parathyroid hormone (PTH) (peptide)	bone, kidney, small intestine/raises serum $[Ca^{2+}]$
Thymus	thymosin (children only) (peptide)	T cell development during childhood
Adrenal medulla	epinephrine (modified amino acid)	sympathetic stress response (rapid)
Adrenal cortex	cortisol ("glucocorticoid") (steroid)	longer-term stress response; ↑ blood [glucose]; ↑ protein catabolism; ↓ inflammation & immunity; many other
	aldosterone ("mineralocorticoid") (steroid)	kidney/↑ Na^+ reabsorption to ↑ b.p.
	sex steroids	not normally important, but an adrenal tumor can overproduce these, causing masculinization or feminization
Endocrine pancreas (islets of Langerhans)	insulin (β cells secrete) (peptide) —absent or ineffective in diabetes mellitus	↓ blood [glucose]/↑ glycogen & fat storage
	glucagon (α cells secrete) (peptide)	↑ blood [glucose]/↓ glycogen & fat storage
	somatostatin (SS—δ cells secrete) (peptide)	inhibits many digestive processes
Testes	testosterone (steroid)	male characteristics, spermatogenesis
Ovaries/placenta	estrogen (steroid)	female characteristics, endometrial growth
	progesterone (steroid)	endometrial secretion, pregnancy
Heart	atrial natriuretic factor (ANF) (peptide)	kidney/↑ urination to ↓ blood pressure
Kidney	erythropoietin (peptide)	bone marrow/↑ RBC synthesis

Chapter 12 Summary

- The neuron is the basic structural and functional unit of the nervous system. It has several specialized structures that allow it to transmit action potentials.

- Neurons receive incoming information via dendrites. Signals are summed by the axon hillock, and if the signal is greater than the threshold, an action potential is initiated.

- The action potential is an all-or-none signal that includes depolarization (via voltage-gated sodium channels) and repolarization (via voltage-gated potassium channels); it begins and ends at the cell's resting potential of −70 mV.

- Since action potentials are all-or-none events, signal intensity is coded by the frequency of the action potentials being fired.

- Neurons communicate with other neurons, organs, and glands at synapses. Most synapses are chemical in nature.

- The central nervous system includes the spinal cord and the brain; specialized areas control specific aspects of human behavior, movement, intelligence, emotion, and reflexes.

- The peripheral nervous system includes the somatic (voluntary) and autonomic (involuntary) subdivisions.

- The sympathetic branch of the autonomic system controls our fight-or-flight response; norepinephrine is the primary neurotransmitter of this system, and it is augmented by epinephrine from the adrenal medulla.

- The parasympathetic branch of the autonomic system controls our resting and digesting state; acetylcholine is the primary neurotransmitter of this system.

- Humans have several types of receptors (mechanoreceptors, chemoreceptors, nociceptors, thermoreceptors, electromagnetic receptors, and proprioceptors) that allow us to detect a variety of stimuli.

- The endocrine system controls our overall physiology and homeostasis by hormones that travel through the bloodstream.

- Peptide hormones are made from amino acids, bind to receptors on the cell surface, and typically affect target cells via second messenger pathways.

- Steroid hormones are derived from cholesterol, bind to receptors in the cytoplasm or nucleus, and bind to DNA to alter transcription.

CHAPTER 12 FREESTANDING PRACTICE QUESTIONS

1. A demyelinating disorder, such as multiple sclerosis, would cause all of the following symptoms EXCEPT:

A) a reduction of white matter in the central nervous system.
B) increased saltatory conduction.
C) slower propagation of signals along the axon.
D) a deficiency of sensation.

2. Which area of the brain is responsible for coordinating complex motor functions?

A) Frontal lobe
B) Occipital lobe
C) Reticular activating system
D) Cerebellum

3. All of the following brain areas are associated with the experience of emotion EXCEPT the:

A) temporal lobes.
B) amygdala.
C) hypothalamus.
D) pons.

4. Acetylcholine is stimulatory to which of the following?

   I.   Skeletal muscle
  II.   Postganglionic neurons
 III.   Cardiac muscle

A) I only
B) I and II only
C) II and III only
D) I, II, and III

5. Cortisol has a direct inhibitory effect on:

A) the posterior pituitary.
B) the hypothalamus.
C) the adrenal cortex.
D) glycogen mobilization.

CHAPTER 12 PRACTICE PASSAGE

Long-term potentiation (LTP) involves communication between two neurons and is a major cellular mechanism underlying learning and memory processes. During LTP, a presynaptic neuron releases the neurotransmitter glutamate, which binds to receptors on the postsynaptic neuron. This leads to an influx of sodium, and ultimately calcium, followed by activation of various genes (see Figure 1). The initial receptor activated by glutamate is the AMPA receptor; the NMDA receptor is blocked by extracellular Mg^{2+} that must be displaced by a sufficient change in membrane potential before that channel will fully open.

LTP has been shown to be disrupted in neurodegenerative disorders, such as Alzheimer's disease, leading to memory deficits. In the brains of Alzheimer's patients, loss of vital neurons occurs in the hippocampus (a region of the brain involved in memory acquisition). Several mechanisms are hypothesized to lead to this neurodegeneration. One involves calcium-mediated toxicity and occurs due to excessive glutamate-induced neuronal excitation.

Another potential contributing factor to this cell loss is exposure to chronic stress, which results in elevated levels of corticosteroids that can influence neuronal activity in the brain. This has led to the formation of the "glucocorticoid hypothesis of aging." The intact hippocampus has an inhibitory effect on the stress axis (hypothalamic-pituitary-adrenal axis) that is responsible for inducing release of cortisol from the adrenal gland during times of stress. Thus, if the hippocampal region is compromised, it could lead to lack of inhibition of the stress axis and further release of cortisol, causing a feed-forward cycle of excessive release of steroids with each stressful event.

Figure 1   Synaptic transmission during LTP

1. In which region of the brain is the hippocampus located?

A) Cerebellum
B) Occipital lobe
C) Temporal lobe
D) Hypothalamus

2. One treatment for Alzheimer's disease involves a drug that blocks NMDA receptors. This treatment could lead to all of the following EXCEPT:

A) a suppression of LTP.
B) a suppression of gene expression.
C) a significant decrease in intracellular sodium.
D) a significant decrease in intracellular calcium.

3. A researcher removes the adrenal glands from a rat and then supplements the rat with baseline levels of steroids for the remainder of its lifespan. Which of the following would be expected?

    I.   Blunted sympathetic nervous system response
    II. Slowing of age-related neurodegeneration
    III. Enhancement of LTP

A) II only
B) II and III
C) I and II
D) I, II, and III

4. Which of the following statements is LEAST likely to be true?

A) Drugs that increase Cl^- influx into the postsynaptic cell could disrupt LTP.
B) Drugs that increase K^+ efflux from the postsynaptic cell would result in hyperpolarization of the cell and would increase LTP.
C) The insertion of new AMPA receptors in the postsynaptic cell membrane would increase the rate at which Mg^{2+} is displaced from NMDA receptors upon subsequent stimulation by glutamate.
D) The influx of Na^+ upon initial stimulation by glutamate depolarizes the postsynaptic cell in order to displace Mg^{2+}.

5. AMPA receptors are found throughout the central nervous system and are comprised of four different subunits. Not all AMPA receptors have all the subunits. If a knockout mouse was made deficient for the gene for one of the AMPA receptor subunits, what would be the expected outcome?

A) An observed deficit only in LTP and the mouse's ability to learn
B) Altered function in any region containing an AMPA receptor
C) No change in LTP function due to the NMDA receptor still being present and functional
D) Altered function and/or compensatory expression of other AMPA receptor subunits in regions with AMPA receptors that lack the affected subunit

6. Based on Figure 1, what is a logical function of CREB?

A) To interact with the genomic DNA to enhance transcription
B) To interact with RNA to enhance translation
C) To bind ribosomes to enhance transcription
D) To bind RNA polymerase to enhance replication

7. Symptoms of Alzheimer's disease include all of the following EXCEPT:

A) disorientation.
B) forgetfulness.
C) mood swings.
D) slow, uncoordinated fine movements.

SOLUTIONS TO CHAPTER 12 FREESTANDING PRACTICE QUESTIONS

1. **B** Myelin is an insulating sheath wrapped around the axons of neurons. White matter in the central nervous system is composed of myelinated axons; thus, a reduction in myelination would result in a decrease in white matter (choice A is a symptom and can be eliminated). Gaps in the myelin sheath (called nodes of Ranvier) allow depolarization of the axon and conduction of neuronal signals along the length of the axon. Myelination speeds the movement of the action potential along the length of the axon (choice C would be a symptom and can be eliminated), in a process called saltatory conduction; a reduction in myelination would decrease (not increase) saltatory conduction (choice B is not a symptom and is the correct answer choice). This would decrease sensation, as sensory information from the peripheral nervous system would be hindered from reaching the central nervous system (choice D is a symptom and can be eliminated).

2. **D** The cerebellum, located behind the pons and below the cerebrum, receives input from the primary motor cortex in the forebrain, and coordinates complex motor function (choice D is correct). The frontal lobe contains the primary motor cortex, which is responsible for initiating movement, but does not coordinate complex motor functions (choice A is wrong). The occipital lobe is responsible for vision (choice B is wrong), and the reticular activating system is responsible for arousal and wakefulness (choice C is wrong).

3. **D** The pons is located below the midbrain and above the medulla oblongata, and connects the brain stem and the cerebellum. Along with the medulla, the pons controls some autonomic functions and plays a role in equilibrium and posture, but it is not associated with the experience of emotion (choice D is correct). The amygdala, located in the temporal lobes, is part of the limbic system and is responsible for processing information about emotion (choices A and B are associated with emotion and can be eliminated). The hypothalamus links the nervous system to the endocrine system and also plays a role in emotion (choice C is associated with emotion and can be eliminated).

4. **B** Item I is true: acetylcholine is the neurotransmitter released by motor neurons onto skeletal muscle to cause contraction (choice C can be eliminated). Item II is true: the preganglionic neurons of both the sympathetic and parasympathetic nervous systems release acetylcholine onto the postganglionic neurons, triggering action potentials (choice A can be eliminated). Item III is false: acetylcholine on cardiac muscle is inhibitory and reduces the heart rate (choice D can be eliminated, and choice B is correct).

5. **B** The hypothalamic-pituitary axis (HPA) regulates the release of cortisol via negative feedback. The hypothalamus releases corticotropin-releasing hormone (CRH), which stimulates the anterior pituitary to release adrenocorticotropic hormone (ACTH), which in turn stimulates the adrenal cortex to release cortisol. Cortisol then inhibits the hypothalamus from releasing further CRH and the anterior pituitary from releasing more ACTH, thus having an inhibitory effect on both (choice B is correct). The posterior pituitary releases oxytocin and antidiuretic hormone; cortisol does not inhibit the posterior pituitary (choice A is wrong). Additionally, cortisol does not inhibit the adrenal cortex directly, but rather inhibits the hypothalamus and anterior pituitary from releasing the hormones that stimulate the adrenal cortex; thus cortisol has an indirect inhibitory effect on the adrenal cortex (choice C is wrong). Cortisol stimulates glycogen mobilization (choice D is wrong).

SOLUTIONS TO CHAPTER 12 PRACTICE PASSAGE

1. **C** The passage states that the hippocampus is involved in memory acquisition; thus, it is likely to be located in the temporal lobe of the cerebrum (choice C is correct). The cerebellum is involved in balance and coordination, not memory (choice A is wrong), the occipital lobe is responsible for vision (choice B is wrong), and the hypothalamus is involved in maintaining homeostasis and hormonal regulation (choice D is wrong).

2. **C** If NMDA receptor activation is necessary for LTP, then blocking this receptor would likely suppress LTP (choice A could occur and can be eliminated). Based on Figure 1, activation of the NMDA receptor triggers an influx of intracellular calcium and a cascade of events resulting in activation of gene expression; thus, blocking this receptor could lead to both a significant decrease in intracellular calcium and a suppression of gene expression (choices B and D could occur and can be eliminated). Since the NMDA receptor allows an influx of sodium, some reduction in intracellular sodium could be expected; however, this is unlikely to be significant since the AMPA receptor would still be functional and is the main source of Na^+ influx (choice C would not occur and is the correct answer choice).

3. **C** Item I is true: The adrenal glands secrete both steroid hormones (from the adrenal cortex) and epinephrine (from the adrenal medulla). If the researcher only replaces the steroids, then the sympathetic response (which relies on epinephrine) could be blunted (choices A and B can be eliminated). Since both remaining answer choices include Item II, then Item II must be true and we only need to evaluate Item III. Item III is false: based on Figure 1, corticosteroids do not seem to play an integral role in LTP. In addition, the passage only discusses their possible involvement in neuronal cell death at high concentrations. Keeping baseline levels may not lead to cell death, but would not necessarily enhance LTP (choice D can be eliminated, and choice C is correct). Note that Item II is in fact true: based on information in the passage (the glucocorticoid aging hypothesis), stress levels of corticosteroids could lead to age-related neurodegeneration. Thus, if the levels of these hormones are kept at baseline throughout the life of the animal, it is possible to attenuate age-related neurodegeneration.

4. **B** The passage states that the NMDA receptor is blocked by extracellular Mg^{2+} that must be displaced by a sufficient change in membrane potential. It is fair to assume that this change must be a depolarization, since the initial receptor activated is the AMPA receptor, and according to the figure, that receptor allows an influx of Na^+ (choice D is likely to be true and can be eliminated). Additional AMPA receptors would increase the rate of depolarization and thus the rate of Mg^{2+} displacement. This is in fact the basis for LTP; the first stimulation leads to the effects shown in the figure, including new receptors in the membrane, thus the effect of subsequent stimulation is enhanced (choice C is likely to be true and can be eliminated). Anything that would lead to a hyperpolarization of the cell would not displace Mg^{2+} and would disrupt the calcium influx and all associated events, including LTP. An increase of Cl^- influx would hyperpolarize the cell and disrupt LTP (choice A is likely to be true and can be eliminated), but an increase in K^+ efflux, while it would hyperpolarize the cell, would not increase LTP (choice B is unlikely to be true and is the correct answer choice).

5. **D** The question states essentially that AMPA receptors can be varied (have variable subunits) and are found throughout the CNS. Certainly if the gene for one of the subunits was deficient, we would expect some deficit to be present. However, because of the widespread location of these receptors, we would not expect the deficit to be limited to only the region of the brain responsible for LTP (choice A is wrong), nor would we expect the deficit to be found in ANY region with receptors, because some regions may have AMPA receptors that do not have the knocked out subunit (choice B is wrong). According to the diagram, the functions of both AMPA and NMDA receptors are required during LTP, so if one of the receptors was compromised, we might expect some alteration in LTP function (choice C is wrong). The most likely outcome is that there would be altered function or potentially compensatory expression of other AMPA receptor subunits in those regions of the CNS that contain an affected AMPA receptor (choice D is correct).

6. **A** In the diagram, CREB is located immediately before gene activation, which would suggest it has something to do with transcription (choices B and D are wrong). Ribosomes do not have anything to do with transcription (choice C is wrong, and choice A is correct). CREB stands for cAMP Response Element Binding and is a transcription factor; thus, it interacts with DNA to enhance transcription.

7. **D** Alzheimer's disease involves the loss of vital neurons throughout the cerebral cortex; symptoms include disorientation (choice A can be eliminated), forgetfulness (choice B can be eliminated), mood swings (choice C can be eliminated), and impairment of other cognitive functions like speaking, writing, thinking, reasoning, and making judgments and decisions. As the disease progresses, it can also lead to changes in personality and behavior, depression, and social withdrawal. However, Alzheimer's disease does not affect fine motor skills (choice D is correct).

Psychology and Sociology Glossary

After each entry, the section number in the *MCAT Psychology & Sociology Review* text where the term is discussed is given.

absolute poverty
The inability to meet a bare minimum of basic necessities. [**Section 5.2**]

acetylcholine (ACh)
The neurotransmitter used at the neuromuscular junction, throughout the parasympathetic nervous system, and by the preganglionic neurons of the sympathetic nervous system. [**Section 12.2**]

acetylcholinesterase
The enzyme that breaks down acetylcholine in the synaptic cleft. [**Section 12.2**]

achieved status
A status due largely to an individual's efforts. [**Section 6.3**]

acquisition
The process of learning the association between a conditioned stimulus and response. [**Section 9.1**]

action potential
A localized change in a neuron's membrane potential that propagates away from its point of origin. [**Section 12.1**]

activation-synthesis theory
The theory that dreams are simply byproducts of brain activation during REM sleep. [**Section 11.5**]

actor-observer bias
The tendency to blame our actions on the situation and blame the actions of others on their personalities. [**Section 6.2**]

addiction
A compulsion to perform an act repeatedly, often with detrimental effects on the individual. [**Section 10.3**]

adrenal cortex
The outer region of the adrenal gland that produces cortisol in response to long-term (chronic) stress and aldosterone in response to low blood pressure or low blood osmolarity. [**Section 12.4**]

adrenal medulla
The inner region of the adrenal gland that releases epinephrine (adrenaline) and norepinephrine into the bloodstream. [**Section 12.3**]

adrenocorticotropic hormone (ACTH)
A tropic hormone produced by the anterior pituitary gland that targets the adrenal cortex, stimulating it to release cortisol and aldosterone. ACTH is part of the stress response. [**Sections 12.4 & 8.2**]

affect
A person's visible emotion in the moment. [**Section 8.1**]

affirmative action
Policies that seek to benefit underrepresented groups in admissions or job hiring decisions. [**Section 6.2**]

aggregate
People who exist in the same space but do not interact or share a common sense of identity. [**Section 6.2**]

aggression
Behavior that is forceful, hostile, or attacking. [**Section 6.3**]

agnosia
The inability to recognize objects through sensory mechanisms despite intact function of the underlying sense itself. [**Section 11.4**]

Ainsworth, Mary
Conducted famous studies on attachment style in infants. [**Section 9.3**]

algorithm
A step-by-step detailing aid to problem-solving. [**Section 11.4**]

alpha waves
Low amplitude, high frequency brain waves present in a relaxed state. [**Section 11.5**]

altruistic behavior
A behavior that benefits others, possibly at the expense of the individual. [**Section 6.3**]

Alzheimer's disease
The most prevalent form of dementia, characterized by severe memory impairment. [**Section 8.1**]

amalgamation
Occurs when majority and minority groups combine to form a new group. [**Section 6.1**]

amygdala
Almond-shaped structure deep within the brain that orchestrates emotional experiences. [**Section 10.3**]

anal stage
The second of Freud's five psychosexual stages, in this stage the child seeks sensual pleasure through control of elimination. [**Section 7.1**]

anterograde amnesia
An inability to form new memories. [**Sections 8.1 & 9.2**]

antisocial personality disorder
A psychological disorder characterized by serious behavior problems beginning in adolescence, including significant aggression against people or animals, property destruction, lying, or theft. [Section 8.1]

anxiety disorder
A psychological disorder characterized by intense, frequent, and uncontrollable anxiety. [Section 8.1]

archival studies
Studies that explore historical records and search for patterns or insight. [Section 3.3]

Asch, Solomon
Conducted important research on conformity and group pressure. [Section 6.2]

ascribed status
A status that is assigned to a person by society regardless of the person's own efforts. [Section 6.3]

assimilation
The process in which an individual forsakes aspects of his or her own cultural tradition to adopt those of a different culture. [Section 6.1]

associative learning
Process of learning in which one event, object, or action is directly connected with another. Two general categories include classical and operant conditioning. [Section 9.1]

attenuation model of selective attention
Model of selective attention in which the mind has an attenuator, like a volume knob, that tunes up attended inputs and tunes down unattended inputs, rather than eliminating them. [Section 11.4]

attitude
A person's feelings and beliefs about other people or events and behavioral tendencies. [Section 7.3]

attribution theory
A theory that attempts to explain behavior by attributing it to either internal or external causes. [Section 6.2]

attrition
Occurs when participants in a study drop out before completion. [Section 3.1]

auditory cortex
The area of the temporal lobe responsible for processing sound information. [Section 11.1]

auditory tube
Functions to equalize middle ear pressure with atmospheric pressure so that pressure on both sides of the tympanic membrane is equal. [Section 11.1]

authoritarian parenting
Parents impose strict rules that are expected to be followed unconditionally. [Section 9.3]

authoritative parenting
Parents place limits on behavior and consistently follow through on consequences, but also allow for two-way communication with children. [Section 9.3]

autonomic nervous system (ANS)
The division of the peripheral nervous system that innervates and controls the visceral organs. It can be subdivided into sympathetic and parasympathetic branches. [Sections 10.3 & 12.3]

availability heuristic
Mental shortcut of making judgments on the frequency of something occurring based on how readily it is available in our memories. [Section 11.4]

avoidance learning
The process by which one learns to ensure that a negative stimulus will not occur. [Section 9.1]

avoidant personality disorder
A psychological disorder characterized by feelings of inadequacy, inferiority, and undesirability, and a preoccupation with fears of criticism. [Section 8.1]

axon
A long projection of the cell body of a neuron down which an action potential can be propagated. [Section 12.1]

back stage
In the dramaturgical perspective, this is where we can "let down our guard" and be ourselves. [Section 6.3]

Bandura, Albert
Famous for his Bobo doll studies that demonstrated observational learning. [Section 9.1]

baroreceptor
A sensory receptor that responds to changes in pressure. [Section 11.2]

basal nuclei, or basal ganglia
Structures that coordinate smooth motion by inhibiting excess movement. [Section 10.2]

basilar membrane
Membrane in the cochlea that supports the organ of Corti, which contains hearing receptors. [Section 11.1]

behavioral genetics
Study of the role of inheritance in interacting with experience to determine an individual's personality and behaviors. [Section 6.4]

behavioral therapy
This type of therapy uses conditioning to shape a client's behaviors in the desired direction. [Section 7.1]

behaviorism
The perspective that personality is a result of learned behavior patterns based on the environment. [Section 7.1]

belief bias
A tendency to draw conclusions based on what one already believes rather than sound logic. [Section 11.4]

belief perseverance
The maintenance of beliefs even in the face of evidence to the contrary. [Section 11.4]

beliefs
The convictions or principles that people within a culture hold. [Section 5.1]

beta waves
Waking EEG waves seen during alert focus with oscillations between 12.5 Hz and 30 Hz. [Section 11.5]

between-subjects design
Comparisons are made between one group and another to test for differences. [Section 3.1]

bilateral descent
A system of lineage in which the relatives on the mother's side and father's side are considered equally important. [Section 4.2]

biofeedback
Means of recording and feeding back information about autonomic responses to an individual in an attempt to train the individual to control previously involuntary responses. [Section 8.2]

biographical studies
Studies that investigate all relevant details of the life of an individual or small group. [Section 3.3]

bipolar disorder
A psychological disorder characterized by cyclic mood episodes of depression and mania. [Section 8.1]

bipolar neuron
A neuron with a single axon and a single dendrite. [Section 12.1]

borderline personality disorder
A psychological disorder characterized by enduring or recurrent instability in impulse control, mood, and image of self and others. [Section 8.1]

bottom-up processing
Sensory processing that begins with sensory receptors and works up to complex integration of information in the brain. [Section 11.2]

Broca's area
Region in the left hemisphere of the frontal lobe involved in language production. [Section 11.6]

bystander effect
The fact that a person is less likely to provide help when there are other people around. [Section 6.2]

Cannon-Bard Theory
Asserts that the physiological and cognitive aspects of emotion occur simultaneously and collectively lead to the behavioral reaction. [Section 7.4]

capitalism
An economic system in which resources and production are mainly privately owned and goods/services are produced for a profit. [Section 4.1]

case studies
Studies that make a deep and comprehensive exploration of a single individual, phenomenon, or disorder. [Section 3.3]

caste system
A closed social stratification where people remain in the category that they are born into. [Section 5.2]

category
People who share similar characteristics but are not otherwise linked as a group. [Section 6.2]

Cattell, Raymond
Psychologist who used factor analysis with hundreds of traits to identify sixteen source traits, then reduced these into five global factors. [Section 6.4]

central executive
Part of working memory that controls the visuospatial sketchpad, phonological loop, and episodic buffer. [Section 11.4]

central nervous system
The subdivision of the nervous system consisting of the brain and spinal cord. [Sections 10.2 & 12.3]

central route
Cognitive route of persuasion based on the content and deeper aspects of an argument. [Section 6.4]

cerebellum
The region of the brain that coordinates and smooths skeletal muscle activity. [Section 10.2]

cerebral cortex
A thin layer of gray matter on the surface of the cerebral hemispheres. [Section 10.2]

cerebrospinal fluid (CSF)
A clear fluid that circulates around and through the brain and spinal cord. [Section 10.2]

charismatic authority
A form of leadership where devotion is reliant upon an individual with exceptional charisma. [Section 4.2]

chemical synapse
Synapse at which a neurotransmitter is released from the axon of a neuron into the synaptic cleft, where it binds to receptors on the next structure. [Section 12.2]

chemoreceptor
A sensory receptor that responds to specific chemicals, for example, gustatory (taste) receptors, and olfactory (smell) receptors. [Section 11.1]

chunking
Memory technique in which information is organized into groups of data, allowing more information to be remembered overall. [Section 9.2]

church
A type of well-integrated religious organization that attempts to provide an all-encompassing worldview for followers. [Section 4.2]

ciliary muscle
Muscle that helps focus light on the retina by controlling the curvature of the lens of the eye. [Section 11.1]

circadian rhythm
The waxing and waning of alertness throughout the 24-hour day. [Section 11.5]

class system
A social stratification where people are grouped together by similar wealth, income, and education, but the classes are open, so people can strive to reach a higher class (or fall to a lower one). [Section 5.2]

classical conditioning
Process in which two stimuli are paired in a way that changes a response to one of them. [Section 9.1]

cochlea
The curled structure in the inner ear that contains the membranes and hair cells used to transduce sound waves into action potentials. [Section 11.1]

cocktail party effect
Phenomenon in which salient information "catches" one's attention. [Section 11.3]

coercive organizations
Organization in which members do not have a choice in joining. [Section 6.3]

cognitive behavioral therapy (CBT)
A type of therapy that addresses thoughts and behaviors that are maladaptive by using goal-oriented and systematic techniques. [Section 7.1]

cognitive dissonance theory
A theory that explains that we feel tension ("dissonance") whenever we hold two thoughts ("cognitions") that are incompatible. [Section 7.3]

cognitive psychology
Tradition of psychology that focuses on the brain, cognitions, and thoughts as mediating learning and stimulus-response behaviors. [Section 9.1]

conditioned response
Previously unlearned response that has become a learned response to a conditioned stimulus. [Section 9.1]

conditioned stimulus
An originally neutral stimulus that is paired until it can produce the conditioned response without the unconditioned stimulus. [Section 9.1]

conduction aphasia
Language dysfunction characterized by poor speech repetition despite intact comprehension and fluent speech. [Section 11.6]

cones
Photoreceptors in the retina of the eye that respond to bright light and provide color vision. [Section 11.1]

confederates
A person who is working with the experimenter and posing as a part of the experiment, but the subjects are not aware of this affiliation. [Section 6.2]

confirmation bias
A tendency to search only for information that confirms a preconceived conclusion. [Section 11.4]

conflict theory
A theory that views society as being in competition for limited resources. [Section 4.1]

conformity
The phenomenon of adjusting behavior or thinking based on the behavior or thinking of others. [Section 6.2]

confounding variables
Variables other than the research variables that would explain an experimental effect if one were found; also known as extraneous variables. [Section 3.1]

consciousness
Awareness of self, internal states, and the environment. [Section 11.5]

construct validity
The extent to which a psychometric instrument measures what it purports to. [Section 3.1]

control group
The group that does not receive the treatment in an experiment, and is used as a point of reference for the experimental group. [Section 3.1]

conversion disorder
A psychological disorder characterized by a change in sensory or motor function that has no discernible physical or physiological cause. [Section 8.1]

cornea
The clear portion of the tough outer layer of the eyeball, found over the iris and the pupil. [Section 11.1]

corpus callosum
The largest bundle of white matter (axons) connecting the two cerebral hemispheres. [Section 10.2]

correlational studies
Studies that measure the quantitative relationship between two variables. [Section 3.3]

cortisol
Steroid hormone released during chronic stress. Prolonged release of cortisol is associated with suppressed immunity and increased illness. [Sections 8.2, 10.3, & 12.4]

cross-sectional study
A study design in which data collection or survey of a population or sample occurs at a specific time. [Section 3.3]

crude birth rate
The annual number of live births per thousand people in a population. [Section 5.1]

crude death rate
The annual number of deaths per thousand people in a population. [Section 5.1]

cult
A religious organization that is far outside society's norms. [Section 4.2]

cultural capital
The non-financial social assets that promote social mobility. [Section 5.2]

cultural relativism
Judging another culture based on its own cultural standards. [Section 6.2]

cultural universals
Patterns or traits that are common to all people, such as securing food and shelter. [Section 5.1]

culture
A shared way of life, including the beliefs and practices that a social group shares. [Section 5.1]

cyclothymic disorder
A psychological disorder that is similar to bipolar disorder but the moods are less extreme. [Section 8.1]

death drive
According to psychoanalytic theory, the death instinct drives aggressive behaviors fueled by an unconscious wish to die or to hurt oneself or others. [Section 7.1]

debriefing
After participants complete a study or some part of a study, researchers thoroughly review the purpose of the study, hypotheses, and implications. [Section 3.2]

deindividuation
An explanation of people's uncharacteristic behavior when situations provide a high degree of arousal and low sense of responsibility. [Section 6.2]

delusion
A false belief that is not due to culture, and is not relinquished despite evidence that it is false. [Section 8.1]

demand characteristics
Researcher expectations that influence participant responses; often, participants subconsciously adapt their behavior and responses to fit with the research hypothesis, which they have guessed. [Section 3.2]

demography
The study of human population dynamics, including the size, structure, and distribution of a population, and changes in the population over time due to birth, death, and migration. [Section 5.1]

dendrite
A projection off the cell body of a neuron that receives nerve impulses from a different neuron and sends the impulse to the cell body. Neurons can have one or several dendrites. [Section 12.1]

dependent personality disorder
A psychological disorder characterized by a need to be taken care of by others and an unrealistic fear of being unable to take care of himself or herself. [Section 8.1]

depersonalization disorder
A psychological disorder characterized by a recurring or persistent feeling of being cut off or detached from one's body or mental processes, as if observing one's self from the outside. [Section 8.1]

depolarization
The movement of the membrane potential of a cell away from the resting potential to a more positive membrane potential. [Section 12.1]

depressant
Class of drugs that depress or slow down neural activity. [Section 11.5]

depth of processing
The idea that information that is thought about at a deeper level is better remembered. [Section 9.2]

deviance
A violation of society's standards of conduct or expectations. [Sections 6.1 & 6.2]

Diagnostic and Statistical Manual (DSM)
The universal authority on the classification and diagnosis of psychological disorders. [Section 8.1]

diencephalon
The portion of the forebrain that includes the thalamus and hypothalamus. [Section 10.2]

difference threshold
The minimum noticeable difference between any two sensory stimuli 50% of the time. [Section 11.2]

disclosure
Before participants take part in a study, researchers must give them an idea of what they will be expected to do, and reinforce the right to discontinue participation in the study at any time. [Section 3.2]

discrimination (scientific)
Occurs when the conditioned stimulus is differentiated from other stimuli. [Section 9.1]

discrimination
Unjust treatment of a group, based on group characteristics. [Sections 5.1 & 6.2]

dishabituation
The restoration to full strength of a response to a stimulus that had previously become weakened through habituation. [Section 9.1]

dissociative amnesia
A psychological disorder characterized by at least one episode of suddenly forgetting some important personal information, usually related to severe stress or trauma. [Section 8.1]

dissociative disorder
A psychological disorder characterized by a person's thoughts, feelings, or behaviors being separated from conscious awareness and control, and not explainable as mere forgetfulness. [Section 8.1]

dissociative fugue
A psychological disorder in which someone goes on a journey, during which he or she cannot recall personal history prior to the journey. [Section 8.1]

dissociative identity disorder
A psychological disorder characterized by alternating between multiple personality states. [Section 8.1]

divided attention
Focusing on multiple tasks simultaneously. [Section 11.3]

downward mobility
A decrease in social class. [Section 5.2]

dramaturgical perspective
Assumes that people are theatrical performers and that everyday life is a stage. [Section 6.3]

drive
An urge originating from a physiological discomfort such as hunger, thirst, or sleepiness. [Section 7.2]

Drive Reduction Theory
A theory that suggests that a physiological need creates an aroused state (drive) that motivates the organism to reduce that drive (satiate the need) by engaging in some behavior. [Section 7.2]

dual coding hypothesis
A hypothesis that it is easier to remember words with associated images than either words or images alone. [Section 9.2]

Durkheim, Émile
Considered the founder of sociology and a major proponent of functionalism. [Section 4.1]

dynamic equilibrium
Occurs when complex societies contain many different but interdependent parts working together to maintain stability. [Section 4.1]

dyssomnias
Disorders that involve abnormalities in the amount, quality, or timing of sleep. [Section 11.5]

dysthymic disorder
A psychological disorder characterized as a less intense, less chronic form of depression. [Section 8.1]

ecclesia
A dominant religious organization that includes most members of a society, and is recognized as the exclusive national religion. [Section 4.2]

echoic memory
Sensory memory for sound. [Section 9.2]

effector
The organ that carries out the command sent along a particular motor neuron. [Section 12.3]

efferent neurons
A neuron that carries information away from the central nervous system; a motor neuron. [Section 12.3]

egalitarian family
A family system where spouses are equals involved in negotiation when making decisions. [Section 4.2]

ego
According to Freud's psychoanalytic theory, the ego is ruled by the reality principle, and uses logical thinking and planning to control consciousness. [Section 7.1]

ego defense mechanisms
According to psychoanalytic theory, mechanisms developed to cope with anxiety and protect the ego, in a way that unconsciously denies or distorts reality. [Section 7.1]

eidetic memory
Ability found in some children to vividly recall an image after brief exposure. [Section 9.2]

elaboration likelihood model
Model that explains whether the content of an argument or some more superficial attribute is more likely to cause persuasion. [Section 6.4]

Electra complex
Occurs during the phallic stage when a female child is sexually attracted to her father and hostile toward her mother, who is seen as a rival. [Section 7.1]

electrical synapse
A type of synapse in which the cells are connected by gap junctions, allowing ions (and therefore the action potential) to spread easily from cell to cell. [Section 12.2]

electroencephalography
Low resolution functional technique that provides real-time data on brain wave synchronization at nodes spread through the scalp. [Section 10.1]

electromyogram (EMG)
Recording of skeletal muscle movements. [Section 11.5]

electrooculogram (EOG)
Recording of eye movements. [Section 11.5]

empathy
The ability to identify with others' emotions. [Section 6.3]

encoding
The process of transferring sensory information into the memory system. [Section 9.2]

endocrine gland
A ductless gland that secretes hormones into the blood. [Section 12.4]

endocrine system
A system of ductless glands that secrete chemical messengers (hormones) into the blood. [Section 12.4]

endogamy
The practice of marrying within a particular group. [Section 4.2]

environmental injustice
When people in poorer communities are more likely to be subjected to negative environmental impacts to their health and well-being. [Section 5.2]

epinephrine
A hormone produced and secreted by the adrenal medulla that prolongs and increases the effects of the sympathetic nervous system. [Section 12.3]

episodic buffer
Part of working memory that interacts with information in long-term memory. [Section 11.4]

episodic memory
Autobiographical memory for information of personal importance. [Section 9.2]

Erikson, Erik
Extended Freud's theory of developmental stages by adding social factors and adding developmental stages in adolescence and adulthood. [Section 7.1]

escape learning
Through operant conditioning, this is the process of learning to engage in a particular behavior in order to get away from a negative or aversive stimulus. [Section 9.1]

ethnicity
A socially defined concept referring to whether a large social group identifies with each other based on culture. [Section 5.1]

ethnocentrism
The tendency to judge people from another culture by the standards of one's own culture. [Section 6.2]

ethnographic studies
Studies that make a deep and comprehensive exploration of an ethnicity or culture. [Section 3.3]

excitatory postsynaptic potential (EPSP)
A slight depolarization of a postsynaptic cell, bringing the membrane potential closer to the threshold for an action potential. [Section 12.2]

executive functions
Higher order thinking processes that include planning, organizing, and decision-making. [Section 10.3]

exocrine gland
A gland, such as a sweat gland, that secretes its product into a duct, which ultimately carries the product to the surface of the body or into a body cavity. [Section 12.4]

exogamy
A requirement to marry outside a particular group, to prohibit sexual relationships between certain relatives. [Section 4.2]

experimental group
The group that receives the treatment in an experiment, in contrast to the control group. [Section 3.1]

experimental hypothesis
The hypothesis that there is an experimental effect and the treatment is responsible for the measured difference. [Section 3.1]

explicit (or declarative) memory
Memories that can be consciously recalled, such as factual knowledge. [Section 9.2]

external locus of control
The belief that outcomes in one's life are determined by outside forces. [Section 6.1]

external validity
The extent to which experimental results can be applied to real-world situations. [Section 3.2]

extinction
In classical conditioning, the unpairing of the conditioned and unconditioned stimuli. [Section 9.1]

extraneous variables
Variables other than the research variables that would explain an experimental effect if one were found; also known as confounding variables. [Section 3.1]

false consensus
Occurs when we assume that everyone else agrees with what we do (even though they may not). [Section 6.2]

false memory
Inaccurate memory created by the power of imagination or suggestion. [Sections 9.2 & 11.5]

feature detection theory
A theory of visual perception that proposes that certain neurons fire for specific features of a visual stimulus, such as shape, color, movement, etc. [Section 11.2]

feral children
Neglected or abandoned children who grow up without human contact or care. [Section 6.1]

filter model
Model of selective attention developed by Donald Broadbent that suggests that information is put through a filter that allows only selected inputs through. [Section 11.3]

Five-Factor Model
A model developed to explain personality using five overarching personality traits. [Section 7.1]

fixed-interval schedule
Reinforcement schedule in which reward is offered after a set period of time has passed. [Section 9.1]

fixed-ratio schedule
Reinforcement schedule in which reward is offered after a set number of instances of a behavior. [Section 9.1]

flashbulb memory
Intense vivid "snapshot" of an emotionally intense experience. [Section 9.2]

folkways
Norms that are more informal, yet shape everyday behavior (styles of dress, ways of greeting). [Section 6.1]

food desert
An area, typically in a highly populated lower-income urban environment, where healthy, fresh food is difficult to find. [Section 4.2]

foot-in-the-door phenomenon
A persuasion strategy that involves enticing people to take small actions, then gradually asking for larger commitments. [Section 7.3]

Freud, Sigmund
An Austrian neurologist who is considered the founder of psychoanalytic theory. [Section 7.1]

front stage
In the dramaturgical perspective, this is where we play a role and use impression management to craft the way we come across to other people. [Section 6.3]

frustration-aggression principle
This principle suggests that when someone is blocked from achieving a goal, this frustration can trigger anger, which can lead to aggression. [Section 6.3]

functional fixedness
A tendency to perceive the functions of objects as fixed and unchanging. [Section 11.4]

functionalism
A theory that conceptualizes society as a living organism with many different parts and organs, each of which has a distinct purpose. [Section 4.1]

fundamental attribution error
The tendency to underestimate the impact of the situation and overestimate the impact of a person's character or personality on their behavior. [Section 6.2]

fundamentalists
People who observe strict adherence to religious beliefs. [Section 4.2]

Gage, Phineas
Famous case of a man who suffered damage to his prefrontal cortex after a railroad tie blasted through his head. [Section 10.1]

game theory
A theory used to predict large, complex systems, such as the overall behavior of a population. [Sections 4.1 & 6.4]

ganglion
A clump of gray matter (unmyelinated neuron cell bodies) found in the peripheral nervous system. [Section 11.1]

gender bias in medicine
Occurs when women and men receive different treatment for the same disease or illness. [Section 5.2]

gender conditioning
The socialization of gender roles is also known as gender conditioning [Section 5.1].

gender schema theory
The study of how gender beliefs become socialized in society. [Section 5.1]

general fertility rate
The annual number of live births per 1000 women of childbearing age within a population. [Section 5.1]

general intelligence
Foundational base of intelligence that supports more specialized abilities. [Section 6.4]

generalization
In classical conditioning, the process by which stimuli similar to a conditioned stimulus elicit the conditioned response. [Section 9.1]

generalized anxiety disorder (GAD)
A psychological disorder characterized by tension or anxiety much of the time about many issues, but without the presence of panic attacks. [Section 8.1]

generalized other
When a person tries to imagine what is expected of them from society, they are taking on the perspective of the generalized other. [Section 6.1]

genotype
The genetic makeup of an organism. [Section 6.4]

gestalt psychology
A theory that the brain processes information in a holistic manner. [Section 11.2]

global inequality
The extent to which wealth is distributed unevenly among the world's population. [Section 5.2]

global stratification
A comparison of the wealth, economic stability, and power of various countries. [Section 5.2]

gray matter
Unmyelinated neuron cell bodies and short unmyelinated axons. [Section 10.2]

group
A collection of people (as few as two) who regularly interact and identify. [Section 6.2]

group polarization
The phenomenon where groups tend to intensify the preexisting views of their members until the average view is more extreme than it initially was. [Section 6.2]

group pressure (or peer pressure)
Pressure exerted by a group that causes one to change behaviors, values, attitudes, or beliefs. [Section 6.2]

groupthink
A phenomenon in which the desire for group harmony results in an easy consensus, even if the final decision is not the best one. [Section 6.2]

growth hormone
Hormone released by the anterior pituitary that causes whole body growth in children and adolescents, and increasing cell turnover rate in adults. [Section 12.4]

gustatory receptors
Chemoreceptors on the tongue that respond to chemicals in food. [Section 11.1]

habit
Action that is performed repeatedly until it becomes automatic. [Section 9.1]

habituation
A decrease in response to a stimulus after repeated presentations. [Section 9.1]

hair cells
Sensory receptors found in the inner ear that respond to vibrations in the cochlea caused by sound waves and changes in position and acceleration (used for balance). [Section 11.1]

hallucination
A false sensory perception that occurs while a person is conscious (not during sleep or delirium). [Section 8.1]

hallucinogens
Class of drugs that distort perceptions in the absence of any sensory input, creating hallucinations or altered sensory perceptions. [Section 11.5]

halo effect
A tendency to believe that people have inherently good or bad natures, rather than looking at individual characteristics. [Section 6.2]

Harlow, Harry and Margaret
Researchers known for their controversial experiments with isolated baby monkeys. [Section 9.3]

health care disparities
The population-specific differences in the presence of disease, health outcomes, and quality of health care across different social groups. [Section 5.2]

heritability
The extent to which a behavior is due to genetic factors. [Section 3.3]

heuristics
Mental shortcuts used for problem-solving; sometimes sacrifices accuracy for speed. [Section 11.4]

hindsight bias
Tendency to believe that an event was predictable after it has already occurred. [Section 6.2]

hippocampus
Brain structure located in the medial temporal lobe; plays a key role in forming memories. [Section 10.3]

histrionic personality disorder
A psychological disorder characterized by a strong desire to be the center of attention. [Section 8.1]

homogenous
The same throughout; often used to describe a sample in which participants have similar characteristics. [Section 3.1]

humanistic psychology
A psychological perspective that emphasizes an individual's inherent drive toward self-actualization. [Section 6.1]

hypnotism
Structured interaction in which an individual is instructed to focus attention a particular way, relax, and let go. [Section 11.5]

hypochondriasis
A psychological disorder characterized by a preoccupation with having a serious illness. [Section 8.1]

hypophysis
The pituitary gland. [Section 12.4]

hypothalamus
Brain structure that is involved in many autonomic processes including body temperature, hunger, thirst, fatigue, and sleep. [Sections 12.4]

iconic memory
The brief photographic memory for visual information, which decays in a few tenths of a second. [Section 9.2]

id
According to Freud's psychoanalytic theory, is the source of energy and instincts that seeks to gain pleasure. [Section 7.1]

ideal self
Constructed out of experiences, expectations, and role models; the person one wishes to be. [Section 6.1]

identity formation (or individuation)
Development of a distinct personality. [Section 6.1]

illusory correlation
A perceived relationship between two things, even when none exists. [Section 6.2]

implicit (or procedural) memory
Memory that involves conditioned associations and knowledge of how to do something. [Section 9.2]

impression management or self-presentation
The process whereby people attempt to manage their images by influencing others' perceptions. [Section 6.3]

in-group
A group that an individual belongs to and believes to be an integral part of who they are. [Section 6.2]

incentive theory
A theory that suggests that incentives (objects that either induce or discourage behaviors) motivate human behavior. [Section 7.2]

inclusive fitness
A theory that suggests that cooperation among organisms promotes genetic success. [Section 6.3]

incongruity
The emotional result when the real self falls short of the ideal self. [Section 6.1]

infantile amnesia
A lack of explicit memory for events that occurred before the age of roughly 3.5 years. [Section 9.3]

information-processing models
Models that use computers as an analogy for understanding cognitive processes such as attention, perception, and memory. [Section 11.4]

informational social influence
The process of complying to do the right thing because others "know something we don't know." [Section 6.2]

Inhibitory postsynaptic potential (IPSP)
Slight hyperpolarization of a postsynaptic cell, moving the membrane potential of that cell further from threshold. [Section 12.2]

insecure attachment
Category of attachment styles in which infants are less likely to explore the environment in the presence of the mother and less likely to be soothed by her. [Section 9.3]

insight learning
Sudden flash of inspiration that provides a solution to a problem. [Section 9.1]

insomnia
Most common sleep disorder, characterized by difficulty falling or staying asleep. [Section 11.5]

instinct
Behaviors that are unlearned and present in fixed patterns throughout a species. [Section 7.2]

institutional discrimination
Unjust practices employed by large organizations that have been codified into operating processes or institutional objectives. [Section 6.2]

instrumental conditioning
See operant conditioning. [Section 9.1]

intellectual disability
Classification for individuals who have an IQ below 70 and functional impairment in their everyday lives. [Section 6.4]

intelligence
The ability to learn from experience, problem-solve, and adapt to new situations. [Section 6.4]

intergenerational mobility
A change (increase or decrease) in social class between parents and children within a family. [Section 5.2]

internal locus of control
An individual's belief that they can affect outcomes through their own actions. [Section 6.1]

internal validity
How "well-designed" a study is; how valid it is to draw conclusions from the research based on the way it was constructed. [Section 3.2]

interneuron
A neuron found completely within the central nervous system. [Section 12.3]

intragenerational mobility
Describes the differences in social class between different members of the same generation. [Section 5.2]

iris
A pigmented membrane found just in front of the lens of the eye. The iris regulates the diameter of the pupil in response to the brightness of light. [Section 11.1]

James-Lange Theory
Theory of emotion in which emotional experience is the result of physiological responses. [Section 7.4]

just world phenomenon
The tendency to believe that the world is fair and people get what they deserve. [Section 6.2]

justification of effort
When people modify their attitudes to match their behaviors, specifically those involving effort. [Section 7.3]

K-complex
Large and slow wave with a duration of a half second that occurs in Stage 2 sleep. [Section 11.5]

kinship
Familial relationships including blood ties, family ties, and common ancestry. [Section 4.2]

Kohlberg's stages of moral development
Six developmental stages of moral reasoning, which form the basis of ethical behavior. [Section 6.1]

language
A symbolic system that is codified for communication. [Section 11.6]

language acquisition
The process by which infants learn to understand and speak their native language. [Section 11.6]

language acquisition device
The Nativist theory proposes that there is a theoretical language acquisition device (LAD) somewhere in our brains that is responsible for learning a language during the critical period of language acquisition (before adolescence). [Section 11.6]

latent content
The unconscious drives and wishes that are difficult to express and underlie dreams. [Section 11.5]

latent functions
The unintended or less recognizable consequences or a social structure. [Section 4.1]

latent learning
Learning that takes place in the absence of any observable behavior to show that it has occurred. [Section 9.1]

learned helplessness
A condition where an individual does not act even though there are opportunities to avoid unpleasant circumstances or gain positive rewards. [Sections 6.1 & 8.2]

libido
The life instinct, which drives behaviors focused on survival, growth, creativity, pain avoidance, and seeking pleasure. [Section 7.1]

life course perspective
Sociological theory that investigates key events in a person's life and how they unfold over time and lead to a person's development. [Section 6.4]

life expectancy
The number of years that an individual at a given age can expect to live at present mortality rates. [Section 5.1]

linguistic relativity hypothesis
Asserts that the language one speaks determines their thoughts and perceptions of the world. [Section 11.6]

long-term memory
Information that is retained long-term, potentially indefinitely. [Section 9.1]

long-term potentiation
An increase in synaptic strength between two neurons following simultaneous firing. [Sections 9.1 & 10.3]

looking glass self
The idea that a person's sense of self develops from interpersonal interactions with others in society and the perceptions of others. [Section 6.1]

major depressive disorder
A psychological disorder characterized by one or more depressive episodes, in which a person has felt worse than usual for most of the day, nearly every day, for at least two weeks. [Section 8.1]

manic episode
An experience of an abnormal euphoric, unrestrained, or irritable mood. [Section 8.1]

manifest content
According to Freud, the overt storylines of dreams. [Section 11.5]

manifest functions
The intended and obvious consequences of a social structure. [Section 4.1]

marginal poverty
Poverty that is due to circumstantial conditions, such as a lack of stable employment. [Section 5.2]

Marx, Karl
Founder of Conflict Theory who argued that societies progress through class struggle between those who control production and those who provide the labor for production. [Section 4.1]

Maslow's Hierarchy of Needs
Abraham Maslow's pyramid of motivational factors from physiological needs, at the base, progressively up to higher level needs such as self-actualization that must be met in order. [Section 7.2]

master status
The status that dominates other statuses and determines an individual's position in society. [Section 6.3]

material culture
Consists of the physical objects that are particular to a culture. [Section 5.1]

matriarchy
A social system where females are the primary authority figures. [Section 4.2]

matrilineal descent
A system of lineage in which the relatives on the mother's side are considered most important. [Section 4.2]

mechanoreceptor
A sensory receptor that responds to mechanical disturbances, such as shape changes (being squashed, bent, pulled). [Section 11.1]

meditation
Mindfulness technique for training attention in a particular way. [Section 11.5]

medulla oblongata
Portion of the hindbrain that controls respiratory rate and blood pressure, and specialized digestive and respiratory functions. [Section 10.2]

melatonin
Hormone produced by the pineal gland that affects sleep/wake cycles and seasonal functions. [Section 11.5]

meninges
The protective connective tissue wrappings of the central nervous system. [Section 12.3]

mental set
A tendency to fixate on ideas and solutions that have worked in the past, even if they may not apply to the current situation. [Section 11.4]

mere exposure effect
The phenomenon where people develop a preference for things because they have been exposed to them. [Section 6.3]

mere presence
The most basic level of "interaction" between individuals; when people are simply in each other's presence. [Section 6.2]

meritocracy
An idealized social stratification in which people's social standings are judged based on merit alone. [Section 5.2]

meta-analysis
An review of many studies to combine results and find emergent patterns in an area of research. [Section 3.1]

method of loci
A memory technique that involves imagining moving through a familiar place, and leaving visual representation topics to be remembered. [Section 9.2]

midbrain
The portion of the brain responsible for visual and auditory startle reflexes. [Section 10.2]

Milgram, Stanley
Conducted research on obedience in which he asked subjects to administer a shock to what they thought was another subject (who was just an actor). [Section 6.2]

Mindfulness-based stress reduction (MBSR)
Protocol involving mindfulness meditation that reduces pain, stress, and anxiety. [Section 11.5]

mindguarding
When dissenting opinions are prevented from permeating a group by filtering out information that goes against group beliefs. [Section 6.2]

mirror neurons
Neurons that fire when a particular behavior or emotion is observed in another. [Sections 9.1 & 10.3]

misinformation effect
A tendency to misremember an event, particularly when misleading information is presented between the event and the mental encoding of the event. [Section 9.2]

mixed methods
Any two types of research methodology are combined in the same study, such as qualitative and quantitative or between-subjects and within-subjects. [Section 3.1]

mnemonic
Any memory technique use to promote the retention and retrieval of information. [Section 9.2]

modeling
Mechanism behind observational learning in which an observer sees a behavior performed, then imitates the behavior. [Section 9.1]

monogamy
A form of marriage in which two individuals are married only to each other. [Section 4.2]

mood
A person's sustained internal emotion that colors his or her view of life. [Section 8.1]

mood-dependent memory
When learning occurs during a particular emotional state, it is most easily recalled when one is again in that emotional state. [Section 9.2]

mood disorder
A psychological disorder, such as bipolar disorder, or depressive disorders, characterized by a persistent pattern of abnormal mood serious enough to cause significant personal distress. [Section 8.1]

mores
Norms that are highly important for the benefit of society and so are often strictly enforced. [Section 6.1]

mortality
The death rate in a population. [Section 5.1]

multiculturalism (also known as pluralism)
A perspective that endorses equal standing for all cultural traditions. [Section 6.1]

multipolar neuron
A neuron with a single axon and multiple dendrites. [Section 12.1]

myelin
An insulating layer of membranes wrapped around the axons of almost all neurons in the body. [Section 12.1]

narcissistic personality disorder
A psychological disorder characterized by grandiosity and inflated sense of self. [Section 8.1]

narcolepsy
Sleep disorder in which an individual experiences short bursts of periodic, overwhelming sleepiness during waking periods. [Section 11.5]

negative feedback
A biological process that maintains homeostasis by feeding back to promote the limitation of a biological product. [Sections 7.2 & 12.4]

negative punishment
The removal of a positive or rewarding stimulus that decreases the likelihood of that behavior. [Section 9.1]

negative reinforcement
The removal of a negative or aversive stimulus following a behavior. Tends to increase the frequency of that behavior. [Section 9.1]

neural plasticity
A process that refers to the malleability of the brain's pathways and synapses based on behavior, the environment, and neural processes. [Section 10.3]

neuron
The basic functional and structural unit of the nervous system. [Section 12.1]

neurotransmitter
A chemical released by a neuron that binds to receptors on the postsynaptic cell and causes it to either depolarize or hyperpolarize. [Sections 10.2, 12.1, & 12.2]

neutral stimulus
A stimulus that does not elicit any intrinsic response. [Section 9.1]

night terror
Occurs during stage 3 sleep when an individual appears terrified and may sit up or walk around. [Section 11.5]

nociceptors
Pain receptors. [Section 11.1]

nodes of Ranvier
Gaps in the myelin sheath of the axons of peripheral neurons that increases the speed of conduction. [Section 12.1]

nonassociative learning
Learning that occurs in the absence of associating specific stimuli or events. [Section 9.1]

nonverbal communication
Involves all the methods of communication that do not include words. [Section 6.3]

norepinephrine (NE)
The neurotransmitter used by the sympathetic division of the autonomic nervous system at the postganglionic (organ-level) synapse. [Section 12.2]

normative organizations
An organization where membership is based on morally relevant goals. [Section 6.3]

normative social influence
When the motivation for compliance is a desire for the approval of others and to avoid rejection. [Section 6.2]

norms
The visible and invisible rules of social conduct within a society. [Sections 5.1 & 6.1]

nucleus accumbens
Structure located in the brainstem that releases dopamine in response to many drugs, contributing to addictive behavior. [Section 10.2]

null hypothesis
The hypothesis that there is no experimental effect and any differences, if measured, are due to chance. [Section 3.1]

object permanence
The understanding that things continue to exist once they are out of sight. [Section 11.4]

observational learning
A type of learning that occurs when a person watches another person. [Section 7.1]

observational studies
A type of research characterized by minimal manipulation in an attempt to investigate phenomena in their naturalistic state. [Section 3.3]

obsessive-compulsive disorder (OCD)
A psychological disorder characterized by repeated, intrusive, uncontrollable thoughts and repeated physical behaviors that are done in response to an obsession. [Section 8.1]

Oedipus complex
This complex occurs during the phallic stage when a male child is sexually attracted to his mother and hostile toward his father, who is seen as a rival. [Section 7.1]

olfactory receptors
Chemoreceptors in the upper nasal cavity that respond to odor chemicals. [Section 11.1]

operant conditioning
A form of associative learning based on consequences, in which rewards increase the frequency of behaviors and punishments decrease their frequency. [Section 9.1]

operational definition
The specifications of experimental variables in terms that can be used by other researchers to replicate methodology. [Section 3.1]

optic disk
The "blind spot" of the eye, where axons of ganglion cells exit the retina to form the optic nerve. [Section 11.1]

optic nerve
The nerve extending from the back of the eyeball to the brain that carries visual information. [Section 11.1]

optimism bias
The belief that bad things happen to other people, but not to us. [Section 6.2]

oral stage
The first of Freud's five psychosexual stages, in this stage the child seeks sensual pleasure through oral activities such as sucking and chewing. [Section 7.1]

organ of Corti
The structure in the cochlea of the inner ear made up of the basilar membrane, the auditory hair cells, and the tectorial membrane. [Section 11.1]

organization
A large group, more impersonal than a network, that comes together to pursue particular activities and meet goals efficiently. [Section 6.3]

ossicles
The three small bones found in the middle ear (the malleus, the incus, and the stapes) that help to amplify the vibrations from sound waves. [Section 11.1]

out-group
A group that an individual does not belong to. [Section 6.2]

outer ear
The portion of the ear consisting of the pinna and the external auditory canal. [Section 11.1]

oval window
The membrane that separates the middle ear from the inner ear. [Section 11.1]

overconfidence
An overestimation of the accuracy of one's knowledge and judgments. [Section 11.4]

p-value
Numerical value that gives the probability that a measured difference occurred due to chance. [Section 3.1]

pain disorder
A psychological disorder characterized by clinically important pain affected by psychological factors. [Section 8.1]

panic disorder
A psychological disorder that is characterized by panic attacks that are cued by certain situations or occur frequently and unexpectedly. [Section 8.1]

parallel processing
A system whereby many aspects of a stimulus are processed simultaneously instead of in a step-by-step or serial fashion. [Section 11.2]

paranoid personality disorder
A psychological disorder characterized by mistrust and misinterpretation of others' motives and actions, and suspicion of harm or betrayal. [Section 8.1]

paranoid-type schizophrenia
A psychological disorder characterized by psychosis is in the form of hallucinations and/or delusions, usually relating to a certain theme. [Section 8.1]

parasomnia
Abnormal behaviors during sleep, including somnambulism and night terrors. [Section 11.5]

parasympathetic nervous system (PNS)
The division of the autonomic nervous system known as the "resting and digesting" system. It causes a general decrease in body activities such as heart rate and blood pressure. [Sections 10.2 & 12.3]

Parkinson's disease
A movement disorder caused by the death of dopamine-releasing cells. [Section 8.1]

patriarchy
A social system where males are the primary authority figures. [Section 4.2]

patrilineal descent
A system of lineage in which the relatives on the father's side are considered most important. [Section 4.2]

Pavlov, Ivan
Famous for naming and describing the process of classical conditioning by training dogs to salivate to the sound of a ringing bell. [Section 9.1]

Pearson correlation
A numerical value between −1 and 1 that indicates how two variables correlate; a negative value indicates an inverse relationship, a positive value indicates a direct relationship, and values further from zero indicate a stronger relationship. [Section 3.3]

peg word method
Mnemonic strategy that involves assigning images to a sequence of numbers. [Section 9.2]

penis envy
Occurs during the phallic stage (the third of Freud's five psychosexual stages), when a female realizes she does not have a penis. [Section 7.1]

peptide hormone
A hormone made of amino acids that is generally hydrophilic and cannot cross the plasma membranes of cells. [Section 12.4]

peripheral nervous system
All the parts of the nervous system except for the brain and spinal cord. [Sections 10.2 & 12.3]

peripheral route
Cognitive route of persuasion that involves more superficial or secondary characteristics. [Section 6.4]

permissive parenting
Parenting style that creates few rules and demands and little discipline. [Section 9.3]

person-situation controversy
A disagreement about the degree to which a person's reaction in a given situation is due to their personality or is due to the situation itself. [Section 7.1]

personal identity
A distinct sense of self, including personally-defined attributes. [Section 6.1]

personality
The nuanced and complex individual pattern of thinking, feeling, and behavior associated with each person. [Section 7.1]

personality disorder
A psychological disorder characterized by an enduring, rigid set of personality traits that deviates from cultural norms, impairs functioning, and causes distress. [Section 8.1]

personality trait
A generally stable predisposition toward a certain behavior. [Section 7.1]

phenomenological method
The use of introspection to explore the nature of phenomena, often related to perception or subjective experience. [Section 3.3]

phenotype
The observable characteristics and traits of an organism. [Section 6.4]

pheromone
A chemical signal that causes a social response in members of the same species. [Section 11.1]

phobia
A strong unreasonable fear that almost always causes either general anxiety or a full panic attack. [Section 8.1]

phonological loop
Part of working memory that allows for repetition of verbal information to aid with encoding. [Section 11.4]

photoreceptor
A receptor that responds to light. [Section 11.1]

physical attractiveness stereotype
The tendency of people to rate attractive individuals more favorably for personality traits. [Section 6.2]

Piaget, Jean
Developmental psychologist who formulated a four-stage theory of development for children. [Section 11.4]

pineal gland
Region of the brain responsible for the production of melatonin, a hormone that influences sleep/wake cycles and seasonal functions. [Section 11.5]

placebo effect
The phenomenon that if a group of participants simply believes that it has been given a treatment, this can lead to a measurable effect. [Section 3.1]

polyandry
A form of marriage in which a woman is married to more than one man. [Section 4.2]

polygamy
A form of marriage in which an individual may have multiple wives or husbands simultaneously. [Section 4.2]

polygyny
A form of marriage in which a man is married to more than one woman. [Section 4.2]

polysomnography (PSG)
Multimodal technique for measuring physiological processes during sleep, including EEG, EMG, and EOG. [Section 11.5]

positive punishment
The introduction of a negative or aversive stimulus following a behavior. Tends to decrease the likelihood of that behavior. [Section 9.1]

positive reinforcement
Reward immediately following a behavior that increases the frequency of that behavior (for example, praise). [Section 9.1]

positive transfer
When old information facilitates the learning of new information. [Section 9.2]

posttraumatic stress disorder (PTSD)
Disorder characterized by re-experiencing a traumatic event through flashbacks or nightmares. [Section 8.1]

posterior pituitary gland
Nervous tissue located at the rear of the pituitary that secretes two hormones made by the hypothalamus: oxytocin and ADH. [Section 12.4]

postganglionic neuron
In the autonomic division of the PNS, a neuron that has its cell body in an autonomic ganglion, and whose axon synapses with the target organ. [Section 12.3]

power
The ability of a study to pick up an effect if one is indeed present; this is related to factors such as large sample size and low variation. [Section 3.1]

predictive validity
The extent to which a psychometric instrument predicts results along a well-known test or in variable of interest. [Section 3.2]

prefrontal cortex
Anterior part of the frontal lobes of the brain involved in complex behaviors such as planning, sequencing, social responses, and decision making. [Sections 10.1 & 10.3]

preganglionic neuron
In the autonomic division of the PNS, neuron that has its cell body located in the CNS, and whose axon extends into the PNS to synapse with a second neuron at an autonomic ganglion. [Section 12.3]

prejudice
Thoughts, attitudes, and feelings someone holds about a group that are based on a prejudgment or biased thinking about a group and its members. [Section 6.2]

primacy effect
A tendency to better recall the first items on a list. [Section 9.2]

primary groups
Groups that play a more important role in an individual's life; these groups are usually smaller and include those with whom the individual engages with in person. [Section 6.2]

primary reinforcers
Unconditioned consequences that are innately satisfying or desirable. May be biologically driven. [Section 9.1]

priming
An effect of implicit memory whereby exposure to a given stimulus "primes" or prepares the brain to respond to a later stimulus. [Section 9.2]

principle of aggregation
The idea that an attitude affects a person's aggregate or average behavior, but cannot necessarily predict each isolated act. [Section 7.3]

proactive interference
A type of memory interference that occurs when previously learned information interferes with the recall of information learned more recently. [Section 9.2]

projection bias
Occurs when we assume others have the same beliefs we do, due to our tendency to look for similarities between ourselves and others. [Section 6.2]

proprioceptor
A receptor that responds to changes in the body position, such as stretch on a tendon, or contraction of a muscle. [Section 11.1]

prospective memory
Remembering to do something in the future. [Section 9.2]

psychoanalytic theory
According to this theory, personality is shaped by a person's unconscious thoughts, feelings, and memories. [Section 7.1]

psychoanalytic therapy
This therapy approach helps a patient become aware of his or her unconscious sources for emotional issues and conflicts that are causing difficulties. [Section 7.1]

psychological disorder
A set of behavioral and/or psychological symptoms that are not in keeping with cultural norms and are severe enough to cause significant personal distress. [Section 8.1]

psychological fixation
Occurs in psychoanalytic theory when parents either frustrate or overindulge a child's expression of sensual pleasure at a certain stage, and as an adult the individual continues to seek sensual pleasure through behaviors related to that stage. [Section 11.4]

psychometrics
The art and science of measuring psychological processes. [Section 3.1]

psychosexual stages
According to Freud's psychoanalytic theory, individuals progress through five psychosexual stages, one corresponding to the part of the body that is the focus of sensual pleasure. [Section 7.1]

punishment
In operant conditioning, a consequence that decreases the likelihood that a preceding behavior will be repeated. [Section 9.1]

pupil
A hole in the center of the iris of the eye that allows light to enter the eyeball. [Section 11.1]

qualitative
Descriptive, as opposed to numerical; often used to refer to data. [Section 3.1]

quantitative
Numerical, as opposed to descriptive; often used to describe data. [Section 3.1]

race
The biological, anthropological, or genetic origin of an individual. [Section 5.1]

racism
Prejudices and discriminatory actions that are based on race (or ethnicity), or hold that one race (or ethnicity) is inferior to another. [Sections 5.1 & 6.2]

randomized block technique
A technique used by researchers who wish to make experimental and control groups similar along a set of variables. [Section 3.1]

rapid eye movement (REM)
Bursts of quick eye movements present in the last stage of sleep. [Section 11.5]

rational-legal authority
A form of leadership that is organized around rational legal rules. [Section 4.2]

recall
Retrieving information from memory.
[Sections 9.2 & 11.4]

recency effect
A tendency to recall the last items presented in a list. [Section 9.2]

reciprocal determinism
A reciprocal interaction between a person's behaviors, personal factors, and environmental factors. [Section 6.4]

recognition
Retrieving information from memory with the use of cues. [Section 9.2]

reconstructive memory
Theory that memory is constructed rather than a perfect recollection of an event. [Section 9.2]

reference group
A group that serves as a standard measure that people compare themselves to. [Section 6.2]

reflex
Automatic behaviors that occur without thinking. [Section 12.3]

reflex arc
A relatively direct connection between a sensory neuron and a motor neuron that allows an extremely rapid response to a stimulus. [Section 12.3]

rehearsal
Technique of repeating verbal information in one's phonological loop to promote the encoding of sensory information into memory. [Section 9.2]

reinforcement
A consequence that increases the likelihood that a preceding behavior will be repeated. Two types are positive and negative reinforcement. [Section 9.1]

reinforcement schedule
The frequency and regularity with which rewards are offered, based on a number of target behaviors (ratio) or on a time interval (interval). [Section 9.1]

relative poverty
An inability to meet the average standard of living within a society. [Section 5.2]

relative refractory period
The period of time following an action potential when it is possible, but difficult, for the neuron to fire a second action potential. [Section 12.1]

relearning
The process of learning material that was originally learned. [Section 9.2]

reliable
The tendency of a survey or other instrument of measurement to produce similar results under similar conditions and measure what they are purported to. [Section 3.1]

religiosity
The extent that religion influences a person's life. [Section 4.2]

REM stage
Final stage of sleep characterized by rapid eye movements (REM) and beta waves, which are seen in individuals when they are awake. [Section 11.5]

replacement fertility rate
The number of children that a woman or couple must have in order to replace the number of the people in the population who die. [Section 5.1]

replicability
Obtaining consistent results across various studies attempting to answer the same scientific question using different data and/or new statistical methods. [Section 3.1]

representativeness heuristic
A mental shortcut in which one judges the likelihood of things based on typical mental representations or examples of those things. [Section 11.4]

reproducibility
Obtaining consistent results using the same data and statistical methods as a prior study. [Section 3.1]

reproductive memory
Theory that suggests memory recall occurs through storage of the original stimulus input and subsequent recall. [Section 9.2]

resource model of attention
States that if multiple tasks exceed the limit of attention, they cannot be done simultaneously. [Section 11.3]

retention interval
The amount of time elapsed since information was learned and when it must be recalled. [Section 9.2]

reticular formation
Also known as the Reticular Activating System. Structures in the brainstem that are important for alertness and arousal (as in wakefulness). [Section 11.5]

retina
The innermost layer of the eyeball. The retina is made up of photoreceptors, bipolar cells, and a layer of ganglion cells. [Section 11.1]

retroactive interference
A type of memory interference that occurs when newly learned information interferes with the recall of information learned previously. [Section 9.2]

retrograde amnesia
Occurs when one is unable to recall information that was previously encoded. [Sections 8.1 & 9.2]

rods
Photoreceptors in the retina that respond to dim light and provide black and white vision. [Section 11.1]

Rogers, Carl
Considered the founder of humanistic psychology who pioneered the person-centered approach to therapy. [Section 6.1]

role conflict
Occurs when there is a conflict in society's expectations for multiple statuses held by the same person (for example "male" and "nurse"). [Section 6.3]

role exit
The process of disengaging from a role that has become closely tied to one's self-identity to take on a new role. [Section 6.3]

role strain
Occurs when a single status results in conflicting expectations. [Section 6.3]

saltatory conduction
A rapid form of neural conduction in which the action potential "jumps" along nodes of Ranvier. [Section 12.1]

sample size
The number of participants in a study. [Section 3.1]

sampling bias
Occurs when some individuals from a population have a greater likelihood of being selected than others. [Section 3.1]

sanctions
Rewards and punishments for behaviors that are in accord with or against norms. [Section 6.1]

scapegoat
The people or group who are unfairly blamed for something, or at whom displaced aggression is directed. [Section 6.2]

Schachter-Singer Theory
Theory of emotion that asserts that the experience of physiological arousal occurs first and is followed by a conscious cognitive interpretation that allows for identification of the emotion. [Section 7.4]

schemas
Mental frameworks or blueprints that shape and are shaped by experience. [Section 11.4]

schizoaffective disorder
A psychological disorder characterized by the combination of mood and psychotic symptoms. [Section 8.1]

schizoid personality disorder
A psychological disorder characterized by little interest or involvement in close relationships, even those with family members. [Section 8.1]

schizophrenia
A psychological disorder that is chronic and incapacitating and is characterized by psychosis and impairment in functioning. [Section 8.1]

schizophreniform disorder
A psychological disorder characterized by symptoms of schizophrenia present for a period of one to six months, during which the symptoms may or may not have interfered with functioning. [Section 8.1]

schizotypal personality disorder
A psychological disorder characterized by constricted or inappropriate affect, magical or paranoid thinking, and odd beliefs, speech, behavior, appearance, and perceptions. [Section 8.1]

Schwann cell
One of the two peripheral nervous system supporting (glial) cells. Schwann cells form the myelin sheath on axons of peripheral neurons. [Section 12.1]

sclera
The white portion of the tough outer layer of the eyeball. [Section 11.1]

secondary group
A larger and more impersonal group than a primary group, which interacts for specific reasons for relatively short periods of time. [Section 6.2]

secondary reinforcers
Conditioned reinforcers that are learned through their relationship with primary reinforcers. [Section 9.1]

sect
A religious organization that is distinct from the parent religion from which it was formed. [Section 4.2]

secure attachment
An attachment style that forms when an infant has caregivers who are sensitive and responsive to needs. [Section 9.3]

selection bias
Nonrandom processes in the selection of participants, experimental groups, or any other process that introduce potential bias into a research study. [Section 3.1]

selective attention
The process by which one input is selected out of the field of environmental stimuli. [Section 11.3]

selective priming
Predisposition to observe something because it has previously been encountered frequently. [Section 11.3]

self-actualization (or actualizing tendency)
According to humanistic psychology, individuals have an innate drive to realize their human potential. [Section 7.1]

self-concept (or self-identity)
The sum of an individual's knowledge and understanding of his- or herself. [Section 6.1]

self-consciousness
Awareness of one's self. [Section 6.1]

self-efficacy
The belief in one's own competence and effectiveness. [Section 6.1]

self-esteem
One's overall self-evaluation of one's self-worth. [Section 6.1]

self-fulfilling prophecy
When stereotypes lead a person to behave in such a way as to affirm the original stereotypes. [Section 6.2]

self-handicapping
A strategy in which people create obstacles and excuses to avoid self-blame when they do poorly. [Section 6.3]

self-reference effect
The tendency to better remember information relevant to ourselves. [Section 9.2]

self-schemas
The beliefs and ideas people have about themselves. [Section 6.1]

self-serving bias
The tendency to attribute our successes to ourselves and our failures to others or the external environment. [Section 6.2]

self verification
Social psychology theory that individuals wish to be understood in terms of their deeply held beliefs in a way that is consistent with their self-concept. [Section 6.1]

semantic memory
Memory for factual information. [Section 9.2]

semicircular canals
Three loop-like structures in the inner ear that contain sensory receptors to monitor balance. [Section 11.1]

sensitization
An increase in the strength of a response with repeated presentations of a stimulus. [Section 9.1]

sensory memory
The initial recording of sensory information in the memory system; sensory memory is a very brief snapshot that quickly decays. [Section 9.2]

serial position effect
When information is presented in a list, individuals are more likely to recall the first and last items presented. [Section 9.2]

shaping
In operant conditioning, the process of reinforcing intermediate, proximal behaviors until a final, desired behavior is achieved. [Section 9.1]

short-term memory
Memory that is limited in duration and in capacity. [Section 9.2]

signal detection theory
A theory that attempts to predict how and when someone will detect the presence of a given sensory stimulus amidst all of the other sensory stimuli in the background (considered the "noise"). [Section 11.2]

significant difference
A difference between two measurements that is unlikely to be due simply to chance, according to a predetermined threshold. [Section 3.1]

Skinner, B.F.
Founder of Behaviorism who measured the effects of reward and punishment on shaping behavior. [Section 9.1]

sleep apnea
Sleep disorder in which the individual intermittently stops breathing during sleep and may wake up gasping for breath. [Section 11.5]

sleep cycle
One progression through sleep stages 1 through 4 in sequence, followed by an ascension from 4 back to 1 and then a transition into REM sleep. Typically takes about ninety minutes. [Section 11.5]

sleep spindle
Bursts of waves present in Stage 2 sleep. [Section 11.5]

social behaviorism
The idea that the mind and self emerge through the process of communicating with others. [Section 6.1]

social capital
The potential for social networks to allow for upward social mobility. [Section 5.2]

social cognition
The ability of the brain to store and process information regarding social perception. [Section 6.2]

social cognitive perspective
According to this perspective, personality is formed by a reciprocal interaction among behavioral, cognitive, and environmental factors. [Sections 6.4 & 7.1]

social constructionism
A social mechanism or practice that is created and sustained by society. [Section 4.1]

social constructionism
A sociological theory that argues that reality is constructed, not inherent. [Section 4.1]

social cues
Verbal or nonverbal hints that guide social interactions. [Section 7.1]

social dysfunction
A process that has undesirable consequences, and may actually reduce the stability of society. [Section 4.1]

social epidemiology
The study of the distribution of health and disease across a population using social concepts to explain patterns of health and illness. [Sections 4.2 & 5.2]

social facilitation effect
The phenomenon that describes how people tend to perform simple, well-learned tasks better when other people are present, while difficult, novel tasks are performed more poorly in front of others. [Section 6.2]

social facts
The elements that serve some function in society, such as the laws, morals, values, religions, customs, rituals, and rules that make up a society. [Section 4.1]

social identity
The social definitions of self, including race, religion, gender, occupation, and the like. [Section 6.1]

social institutions
A complex of roles, norms, and values organized into a relatively stable form that contributes to social order by governing the behavior of people. [Section 4.2]

social loafing
The phenomenon where people tend to exert less effort if they are being evaluated as a group than if they are individually accountable. [Section 6.2]

social mobility
The ability to move up or down within the social stratification system. [Section 5.2]

social network
A web of social relationships, including those in which a person is directly linked as well as indirectly connected to people. [Section 6.3]

social perception
The ability to understand others in our social world. [Section 6.2]

social phobia
An unreasonable, paralyzing fear of feeling embarrassed or humiliated while one is watched by others. [Section 8.1]

social reproduction
The phenomenon of social inequality transmitted from one generation to the next. [Section 5.2]

social roles
Expectations for people of a given social status. [Section 6.3]

social stratification
The way that people are categorized in society. [Section 5.2]

social support
The perception that one is cared for and part of a social network; supportive resources can be tangible or emotional. [Section 6.3]

socialism
An economic system where resources and production are collectively owned. [Section 4.1]

socialization
The process through which people learn to be proficient members of society. [Section 6.1]

society
A group of people who share a culture and live/interact with each other within a definable area. [Section 4.1]

sociobiology
The study of how biology and evolution have affected human social behavior. [Section 5.1]

socioeconomic status (SES)
Prestige and power associated with one's standing in society due to income, and other factors. [Section 5.2]

sociology
The study of how individuals interact with, shape, and are subsequently shaped by society. [Section 4.1]

soma
The cell body of a neuron. [Section 12.1]

somatization disorder
A psychological disorder characterized by a variety of physical symptoms over an extended time period. [Section 8.1]

somatoform disorder
A psychological disorder characterized primarily by physical symptoms and concerns, but the symptoms are not explainable medically and do not improve with medical treatment. [Section 8.1]

somnambulism
Sleepwalking. [Section 11.5]

source monitoring error
A specific type of error of recollection where a memory is incorrectly attributed to the wrong source. [Section 9.2]

source traits
The factors underlying human personality and behavior. [**Section 7.1**]

spatial summation
Integration by a postsynaptic neuron of inputs (EPSPs and IPSPs) from multiple sources. [**Section 12.2**]

specific phobia
A persistent, strong, and unreasonable fear of a certain object or situation. [**Section 8.1**]

spontaneous recovery
In classical conditioning, a reoccurrence of a previously extinct conditioned response in the presence of a conditioned stimulus. [**Section 9.1**]

spotlight model
Model for visual attention, with a spotlight representing one's attention and its ability to move focus onto different targets. [**Section 11.3**]

spreading activation theory
A theory of information retrieval that involves a search process where specific nodes are activated, which leads to the activation of related nodes, and so on. [**Section 10.3**]

state
Situational factors that can influence personality and behavior; states are unstable, temporary, and variable. [**Section 7.1**]

state capitalism
A system in which companies are privately run, but work closely with the government in forming laws and regulations. [**Section 4.2**]

status
A sociological term that refers to all the socially defined positions within a society. [**Section 6.3**]

stereotype threat
Refers to a self-fulfilling fear that one will be evaluated based on a negative stereotype. [**Section 6.2**]

stereotypes
Oversimplified ideas about groups of people, based on characteristics. [**Section 6.2**]

steroid hormone
A hormone derived from cholesterol that is hydrophobic and can easily cross the cell membrane, thus receptors for steroids are found intracellularly. [**Section 12.4**]

stigma
Extreme disapproval of a person or group based on the person or groups actual or perceived deviance from society. [**Section 6.2**]

stimulants
Class of drugs that speed up body functions and neural activity. [**Section 11.5**]

stranger anxiety
Developmentally typical anxiety displayed by children aged eight to twelve months toward strangers. [**Section 9.3**]

structural poverty
Poverty due to structural effects such as systemic oppression or lack of infrastructure and reliable social institutions. [**Section 5.2**]

subculture
A segment of society that shares a distinct pattern of traditions and values that differs from that of the larger society. [**Section 6.1**]

summation
The integration of input from many presynaptic neurons by a single postsynaptic neuron, either temporally or spatially. [**Section 12.2**]

superego
According to Freud's psychoanalytic theory, the superego inhibits the id and influences the ego to follow moralistic rather than realistic goals. [**Section 7.1**]

survey studies
Studies that use questionnaires to explore a research variable. [**Section 3.3**]

symbolic culture
Consists of symbols that carry a particular meaning and are recognized by people of the same culture. [**Section 5.1**]

symbolic interactionism
A micro-level theory in sociology which examines the relationship between individuals and society by focusing on communication, the exchange of information through language and symbols. [**Section 4.1**]

sympathetic nervous system (SNS)
Subdivision of the autonomic nervous system directing the "fight or flight" response to prepare the body for action. It increases heart rate, blood pressure, and directs the adrenal glands to release stress hormones. [**Sections 8.2 & 12.4**]

synapse
A neuron-to-neuron, neuron-to-organ, or muscle cell-to-muscle cell junction. [**Section 12.2**]

synaptic cleft
A microscopic space between the axon of one neuron and the cell body or dendrites of a second neuron, or between the axon of a neuron and an organ. [**Section 12.2**]

telencephalon
The cerebral hemispheres. [Section 10.2]

temperament
Dispositional emotional excitability. [Section 6.4]

temporal summation
Summation by a postsynaptic cell of input from a single source over time. [Section 12.2]

thalamus
A relay station and major integrating area for sensory impulses. [Section 10.2]

thermoreceptor
A receptor that responds to changes in temperature. [Section 11.1]

theta waves
Waves of low to moderate intensity and intermediate frequency present during Stage 1 of sleep. [Section 11.5]

top-down processing
A type of information processing that occurs when the brain applies experience and expectations to interpret sensory information. [Section 11.2]

traditional authority
A form of leadership where power is due to custom, tradition, or accepted practice. [Section 4.2]

trait
Internal, stable, and enduring aspects of personality that should be consistent across most situations. [Section 7.1]

trial and error
Strategy of problem-solving that involves trying different alternatives sequentially until success is achieved. [Section 11.4]

tropic hormone
A hormone that controls the release of another hormone. [Section 12.4]

twin studies
Studies that incorporate research into different types of twins to gain insight into heritability. [Section 3.3]

tympanic membrane
The membrane that separates the outer ear from the middle ear. The tympanic membrane is also known as the eardrum. [Section 11.1]

type 1 error
Researchers incorrectly reject the null hypothesis, also known as false positive. [Section 3.1]

type 2 error
Researchers accept the null hypothesis when in fact it is false, also known as false negative. [Section 3.1]

unconditioned response
A response that automatically follows an unconditioned stimulus, without necessitating learning and conditioning to create the link. [Section 9.1]

unconditioned stimulus
A stimulus that elicits an unconditioned response automatically, without necessitating learning and conditioning to create the link. [Section 9.1]

undifferentiated-type schizophrenia
A psychological disorder characterized by the basic criteria for schizophrenia, but symptoms that do not fit into one of the other subtypes. [Section 8.1]

universal emotions
Six major emotions that appear to be universal across cultures: happiness, sadness, surprise, fear, disgust, and anger. [Section 7.4]

universal grammar
Basic rules of language, presumed to be innate, that allow the human mind to gain mastery of language from limited exposure during sensitive developmental years in early childhood. [Section 11.6]

upward mobility
An increase in social class. [Section 5.2]

urbanization
The growth of urban areas as the result of global change. Urbanization is tied to industrialization. [Section 5.1]

utilitarian organization
An organization in which members get paid for their efforts, such as businesses. [Section 6.3]

vagus nerves
Very large mixed nerves that innervate virtually every visceral organ. They are especially important in transmitting parasympathetic input to the heart and digestive smooth muscle. [Section 12.3]

values
A culture's standard for evaluating what is good or bad. [Section 5.1]

variable-interval schedule
Reinforcement schedule in which reward is offered after an unpredictable time interval. [Section 9.1]

variable-ratio schedule
Reinforcement schedule in which reward is offered after an unpredictable number of occurrences of a behavior. [**Section 9.1**]

visual cortex
The area of the occipital lobe responsible for processing visual information. [**Section 11.1**]

visuospatial sketchpad
Allows for the repetition of visuospatial information (images) to aid with encoding it into memory. [**Section 11.4**]

Weber, Max
Conflict theorist who modified and tempered many of Marx's ideas on society. [**Section 4.1**]

Weber's law
This law pertains to sensory perception and dictates that two stimuli must differ by a constant proportion in order for their difference to be perceptible. [**Section 11.2**]

welfare capitalism
A system in which most of the economy is private with the exception of extensive social welfare programs to serve certain needs within society. [**Section 4.2**]

Wernicke's area
The area of the brain, located in the posterior section of the temporal lobe, that is involved with the comprehension of speech and written language. [**Section 11.6**]

white matter
Myelinated axons. [**Section 10.2**]

withdrawal
An uncomfortable and often painful experience that may accompany the discontinuing of a drug. [**Section 11.5**]

within-subjects design
Comparisons are made at different time points for the same group. [**Section 3.1**]

working memory
Short-term memory for information in immediate awareness, consisting of four components: a central executive, a phonological loop, a visuospatial sketchpad, and an episodic buffer. [**Sections 9.2 & 11.4**]

Yerkes-Dodson law
Law that asserts that a moderate level of arousal creates optimal performance. Too little arousal leads to complacency and too much arousal can be overwhelming. [**Section 7.4**]